ASPEN
Ente
Handbook Second Edition

Editors

Ainsley Malone,
MS, RD, LD, CNSC, FAND, FASPEN

Liesje Nieman Carney,
RD, CSP, LDN

Amy Long Carrera,
MS, RD, CNSC, CWCMS

Andrew Mays,
PharmD, BCNSP, CNSC

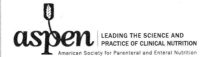

LEADING THE SCIENCE AND
PRACTICE OF CLINICAL NUTRITION
American Society for Parenteral and Enteral Nutrition

The American Society for Parenteral and Enteral Nutrition (ASPEN) is a scientific society whose members are healthcare professionals—physicians, dietitians, nurses, pharmacists, other allied health professionals, and researchers—dedicated to ensuring that every patient receives safe, efficacious, and high-quality patient care.

ASPEN's mission is to improve patient care by advancing the science and practice of clinical nutrition and metabolism.

Suggested citation: Malone A, Carney LN, Carrera AL, Mays A, eds. *ASPEN Enteral Nutrition Handbook.* 2nd ed. Silver Spring, MD: American Society for Parenteral and Enteral Nutrition; 2019.

Printed in the United States.

Contents

Preface

We are pleased to present the second edition of the *ASPEN Enteral Nutrition Handbook*, a comprehensive guide with up-to-date, specific information on how to safely, effectively, and confidently care for patients receiving enteral nutrition (EN). Like its predecessor, this new edition features best-practice recommendations based on the most current research and provides a wide variety of practical tools and tips to save time and elevate the quality of care.

This edition has been completely revised to reflect the many recent advancements in the science and practice of EN therapy. For example, you will find guidance on using ENFit® devices for tube feeding and medication administration, coverage of the indicators of malnutrition in adult and pediatric patients, and the latest recommendations regarding the use of specialty formulas and blenderized tube feedings. There is a new chapter focused on the preparation, labeling, and dispensing of EN, and this edition has divided the discussion of adult and pediatric/infant formulas into separate chapters.

The content in this handbook is aligned with ASPEN's evidence-based guidelines, core curriculum, practice recommendations, and standards. The book is an invaluable resource for students and trainees in dietetics, medicine, nursing, and pharmacy. Its "pocket guide" format and easy-to-follow clinical information will appeal to everyone from the novice to the advanced practitioner.

We thank the many contributors and reviewers who shared their knowledge, analysis of the literature, and clinical expertise in the area of EN support. It is our hope that this handbook improves the ordering, administration and safety of EN support to patients.

Ainsley Malone, MS, RD, LD, CNSC, FAND, FASPEN
Liesje Nieman Carney, RD, CSP, LDN
Amy Long Carrera, MS, RD, CNSC, CWCMS
Andrew Mays, PharmD, BCNSP, CNSC

Editors, Contributors, and Reviewers

Editors

Ainsley Malone, MS, RD, LD, CNSC, FAND, FASPEN
Clinical Practice Specialist
The American Society for Parenteral and Enteral Nutrition
Nutrition Support Dietitian
Mt. Carmel West Hospital
Columbus, OH

Liesje Nieman Carney, RD, CSP, LDN
Clinical Dietitian IV, Publication Specialist
Children's Hospital of Philadelphia
Philadelphia, PA

Amy Long Carrera, MS, RD, CNSC, CWCMS
Lead Clinical Dietitian
Pacifica Hospital of the Valley
Los Angeles, CA

Andrew Mays, PharmD, BCNSP, CNSC
Clinical Pharmacy Specialist–Nutrition Support
University of Mississippi Medical Center
Jackson, MS

Contributors

Phil Ayers, PharmD, BCNSP, FASHP
Chief, Clinical Pharmacy Services, Mississippi Baptist
    Medical Center
Clinical Associate Professor, University of Mississippi
    School of Pharmacy
Jackson, MS

Lillian Harvey Banchik, MD, FACS, CNSC, FASPEN
North Shore University Hospital, Manhasset, NY
Assistant Clinical Professor, Donald and Barbara Zucker
    School of Medicine at Hofstra/Northwell
Long Island, NY

Sarah Ann Borowicz, MS, RDN, LDN
Clinical Pediatric Dietitian
Children's Hospital of Philadelphia
Philadelphia, PA

Kelly Green Corkins, MS, RD-AP, CSP, LDN, FAND
Pediatric/CVICU Clinical Dietitian III
Department of Nutrition Therapy, Le Bonheur Children's
    Hospital
Memphis, TN

Wendy Cruse, MMSc, RDN, CSPCC, CLS, CD
Pediatric/NICU Clinical Dietitian Senior
Riley Hospital for Children at Indiana University Health
Indianapolis, IN

Kathryn Drogan, MS, NP, ANP-BC
Nurse Practitioner
University of Rochester
Rochester, NY

Arlene A. Escuro, MS, RD, LD, CNSC, FAND
Advanced Practice II Dietitian
Cleveland Clinic
Cleveland, OH

John C. Fang, MD
Freston Takeda Professor of Medicine
Chief, Division of Gastroenterology, Hepatology, and
    Nutrition
Department of Internal Medicine, University of Utah
    Health
Salt Lake City, UT

Audrey Foster, MS, RDN, CNSC
Clinical Dietitian
Children's Hospital of Philadelphia
Philadelphia, PA

Kimberly Gorsuch, BSN, RN
Gastroenterology/Nutrition Metabolic Support Care
    Manager
Cancer Treatment Centers of America
Comprehensive Care Network Chicago
Zion, IL

June Greaves, RD, CNSC, CDN, LD, LDN

A. Christine Hummell, MS, RD, LD, CNSC
Clinical Dietitian, Advanced Practitioner
Cleveland Clinic
Cleveland, OH

Deb Hutsler, MS, RD, LD
Manager of Nutrition Services
Akron Children's Hospital
Akron, OH

Andrea K. Jevenn, MEd, RD, LD, CNSC
Advanced Practice II Dietitian
Cleveland Clinic Digestive Disease and Surgical Institute
Cleveland, OH

Merin Kinikini, DNP, FNP, RD, CNSC
Nurse Practitioner for Metabolic Nutrition Support
    Clinic, Intermountain Medical Center
Adjunct Faculty, University of Utah, College of Nursing
Salt Lake City, UT

Mary Kuehl, MS, RD, CNSC
Registered Dietitian
Shield HealthCare

Carolyn Kusenda, MS, RD, LD, CNSC, CSP
Clinical Nutrition Lead
Children's Healthcare of Atlanta
Atlanta, GA

Rachel Larry, PharmD candidate
Student Pharmacist
University of Mississippi
Jackson, MS

Linda M. Lord, NP, ACNP-BC, CNSC
Nutrition Support Nurse Practitioner
University of Rochester Medical Center
Rochester, NY

Beth Lyman, MSN, RN, CNSC
Senior Clinical Program Coordinator, Nutrition Support,
  Co-Director of Nutrition Support
Children's Mercy Kansas City
Kansas City, MO

Mary Marian, DCN, RDN, CSO, FAND
Assistant Professor of Practice and Director, Didactic
  Program in Dietetics
College of Agriculture and Life Sciences
Department of Nutritional Sciences
University of Arizona
Nutrition Consultant, AZ Oncology
Tucson, AZ

Karen Martin, MA, RDN, LD, FAND
Nutrition Support Specialist, Amerita Specialty Infusion
Neuromuscular Dietitian, UT Health San Antonio
San Antonio, TX

Mary S. McCarthy, PhD, RN, CNSC, FAAN
Nurse Scientist
Center for Nursing Science & Clinical Inquiry
Madigan Army Medical Center
Tacoma, WA

Jessica Monczka, RD, CNSC
Nutrition Support Specialist
Option Care Home Infusion
Denver, CO

Katina Rahe, BSN, RN, CPN
Enteral Access Team Nursing Program Coordinator
Children's Mercy Kansas City
Kansas City, MO

Christina Ritchey, MS, RD, LD, CNSC
Consultant
Camarillo, CA

Caroline Steele, MS, RD, CSP, IBCLC, FAND
Director, Clinical Nutrition and Lactation Services
Children's Hospital of Orange County
Orange, CA

Jacqueline Sullivan, MS, RD
Clinical Dietitian
SSM St Mary's Hospital, Nutrition Services
Madison, WI

Reviewers

Anastasia E. Arena, BS, RD, LDN
Clinical Nutrition Specialist
Critical Care Medicine/Home Parenteral Nutrition
    Program
Boston Children's Hospital
Boston, MA

Meg Begany, RD, CSP, CNSC, LDN
Neonatal Dietitian/Nutrition Support Service Specialist
Children's Hospital of Philadelphia
Philadelphia, PA

Stephanie Dobak, MS, RD, LDN, CNSC
Clinical Dietitian
Thomas Jefferson University Hospital
Philadelphia, PA

June Garrett, MS, RDN-AP, CNSC, CLC
Clinical Dietitian
Children's Hospital of Los Angeles
Los Angeles, CA

Peggi Guenter, PhD, RN, FAAN, FASPEN
Senior Director of Clinical Practice, Quality, and Advocacy
American Society for Parenteral and Enteral Nutrition
Silver Spring, MD

Lauren M. Hudson, MS, RD, LDN
Director, Clinical Nutrition Support Services
Hospital of the University of Pennsylvania
Philadelphia, PA

Carol Ireton-Jones, PhD, RDN, LD, CNSC, FASPEN
Nutrition Therapy Specialist
Good Nutrition for Good Living
Dallas, TX

Rachelle Kirsch, RD, LD, CNSC
Clinical Dietitian–Trauma
Baylor University Medical Center
Dallas, TX

Mark Klang, MS, PhD, RPh, BCNSP
Core Manager, Research Pharmacy
Memorial Sloan Kettering Cancer Center
New York, NY

Carolyn Kusenda, MS, RD, CNSC, CSP, LD
Clinical Nutrition Lead
Children's Healthcare of Atlanta
Atlanta, GA

Carol McGinnis, DNP, APRN-CNS, CNSC
Clinical Nurse Specialist, Nutrition Support
Sanford USD Medical Center
Sioux Falls, SD

Kris M. Mogensen, MS, RD-AP, LDN, CNSC
Team Leader Dietitian Specialist
Department of Nutrition
Brigham and Women's Hospital
Boston, MA

Susan Roberts, DCN, RDN, LD, CNSC, FAND
Area Director of Clinical Nutrition/Dietetic Internship
    Director
Baylor Scott & White Health/Aramark Healthcare
Dallas, TX

Carol J. Rollins, MS, RD, PharmD, CNSC, BCNSP,
    FASPEN
Clinical Professor
University of Arizona, College of Pharmacy, Department
    of Pharmacy Practice and Science
Tucson, AZ

David S. Seres, MD, ScM, FASPEN
Director of Medical Nutrition, Associate Clinical Ethicist,
    and Associate Professor of Medicine
Institute of Human Nutrition
Columbia University Irving Medical Center
NewYork-Presbyterian Hospital
New York, NY

Wednesday Marie A. Sevilla, MD, MPH, CNSC
Assistant Professor of Pediatrics
UPMC Children's Hospital of Pittsburgh
Division of Pediatric Gastroenterology, Hepatology and
    Nutrition
Pittsburgh, PA

Allison Shaffer, RD, LDN
Registered Dietitian/Clinical Nutrition Specialist
Boston Children's Hospital
Boston, MA

Erin Sullivan, RD, LDN
Pediatric Critical Care Dietitian
The Children's Hospital of Philadelphia
Philaelphia, PA

Laura J. Szekely, MS, RD, LD
Supervisor, Nutrition Services
Akron Children's Hospital
Akron, OH

Abby Wood, MS, RDN, CSO, LD, CNSC
Clinical Dietitian Specialist
Baylor University Medical Center
Dallas, TX

CHAPTER 1

Nutrition Screening, Assessment, and Care Plan Development

The Nutrition Care Pathway

In clinical practice, the nutrition screening and assessment processes focus on parameters that are easy to obtain, cost effective, age appropriate, and clinically relevant. A complete nutrition assessment involves integrating objective measures including growth history (for pediatric patients) and physical exam findings with subjective clinical judgment to best identify patients who have or are at risk for malnutrition. Although the criteria for identifying and diagnosing both adult and pediatric malnutrition have evolved over the last several decades, the literature consistently demonstrates the need to assess information from the following 5 domains: (a) anthropometrics, (b) etiology and chronicity (with or without inflammation), (c) mechanism, (d) nutrient imbalance, and (e) functional/developmental outcomes. The ability to collect and appropriately assess these data is an important proficiency in any clinician's skill set and has remained an integral component within the scope of practice of clinical nutrition professionals.

While pediatric and adult nutrition assessment share many of the same foundational requirements, pediatric assessment also encompasses two additional pivotal concepts: oral motor skills and optimal growth. The latter is the most important marker for assessing the nutrition status of a pediatric patient.

Nutrition screening and assessment are part of the nutrition care pathway and comprise a series of steps with built-in feedback (see Figures 1-1 and 1-2).[1–4] The information from the screening and assessment steps are used to make a nutrition diagnosis and plan the intervention. Nutrition monitoring involves periodic measurement and review of the individual's assessment data for the purpose of modifying interventions to achieve desired clinical outcomes.[1,5]

Nutrition Screening

Nutrition screening is the first step in the process to evaluate whether an individual is at risk of becoming malnourished or is already malnourished. Screening thereby serves the purpose of identifying who would benefit from a full nutrition assessment to determine appropriate interventions to minimize comorbidities and promote improved patient outcomes.[2,6,7] An effective nutrition screening tool should be valid and reliable, concise, and easy to use by any clinician trained to screen the particular patient population.[7]

Information collected in a nutrition screening varies depending on the population and setting.[2] Nutrition screenings may solicit a wide range of information about the patient, including height (or length), recent weight history, past and current nutrition interventions, clinical and diagnostic information, medical history, functional status, and

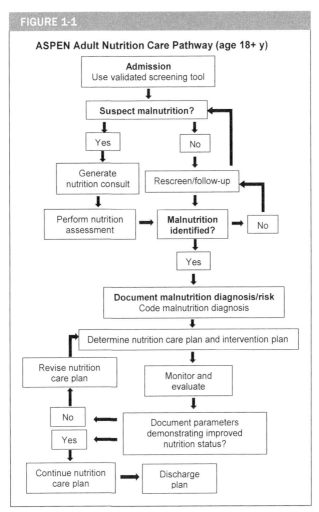

Adult screening and assessment algorithm. Adapted with permission from reference 3: American Society for Parenteral and Enteral Nutrition. *Improve Patient Outcomes: A.S.P.E.N.'s Step-by-Step Guide to Addressing Malnutrition.* Silver Spring, MD: American Society for Parenteral and Enteral Nutrition; 2015.

FIGURE 1-2

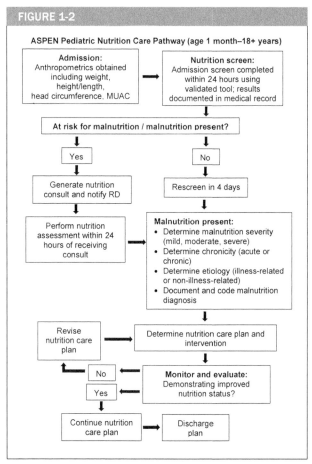

Pediatric nutrition screening and assessment algorithm. MUAC, mid–upper arm circumference; RD, registered dietitian. Adapted with permission from reference 4: A.S.P.E.N. pediatric nutrition care pathway (age 1 month–18 years) (infographic). Malnutrition Solution Center. American Society for Parenteral and Enteral Nutrition website. https://www.nutritioncare.org/Continuing_Education/Programs /Malnutrition_Awareness/Malnutrition. Accessed November 17, 2018.

psychological and social status.[6] Such information helps clinicians determine an individual's nutrition status and the likelihood that he/she will develop nutrient deficits during a course of treatment or hospitalization. While informative, the interpretation of screening parameters often employs clinical judgment and therefore is primarily subjective.[1]

A number of nutrition screening tools have been reviewed in the literature (see Tables 1-1 and 1-2 for examples).[6,8–18] Despite the variety of available tools, most have limitations. For example, they may not have been evaluated for use in long-term care facilities or outpatient clinics; they may not address the screening needs of obese patients; or they could have the potential for error if the necessary components are not readily available.[19] Constraints in using existing screening tools for critically ill adults have led to the recommendation to use the Nutrition Risk in Critically Ill (NUTRIC) tool or the Nutrition Risk Score (NRS-2002).[20] Although there is a need for valid and reliable tools, limited data demonstrating their effectiveness are currently available.[6,8]

Nutrition Assessment and Indicators of Malnutrition

The nutrition assessment process identifies patients with malnutrition or other nutrition-related problems that may require intervention. Alterations in nutrition status can be caused by altered nutrient intake, malabsorption, or altered metabolism.[21] Uncomplicated malnutrition is caused by an imbalance between nutrient intake and nutrient requirements in the absence of disease or trauma.[22]

In the nutrition assessment, the clinician obtains and interprets information that can shed light on the patient's nutrition status. This information includes the patient's medical and social history, food and nutrition-related

TABLE 1-1. Selected Adult Nutrition Screening Instruments

Instrument (Evidence Grade)[a]	Description
NRS-2002 (Grade I)	**Intended population**: Hospitalized medical-surgical and acute patients **Parameters used**: • Recent unintentional weight loss • BMI • Disease severity • Impaired general condition • Age >70 y **Purpose**: Originally designed as a tool to identify patients who would benefit from nutrition support; also used to assess nutrition status and predict clinical outcomes **Comments**: • Good validity against nutrition assessment/body composition • Good to fair validity against SGA • Poor validity against MNA • Good to fair predictive validity for mortality, LOS, and complications
MST (Grade II)	**Intended populations**: Oncology patients; acute and elderly hospitalized patients **Parameters used**: Appetite, unintentional weight loss **Purpose**: Quick to administer tool for screening/assessing nutrition status and predicting clinical outcomes **Comments**: • Only tool available that is both valid and reliable for acute care/hospital-based ambulatory care patients • Good validity against SGA • Performs poorly in predicting clinical outcomes

(continued)

TABLE 1-1. *(Continued)*

Instrument (Evidence Grade)[a]	Description
MUST (Grade II)	**Intended populations**: Hospitalized medical-surgical patients; elderly hospitalized patients **Parameters used**: • BMI • Recent unintentional weight loss • Problems with food intake • Disease severity **Purpose**: Developed for screening in community settings; widely used in Europe; for screening and assessing nutrition status and predicting clinical outcomes **Comments**: • Good validity (by kappa) against SGA, NRS, assessment by dietitian • Good to fair validity in multiple studies • Good to fair predictor of LOS and mortality in malnourished patients
MNA-SF (Grade II)	**Intended population:** Ambulatory, subacute, hospitalized elderly patients **Parameters used**: • Unintentional weight loss • Appetite • Food intake problem • Disease severity • Homebound • Dementia/depression **Purpose**: Easy and simple substitution for full MNA to screen and assess nutrition status of older adults **Comments**: • Excellent validity against MNA (likely because of incorporation bias)

(continued)

TABLE 1-1. *(Continued)*	
Instrument (Evidence Grade)[a]	**Description**
	• Excellent sensitivity but poor specificity against nutrition assessment or assessment by professional (too many false positives for malnutrition) • Does not predict outcomes well in elderly patients
NUTRIC Score (not graded)	**Intended population**: Critically ill adult and elderly patients **Parameters used**: • APACHE II • SOFA (with or without IL-6) • Number of comorbidities • Days from hospital to ICU admission **Purpose**: Quantification of risk of adverse outcomes that may be positively affected by nutrition therapies **Comments**: • Higher scores correlated with increased mortality and longer duration of mechanical ventilation • Predictive of 28-day mortality

Abbreviations: APACHE, Acute Physiology and Chronic Health Evaluation; BMI, body mass index; ICU, intensive care unit; IL-6, interleukin-6; LOS, length of stay; MNA, Mini Nutritional Assessment; MNA-SF, Mini Nutritional Assessment–Short Form; MST, Malnutrition Screening Tool; MUST, Malnutrition Universal Screening Tool; NRS-2002, Nutritional Risk Screening 2002; NUTRIC, Nutrition Risk in Critically Ill; SGA, subjective global assessment; SOFA, sequential organ failure assessment.

[a]Evidence grades are from reference 6. Refer to the original article for additional information on the grades.

Source: Information is from references 6, 8, 10, and 11.

TABLE 1-2. Validated Nutrition Screening Tools for Hospitalized Pediatric Patients	
Instrument	**Description**

PNST	**Intended population**: Hospitalized, full-term children (all ages)
	Parameters used:
	• Simple questionnaire; caregiver can answer with a yes or no:
	  ◦ Weight loss?
	  ◦ Poor weight gain in last few months?
	  ◦ Decreased intake/appetite in last few weeks?
	  ◦ Is the child overtly underweight?
	Comments:
	• Avoids anthropometric measures and growth references
	• Reliability and reproducibility are limited
	• Easy and simple

PYMS	**Intended population**: Hospitalized children **Parameters used**: 5-step scoring system: 1. BMI below the cutoff? 2. Weight loss? 3. Decreased intake? 4. Nutrition affected by recent admission/condition? 5. Calculate score **Comments**: • Identifies patients as at high, medium, or low risk of malnutrition • Studies find to be the most accurate and most reliable in clinical settings • Does not include impact of underlying disease • Recommends a nutrition intervention for each risk

(continued)

TABLE 1-2. *(Continued)*

Instrument	Description
STAMP	**Intended population**: Hospitalized children, ages 2–17 y **Parameters used**: 5-step scoring system: 1. Diagnosis (with nutritional implication) 2. Nutrition intake 3. Weight and height 4. Overall risk of malnutrition 5. Care plan **Comments**: • Identifies patients as at high, medium, or low risk of malnutrition • Available for download from www.stampscreeningtool.org • Recommends a nutrition intervention for each risk
SCAN	**Intended population**: Children with cancer **Parameters used**: • Height • Weight • BMI • Body composition **Comment**: Identifies children with cancer who are at risk for malnutrition
STRONG$_{kids}$	**Intended population**: Hospitalized children, ages 3–18 y **Parameters used**: • Subjective clinical assessment • High-risk diseases • Nutritional intake and losses (excessive diarrhea or vomiting) • Weight loss or poor weight gain **Comments**: • Identifies risk of malnutrition in hospitalized patients • Quick, reliable, and practical tool

(continued)

TABLE 1-2. *(Continued)*	
Instrument	**Description**
SGNA	**Intended population**: General pediatric population
	Parameters used:
	• Detailed questionnaire including gender, age, underlying disease, anthropometrics (including weight, height, BMI), nutrition-related medical history, and a complete physical examination
	Comments:
	• Identifies malnourished children at higher risk of nutrition-associated complications and prolonged hospitalization classifying patient as normal, moderate, or severely malnourished
	• Consists of both subjective and objective components

Abbreviations: BMI, body mass index; PNST, Pediatric Nutrition Screening Tool; PYMS, Pediatric Yorkhill Malnutrition Score; SCAN, Screening Tool for Childhood Cancer; SGNA, Subjective Global Nutritional Assessment; STAMP, Screening Tool for Assessment of Malnutrition in Paediatrics; STRONG$_{KIDS}$, STRONG$_{kids}$ Nutritional Risk Screening Tool.

Source: Information is from references 12–18.

history, anthropometric data, laboratory test findings, results of medical tests and procedures, and the nutrition-focused physical exam. To obtain information for the nutrition assessment, the clinician will review medical records, nutrient intake records, diet histories, and available laboratory test data; interview the patient; and complete a physical assessment.

Adult Malnutrition

Two important nutrition assessment tools used to identify malnutrition in adult patients are the subjective global assessment (SGA) and the clinical characteristics of malnutrition described by the American Society for Parenteral and Enteral Nutrition (ASPEN) and the Academy of Nutrition and Dietetics (AND). SGA is a well-tested and widely accepted nutrition assessment tool that relies on weight history and dietary change, persistent gastrointestinal (GI) symptoms, functional capacity, effects of disease on nutrition requirements, and changes in appearance as determined by a physical exam (see Figure 1-3).[23,24] On the basis of these parameters, clinicians categorize a patient's nutrition status as well nourished, moderate or suspected malnutrition, or severe malnutrition.

In an effort to encourage consistency and promote objectivity for the diagnosis of malnutrition in hospitalized patients, ASPEN and AND have published a list of specific malnutrition criteria within an etiology-based system that account for a modern understanding of the effects of the inflammatory process.[25,26] In many ways, the ASPEN/AND criteria are similar to those used in the SGA (see Table 1-3).[27] However, the ASPEN/AND method identifies markers that may be used to analyze proinflammatory states during an acute illness or injury or during chronic illness.[25,27] Examples of diseases and conditions categorized as acute illness or injury include sepsis, closed head injury, major abdominal surgery, or multiple trauma; these are associated with marked inflammatory response. Inflammation of lesser intensities tends to be affiliated with chronic illnesses, such as chronic obstructive pulmonary disease, organ failure, diabetes mellitus, obesity, or cancer.[28,29] Although they are not all-inclusive listings, Tables 1-4, 1-5, and 1-6 highlight practical indicators to assist the clinician in evaluating the presence and intensity of inflammation in complex patient scenarios.[23,25,27–38] The ASPEN/AND method also highlights risk factors for malnutrition independent of inflammation—including

FIGURE 1-3

Select appropriate category with a checkmark, or enter numerical value where indicated by "#".

A.   History

    1. Weight change

        Overall loss in past 6 mos:

        amount = # _____ kg; % loss = # _____

        Change in past 2 wks:

        _____ increase, _____ no change, _____ decrease

    2. Dietary intake change (relative to normal)

        _____ No change

        _____ Change

        _____ duration = # _____ wks

        Type: _____ suboptimal solid diet

               _____ full liquid diet

               _____ hypocaloric liquids

               _____ starvation

    3. Gastrointestinal symptoms (that persisted for >2 wks)

        ___ none ___ nausea ___ vomiting

        ___ diarrhea ___ anorexia

    4. Functional capacity

        _____ No dysfunction (eg, full capacity)

        _____ Dysfunction _____ duration = # _____ wks

        Type:

        _____ working suboptimally

        _____ ambulatory

        _____ bedridden

    5. Disease and its relation to nutritional requirements

        Primary diagnosis (specify) _____

        Metabolic demand (stress):

        _____ no stress

        _____ low stress

        _____ moderate stress

        _____ high stress

(continued)

FIGURE 1-3 (Continued)

B. Physical
(for each trait specify 0 = normal, 1+ = mild,
2+ = moderate, 3+ = severe)

\# _____ loss of subcutaneous fat (triceps, chest)

\# _____ muscle wasting (quadriceps, deltoids)

\# _____ ankle edema

\# _____ sacral edema

\# _____ ascites

C. SGA rating (select one)

_____ A = Well nourished

_____ B = Moderately malnourished
(or suspected of being malnourished)

_____ C = Severely malnourished

Subjective global assessment (SGA) for adult nutrition assessment. Reprinted with permission from reference 23: Detsky AS, McLaughlin JR, Baker JP, et al. What is Subjective Global Assessment of nutritional status? *JPEN J Parenter Enteral Nutr.* 1987;11:8–13. doi:10.1177/014860718701100108.

social, environmental, and behavioral circumstances—that may be found in patients with conditions such as anorexia nervosa.[25]

Once the contextual influence of the inflammatory state is understood within an individual case, the ASPEN/AND criteria can be evaluated (see Tables 1-7 and 1-8).[25,39] Presentation of at least 2 of the 6 criteria establishes the existence of malnutrition.[25] The severity of those characteristics then determines whether the condition is severe or nonsevere.[25,40]

The ASPEN/AND criteria for severe malnutrition in adults may be used when assigning the *International Classification of Diseases*, 10th edition, Clinical Modification (ICD-10-CM) diagnosis code E43, Severe protein-energy malnutrition, to patient documentation, and the ASPEN/AND criteria for nonsevere/moderate malnutrition may map to the ICD-10-CM code E44.0, Malnutrition of

TABLE 1-3. Comparison of the SGA and ASPEN/AND Nutrition Assessment Methods

SGA	ASPEN/AND Malnutrition Clinical Characteristics
Medical/nutrition history	
• Weight changes	• Unintentional weight loss
• Nutrition intake	• Nutrition intake
• GI symptoms	• No specific GI symptom review
• Functional status	• Functional status
• Metabolic stress from current disease state	• Chronic illness, acute illness, or social/behavioral/environmental circumstances
Physical exam	
• Muscle wasting[a]	• Muscle wasting[a]
◦ Quadriceps	◦ Temporalis
◦ Deltoids	◦ Pectoralis
	◦ Deltoids
	◦ Scapular
	◦ Interosseous
	◦ Quadriceps
	◦ Gastrocnemius
• Loss of subcutaneous fat[a]	• Loss of subcutaneous fat[a]
◦ Triceps	◦ Orbital
◦ Chest	◦ Triceps
	◦ Midaxillary line/iliac crest
• Edema	• Fluid accumulation
◦ Effect on weight	• Nutrition-related edema
◦ Ankles	◦ Effect on weight
◦ Sacral area	◦ Upper/lower extremities
• Ascites	◦ Vulvar/scrotal edema
	• Ascites
Laboratory data	
• Not used	• Used to determine presence and severity of inflammatory process

Abbreviations: AND, Academy of Nutrition and Dietetics; ASPEN, American Society for Parenteral and Enteral Nutrition; GI, gastrointestinal; SGA, subjective global assessment.

[a]Evaluation of muscle wasting and fat loss areas as described by the original methodologies.

Source: Information is from references 23, 25, and 27.

TABLE 1-4. Potential Inflammatory Markers

Examples	Indicators of Infectious Process	Alternate Interpretations
Biochemical markers		
Serum proteins	• Low albumin • Low prealbumin • Low transferrin • Elevated ferritin • Elevated CRP	• Albumin: overhydration, nephrotic syndrome, liver disease, heart failure • Transferrin: anemia, excess excretion from kidneys • Ferritin: frequent blood transfusions, porphyria, hemochromatosis, alcohol abuse
Blood glucose	• Hyperglycemia	• IV fluids with dextrose, medications (eg, steroids)
White blood cells	• Leukocytosis • Leukopenia	• Leukocytosis: medications, normal life-cycle variations (eg, pregnancy, newborn infant) • Leukopenia: medications, congenital problems, autoimmune disorders, vitamin deficiencies
Microbiological markers		
Urine, fecal, blood, or other body fluid cultures	• Results positive for fungal, bacterial, viral microbes	• n/a

Vital signs

Blood pressure	• Hypotension	• Hypotension: dehydration, medications, heart disease, pregnancy, blood loss
	• Hypertension	• Hypertension: pain, medications, underlying disease/condition, physical inactivity
Heart rate	• Tachycardia	• Tachycardia: uncontrolled pain, heart conditions, dehydration, tumors, hypertension, medications, drug/alcohol abuse
	• Bradycardia	• Bradycardia: hypothyroidism, heart damage/disorder, COPD, medications
Temperature	• Fevers	• Fevers: heat exhaustion, medications
	• Hypothermia	• Hypothermia: cold exposure, CNS or endocrine dysfunction, metabolic derangements

Abbreviations: CNS, central nervous system; COPD, chronic obstructive pulmonary disease; CRP, C-reactive protein; IV, intravenous; n/a, not applicable.

Source: Information is from references 25 and 28–38.

TABLE 1-5. Imaging Study and Procedure Results That May Indicate Inflammation

Study/Procedure	Findings Indicative of Inflammatory Process
Chest X-ray	• Inflammation • Pneumonia • Pulmonary fistula • Mass, nodule
CT scans	• Abscess • Pancreatitis • Inflammation • Cancer • Mass • Obstruction
Echocardiogram	• Endocarditis • Vegetations
Endoscopy (eg, colonoscopy, upper GI)	• Radiation enteritis • Esophagitis • Gastritis • Graft-versus-host disease • Ulcers • Fistula • Enteritis • Colitis • Cancer

Abbreviations: CT, computed tomography; GI, gastrointestinal.

Source: Information is from references 27 and 28.

moderate degree. Clinicians should consult with the health information management or coding department about the use of ICD-10 codes.

Figure 1-4 provides a step-by-step schematic that can be used to apply the ASPEN/AND criteria.[25,41] Two studies published in 2018 concluded that adult patients identified with malnutrition by the ASPEN/AND criteria have

TABLE 1-6. Potential Signs of Inflammation from Clinical Inspection

Parameter for Inspection	Potential Indicators of Inflammation
Skin	• Burns • Rashes • Wounds • Erythema • Swelling • Pain
Eyes	• Red, swollen • Tenderness, pain • Drainage
Nose	• Drainage
Mouth/gums	• Swelling • Erythema • Sores • Pain
Miscellaneous	• Chills • Night sweats • Productive cough • Painful urination

Source: Information is from reference 27.

higher hospital mortality rates, longer lengths of stay, and increased likelihood of 30-day hospital readmission.[42,43]

Pediatric Malnutrition

Pediatric malnutrition is defined as "an imbalance between nutrient requirements and intake that results in cumulative deficits of energy, protein, or micronutrients that may negatively affect growth, development and other relevant outcomes."[44] After releasing the adult malnutrition criteria,

TABLE 1-7. ASPEN/AND Assessment Criteria for Severe Malnutrition (Adults)

Criteria	Etiology of Malnutrition		
	Acute Illness/Injury	**Chronic Illness**	**Social/Environmental Circumstances**
Weight loss	>2% in 1 week >5% in 1 month >7.5% in 3 months	>5% in 1 month >7.5% in 3 months >10% in 6 months >20% in 12 months	>5% in 1 month >7.5% in 3 months >10% in 6 months >20% in 12 months
Energy intake	≤50% energy intake compared to estimated energy needs for ≥5 days	≤75% energy intake compared to estimated energy needs for ≥1 month	≤50% energy intake compared to estimated energy needs for ≥1 month

Physical exam findings:

• Body fat	• Moderate loss	• Severe loss
• Muscle mass	• Moderate loss	• Severe loss
• Fluid accumulation	• Moderate to severe	• Severe
Functional status	Measurably diminished[a,b]	Measurably diminished[a]	Measurably diminished[a]	Measurably diminished[a]

Abbreviations: AND, Academy of Nutrition and Dietetics; ASPEN, American Society for Parenteral and Enteral Nutrition.

[a]Demonstration of reduced functional status using dynamometer to measure handgrip strength or an alternate validated method.

[b]Handgrip strength is not recommended for assessment in intensive care settings.[40]

Source: Adapted with permission from reference 25: White JV, Guenter P, Jensen G, et al. Consensus statement: Academy of Nutrition and Dietetics and American Society for Parenteral and Enteral Nutrition: characteristics recommended for the identification and documentation of adult malnutrition (undernutrition). JPEN J Parenter Enteral Nutr. 2012;36(3):275–283. doi:10.1177/0148607112440285.

TABLE 1-8. ASPEN/AND Assessment Criteria for Nonsevere/Moderate Malnutrition (Adults)

Criteria	Acute Illness/Injury	Etiology of Malnutrition	
		Chronic Illness	Social/Environmental Circumstances
Weight loss	1%–2% in 1 week 5% in 1 month 7.5% in 3 months	5% in 1 month 7.5% in 3 months 10% in 6 months 20% in 12 months	5% in 1 month 7.5% in 3 months 10% in 6 months 20% in 12 months
Energy intake	<75% energy intake compared to estimated energy needs for >7 days	<75% energy intake compared to estimated energy needs for ≥1 month	<75% energy intake compared to estimated energy needs for ≥3 months
Physical exam findings: • Body fat • Muscle mass • Fluid accumulation	 • Mild loss • Mild loss • Mild	 • Mild loss • Mild loss • Mild	 • Mild loss • Mild loss • Mild
Functional status	n/a	n/a	n/a

Abbreviations: AND, Academy of Nutrition and Dietetics; ASPEN, American Society for Parenteral and Enteral Nutrition; n/a, not applicable.

Source: Adapted with permission from reference 25: White JV, Guenter P, Jensen G, et al. Consensus statement: Academy of Nutrition and Dietetics and American Society for Parenteral and Enteral Nutrition: characteristics recommended for the identification and documentation of adult malnutrition (undernutrition). *JPEN J Parenter Enteral Nutr.* 2012;36(3):275–283. doi:10.1177/0148607112440285.

FIGURE 1-4

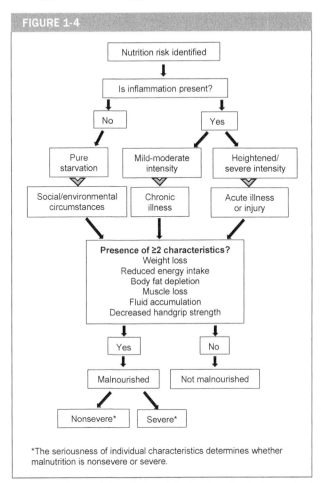

Decision tree for practical application of the American Society for Parenteral and Enteral Nutrition and Academy of Nutrition and Dietetics characteristics to determine the presence and severity of malnutrition in adults. Information is from references 25 and 41.

ASPEN and AND developed a standardized set of indicators to identify and document pediatric malnutrition (Table 1-9).[45] Indicators of malnutrition in pediatric patients include insufficient weight gain velocity and weight-for-length z scores in children under the age of 2 years; weight loss and BMI-for-age z scores are more appropriate indicators in children older than 2 years. Mid–upper arm circumference (MUAC) z scores may be used as an indicator of malnutrition in children ages 6–59 months. Deceleration in either weight-for-length or BMI-for-age z scores and inadequate nutrient intake may be malnutrition indicators from birth to adulthood. Accounting for the general aim for continued growth and development, identification of 1 indicator is sufficient to establish the presence of malnutrition in pediatric patients (vs the adult requirement for 2 indicators).[45] Additionally, a deceleration or deviation from an initially established trend using serial data points (>2) generally captures malnutrition status in pediatric patients better than a single data point.[45]

In pediatrics, malnutrition status is typically identified by the degree of severity and degree of chronicity. As in the adult criteria, the degree of malnutrition severity in pediatrics can range from mild to moderate to severe. Once a degree of malnutrition is identified, the chronicity is then classified based on duration as either acute or chronic. Acute malnutrition is defined as occurring in less than a 3-month span and typically results in a decline in weight and often a correlating deceleration in weight for length (ages 0–2 years) or BMI (ages 2–20 years). In contrast, chronic malnutrition is defined by duration longer than 3 months and often involves a correlating deceleration in linear growth velocity (commonly referred to as "stunting").[45]

The etiology of malnutrition should also be identified as part of the assessment. Malnutrition can be classified as illness

TABLE 1-9. ASPEN/AND Classifications of Pediatric Malnutrition

Primary indicators for malnutrition when a single data point is available

Indicator	Mild Malnutrition	Moderate Malnutrition	Severe Malnutrition
Weight-for-height z score	−1 to −1.9	−2 to −2.9	−3 or less
BMI-for-age z score	−1 to −1.9	−2 to −2.9	−3 or less
Length/height-for-age z score	No data	No data	−3 or less
Mid–upper arm circumference z score	−1 to −1.9	−2 to −2.9	−3 or less

Primary indicators for malnutrition when ≥2 data points are available

Indicator	Mild Malnutrition	Moderate Malnutrition	Severe Malnutrition
Weight gain velocity (ages <2 y)	<75% of norm for expected weight gain[a]	<50% of norm for expected weight gain[a]	<25% of norm for expected weight gain[a]
Weight loss (ages 2–20 y)	5% of usual body weight	7.5% of usual body weight	10% of usual body weight
Decline in weight-for-length z score	Decline of 1 z score	Decline of 2 z scores	Decline of 3 z scores
Inadequate nutrient intake	51%–75% estimated energy/protein needs	26%–50% of estimated energy/protein needs	≤25% of estimated energy/protein needs

Abbreviations: AND, Academy of Nutrition and Dietetics; ASPEN, American Society for Parenteral and Enteral Nutrition; BMI, body mass index.

[a]Growth velocity norms or standards according to World Health Organization data for patients ages <2 years.

Source: Adapted with permission from reference 45: Becker P, Carney LN, Corkins M, et al. Consensus statement of the Academy of Nutrition and Dietetics/American Society of Parenteral and Enteral Nutrition: indicators recommended for the identification and documentation of pediatric malnutrition (undernutrition). *Nutr Clin Pract.* 2015;30(1):147–161. doi:10.1177/0884533614557642.

related or non–illness related. Mechanisms that may lead to malnutrition include decreased intake, increased requirements, excessive losses, and impaired nutrient utilization.[44,45]

Components of the Nutrition Assessment

Medical and Nutrition History

Obtaining and evaluating detailed medical and nutrition histories is paramount to the nutrition assessment. Clinicians can use information from these histories to determine how suboptimal nutrition status relates to intake deficits, absorption/digestion issues, or both.[22] The clinician conducting the nutrition assessment should therefore review a patient's medical history for relevant information about past and present acute and chronic diseases, medications, diagnostic procedures, surgeries, and other therapies (eg, radiotherapy).[2,5,46] The review of medications should include prescription and nonprescription/over-the-counter drugs, vitamin and mineral supplements, and herbal supplements. Whenever possible, information about complementary and alternative medical treatments and the patient's socioeconomic and psychosocial status should also be assessed.

Medical history information specific to pediatrics includes the mother's health history during the pregnancy; the patient's prenatal and perinatal history; gestational age; history of prematurity; birth weight; classification as either small or large for gestational age; and growth patterns for weight, length, and head circumference. If growth history data are not included in the patient's records, they can typically be obtained with permission of the guardian/caregiver from the primary care physician. Other components of the history address the patient's developmental history, including problems with hypotonia or hypertonia as well as any delays in achieving developmental milestones.

To best capture a patient's nutrition history, the clinician must evaluate a variety of information, including recent changes in appetite, ability to eat (or coordinate the suck/swallow/breathe pattern), bowel patterns, activity level, nutrient intake, use of fad diets, feeding skills, types of feeding equipment used, food allergies and intolerances, and use of oral supplements (Table 1-10). Additional components in the nutrition history for pediatric patients may include maternal and infant issues related to breastfeeding; the adequacy of the human milk supply; the patient's overall tolerance of human milk or formula; the patient's interest in feeding or refusal to eat or drink; duration, frequency, and times of feedings; infant sleeping patterns; food-texture aversions; suck and swallow quality; and symptoms of gastroesophageal reflux.

Nutrition-Focused Physical Exam

The nutrition-focused physical exam (NFPE) is an excellent way to help evaluate nutrition status and has been included in assessment criteria for SGA and the ASPEN/AND characteristics.[23,25] The NFPE uses a body-systems approach and includes a logical assessment from head to toe of muscle mass, subcutaneous fat stores, fluid status, and vitamin and mineral abnormalities. NFPE techniques include visual inspection, palpation of specific body areas, auscultation, and interviewing the patient and caregiver for further information and confirmation of findings.[47] See Tables 1-11, 1-12, and 1-13 for NFPE guidelines and suggested areas of the body that are conducive to evaluating muscle mass, fat stores, and fluid accumulation.[25,28,48,49]

The assessment of sexual maturation, using Tanner staging (see Table 1-14), is a physical exam component of the nutrition assessment unique to pediatrics. Tanner staging is based on the development of secondary sex

TABLE 1-10. Components of the Medical and Nutrition History

Component	Examples
Diet	History (food records, diet recall, or feeding practices), dietary restrictions, alternative and/or complementary practices
Intolerances	Drug allergies, food allergies, food intolerances, food avoidances
Supplementation	Vitamin, mineral, or herbal supplements; oral nutrition drinks; other products
Weight	Recent intentional or unintentional changes; growth trends for infants and children[a]
Dental/oral health	Chewing and swallowing abilities, salivation, dentition, pain, aphthous ulcers, other oral lesions, taste changes
Mental status	Altered mental status, delirium, dementia
Gastrointestinal problems	Nausea, vomiting, heartburn, bloating, dyspepsia, gas, diarrhea, constipation, steatorrhea
Chronic disease	Long-term diseases affecting utilization of nutrients
Surgery	Surgical resection or disease of gastrointestinal tract, procedures involving other major organs (eg, organ transplant)

(continued)

TABLE 1-10. *(Continued)*

Component	Examples
Medications	Prescription and over-the-counter drugs, natural health products, other dietary supplements; side effects of medications and supplements; drug-nutrient interactions
Illicit drugs and alcohol	Use, amount, frequency
Socioeconomic factors	Food procurement, food preparation techniques, physical limitations affecting food preparation; use of/need for public aid assistance; level of education; income level
Cultural factors	Religion, customs, and their influence on eating patterns
Physical activity	Occupation, exercise regimen, sleep/rest pattern, dependence on a wheelchair, hypotonic vs hypertonic conditions

[a]See "Interpretation of Weight Data" later in this chapter.

characteristics. In nutrition assessment of children and adolescents, the clinician should interpret findings related to weight changes and growth patterns in the context of the patient's stage of sexual maturity. In boys, the peak of the rapid height growth occurs in Tanner stage 4. In girls, most linear growth is usually completed by the onset of menarche. However, girls who enter puberty early may have more linear growth after menarche than girls who enter puberty later. In pediatric patients, the rate of weight gain generally approximates the velocity of linear growth;

TABLE 1–11. Assessment of Body Areas for Fat Loss

Adult patients

Body Areas	Nutrition Status
Orbital region: Orbital fat pads	• **Well nourished/normal**: Soft, slightly bulging fat tissue • **Mild to moderate loss**: Faint to marginally dark circles, fairly hollow look • **Severe loss**: Deep depressions and sharp features appearing hollow; dark circles; loose skin
Upper arm region: Under triceps muscle	• **Well nourished/normal**: Plentiful fat tissue can be grasped using the forefinger and thumb • **Mild to moderate loss**: Some tissue can be grasped, but it is not abundant • **Severe loss**: Very little tissue can be grasped; examiner's forefinger and thumb touch
Thoracic and lumbar region: Midaxillary line, ribs, lower back, iliac crest	• **Well nourished/normal**: Iliac crest, spine, and ribs are well covered; clinician cannot see/feel individual bones well; chest is full • **Mild to moderate loss**: Iliac crest, spine, and rib bones are more apparent; some depressions are visible between bones • **Severe loss**: Iliac crest, spine, and rib bones are very apparent/prominent, easily visible; deep depressions between bones

(continued)

TABLE 1-11. *(Continued)*

Pediatric patients

Body Areas	Nutrition Status
Facial cheeks (buccal pads)	• **Well nourished/normal**: Rounded, full • **Mild to moderate loss**: Pads are flat • **Severe loss**: Face is hollow-looking, narrow
Upper arm region: Biceps/triceps	• **Well nourished/normal**: Plentiful fat tissue can be grasped using the forefinger and thumb • **Mild to moderate loss**: Some tissue can be grasped, but it is not abundant • **Severe loss**: Very little tissue can be grasped; inspector's forefinger and thumb touch
Thoracic and lumbar region: Midaxillary line, ribs, lower back	• **Well nourished/normal**: Ribs do not show; chest is full • **Mild to moderate loss**: Spine and rib bones are more apparent; some depressions are visible between bones • **Severe loss**: Spine and rib bones are very apparent/prominent, easily visible; deep depressions between bones
Buttocks (in infants)	• **Well nourished/normal**: Rounded, full • **Mild to moderate loss**: Slight curvature, not rounded • **Severe loss**: Flat, wasted-appearing; skin may look wrinkled

Source: Information is from references 28, 48, and 49.

TABLE 1–12. Assessment of Body Area for Muscle Loss

Body Areas	Nutrition Status

Clavicle bone region: Pectoralis major, deltoid, trapezius muscles	• **Well nourished/normal**:
	  ◦ Adults: Bones are not evident in males; may be visible/somewhat noticeable in females
	  ◦ Pediatrics: Bones are possibly visible but not prominent
	• **Mild to moderate loss**:[a]
	  ◦ Adults: Observable definition of bones in males; bones are more prominent than normal in females
	  ◦ Pediatrics: Some protrusion of bones
	• **Severe loss**: Obviously protruding bones, sharp edges

Acromion bone region: Deltoid muscle and shoulders	• **Well nourished/normal**: Soft, rounded features; curves at neck, shoulders, and upper arms • **Mild to moderate loss**:[a] Acromion process starting to look square, slightly protruding • **Severe loss**: Shoulder-to-arm joint is square; bone edges and acromion process are easily observed, rigid/solid to touch
Scapular bone region: Trapezius, supraspinatus, infraspinatus muscles	• **Well nourished/normal**: No significant or obvious depressions; bones are not noticeable • **Mild to moderate loss**:[a] ◦ Adults: Mild depressions, bones may be more prominent

(continued)

TABLE 1-12. *(Continued)*	
Body Areas	**Nutrition Status**
	○ Pediatrics: Degree of wasting is variable, may not be readily seen in all areas • **Severe loss**: Protruding, visible bones; readily observed depressions between shoulder and spine or ribs and scapula
Hand: Interosseous muscle	• **Well nourished/normal**: ○ Adults: Soft, bulging muscle, easy to grasp; potentially flat in some individuals ○ Pediatrics: n/a • **Mild to moderate loss**:[a] ○ Adults: Slight depressions; dorsal bones may be more prominent ○ Pediatrics: n/a • **Severe loss**: ○ Adults: Hollowed areas at base of thumb-forefinger intersection and along dorsal side of hand ○ Pediatrics: n/a
Patellar region: Knee, quadriceps muscles	• **Well nourished/normal**: Muscles add soft, rounded features; bones are not prominent • **Mild to moderate loss**:[a] Kneecap and bones are more noticeable, developing sharper edges due to diminished muscle coverage • **Severe loss**: Bones are sharply prominent/square; minimal muscle is appreciable around knee

(continued)

TABLE 1-12. *(Continued)*	
Body Areas	**Nutrition Status**
Anterior thigh: Quadriceps muscles	• **Well nourished/normal**: Well-rounded muscles; bone structure is not visible • **Mild to moderate loss**:[a] Mild depression visible in inner thighs • **Severe loss**: Inner thighs do not touch when knees are pressed together and are visibly thin
Posterior calf: Gastrocnemius muscle	• **Well nourished/normal**: Firm, well-developed, easy-to-grasp muscle; potentially flat in some adults • **Mild to moderate loss**:[a] Poorly developed muscle; thinner than usual • **Severe loss**: Very little to no muscle definition; thin, flat

Abbreviation: n/a, not applicable.

[a]In pediatric patients, the described characteristics are for moderate loss only; in adults, the characteristics are found in both mild and moderate losses.

Source: Information is from references 28, 48, and 49.

however, in females, the peak weight gain velocity occurs 6 to 9 months before the peak height change.[50,51]

Anthropometric Assessment

Using Growth Charts

In pediatric practice, growth is the most important parameter for assessing the nutrition status of a pediatric patient. It is assessed and monitored by plotting serial measurements of the patient's anthropometric data, including weight, length/height, BMI, and head

---

TABLE 1-13. Assessment of Edema and Fluid Accumulation[a]

Examination method:

- Adults: Inspect upper thighs/flanks (or possibly scrotum/vulva) in the activity-restricted patient; inspect ankles/calves in the mobile patient; in all patients, note ascites or anasarca.
- Pediatric patients: Use thumb to press on distal anterior foot (dorsal side) for 5 sec.

Status:

- **Normal**: No visual or palpable evidence of fluid accumulation
- **Mild (1+) edema**: Slight pitting (≤ 2 mm); no distortion when thumb is pressed into skin on lower extremity; pitting rapidly rebounds
- **Moderate (2+) edema**: Deeper pitting (2–4 mm) with pressure applied by thumb; slight swelling of the extremity; indentation resolves after several seconds
- **Severe (3–4+) edema**: Deep (4–6 mm) to very deep (>6 mm) pitting when skin is pressed by thumb; depression lasts for at least 1 min; extremity is obviously engorged

---

[a]Causes of edema unrelated to nutrition must be ruled out to use this parameter as a criteria for malnutrition. Fluid accumulation masks weight loss, and dehydration may artificially enhance loss of weight; therefore, nutrition assessment should be modified accordingly.

Source: Information is from references 25, 28, 48, and 49.

circumference, as well as (when appropriate) MUAC and triceps skinfold (TSF) thickness, on sex- and age-specific growth charts.[52]

In the United States, the World Health Organization (WHO) growth charts are used for term infants up to 2 years of age.[53] WHO growth standards are based on optimal growth of exclusively breastfed children.[54] Centers for Disease Control and Prevention (CDC) growth charts, which use data from 5 cross-sectional, nationally representative health examination surveys, are used to plot weight, height, and BMI in patients ages 2 through 20 years.[53]

TABLE 1–14. Tanner Stages of Development

Stage	Girls	Boys
1	Prepubescent	Prepubescent
2	Pubic hair and breast buds appear, increased activity of sweat glands	Pubic hair appears, growth of genitalia, increased activity of sweat glands
3	Breast enlargement, axillary hair present	Continued enlargement of genitalia, changes in voice, faint moustache/facial hair begins, axillary hair present
4	Nipple and areola become more pronounced, menarche begins	Pubic hair thickens, voice deepens, facial hair increases, hair on legs becomes darker
5	Breasts fully mature	Genitalia fully mature

Source: Information is from references 50 and 51.

Specialized growth curves are available for premature infants[55,56] and children with diagnoses such as Down syndrome (trisomy 21),[57] Turner syndrome,[58] Williams syndrome,[59] Prader-Willi syndrome,[60] and cerebral palsy.[61–63] Clinical judgment is particularly important when considering the use of such charts, which may be dated or based on small, nongeneralizable sample populations.[64] Specialized growth charts should be used in conjunction with WHO and CDC growth charts to monitor a patient's growth trends.[64] See Table 1-15 for more information on selected growth charts.[53–56,62,63]

Measuring Body Weight

Body weight measurement can be accomplished in a variety of ways depending on the condition and age of the patient.[65,66] Methods include the following:

TABLE 1-15. Examples of Growth Charts

Author	Description
WHO[54]	**Target population**: Infants and children from birth to age 24 months (should reflect corrected age up to age 3 years) **Parameters assessed**: • Weight for age • Length for age • Weight/length for age • Head circumference for age **Comments**: Based exclusively on data from breastfed infants; growth as the standard
CDC[53]	**Target population**: Children ages 2–20 years **Parameters assessed**: • Weight for age • Length for age • BMI for age • Head circumference for age (to age 36 months) **Comments**: Growth as reference, not a standard
Olsen[55]	**Target population**: Premature infants born at ≥23 weeks' gestational age **Parameters assessed**: • Weight for age • Length for age • Head circumference for age **Comments**: Based on large US population; separate charts for males and females
Fenton[56]	**Target population**: Premature infants born at 22 to <37 weeks' gestational age **Parameters assessed**: • Weight for age • Length for age • Head circumference for age **Comments**: 2003 Fenton growth chart postnatal data matches WHO data

(continued)

TABLE 1-15. *(Continued)*	
Author	**Description**
Brooks et al[62]	**Target population**: Children ages 2–20 years with cerebral palsy **Parameters assessed:** • Weight for age • Length for age • BMI for age **Comments**: 5 different charts based on gross motor function

Abbreviations: BMI, body mass index; CDC, Centers for Disease Control and Prevention; WHO, World Health Organization.

Source: Information is from references 53–56, 62, and 63.

- Standing weight: Assess the patient's ability to stand. Balance or recalibrate the scale and position the patient on the center of the scale base. Obtain the measurement from the balance scale or digital readout. The clothing worn by the patient, measuring equipment, and the time of day should all be uniform across measurements, and these data should be documented along with the weight.

- Built-in bed scale weight: If patients have difficulty with balance while standing or have limited mobility, a bed with a built-in scale can be used to measure weight. Before placing the patient in the bed, remove all unnecessary pillows, blankets, and medical devices. Zero the bed scale, making sure to follow bed-specific guidelines for accuracy. Transfer the patient to the center of the bed, without excessive clothing and shoes, and follow the manufacturer's instructions for measuring weight.[67]

- Sling weight: Roll the patient to one side and place the sling under the patient. Position the sling under the patient evenly. Attach the sling to the scale and record the weight measurement.

- Wheelchair weight: Position the ramp for wheelchair access. Weigh the empty wheelchair and record the weight of the chair. Repeat the procedure with the patient in the chair and deduct the chair weight from the total weight.

- Infant gram scale or platform beam balance scale (for pediatric patients): It is preferable to weigh infants and toddlers in the nude without clothing. Older children may be weighed while wearing underwear.

Body Mass Index and Weight for Length

BMI is a calculated measure using a person's weight and height to estimate body mass.

$$BMI = \text{Weight (kg)}/(\text{Height [m]})^2$$

BMI measures are classified as underweight, normal, overweight, or obese. In adults, BMI ≤ 18.4 is considered underweight and BMI ≤ 17 indicates moderate or severe underweight.[68] Of note, morbidity increases significantly with BMI ≤ 16.[69] Normal BMI ranges between 18.5 and 24.9, BMI between 25 and 29.9 is classified as overweight, and BMI ≥ 30 is classified as obesity.[68] In healthy older adults, the optimal BMI range is between 22 and 27.[70]

In pediatrics, a patient's weight for length or BMI is assessed using sex- and age-specific growth charts or z scores. For children ages 0 to 2 years, the CDC recommends plotting weight-for-length measurements on sex-specific WHO weight-for-length growth curves.[53] These curves reflect standards for how young children should grow in ideal conditions.[54] To assess weight in relation to height in children 2 to 29 years of age, BMI should be plotted on the CDC's sex-specific BMI-for-age growth charts.[53]

In children, BMI for age <5th percentile is classified as underweight, BMI for age between the 85th and 94th percentile is classified as overweight, and obesity is defined as BMI for age ≥95th percentile or BMI ≥30. BMI for age >99th percentile is considered severe obesity.[71]

There are limitations to the use of BMI in nutrition assessment. BMI does not differentiate fat mass, muscle mass, and skeletal mass, and the calculation may be skewed by weight data that reflect fluid shifts in the setting of critical or chronic illness.[72] For example, older, athletic children with increased muscle mass may be misclassified as overweight based on their BMI for age; therefore, other nutrition parameters may need to be used to assess body composition.[68]

Waist Circumference

In adults, waist circumference is used to predict abdominal obesity and correlates with comorbid medical conditions associated with increased visceral fat deposits or adipose tissue, including cardiovascular disease.[68] To measure weight circumference, use a flexible tape measure to measure the distance around the waist at the smallest area immediately below the rib cage and directly above the umbilicus.

Ideal Body Weight

Ideal body weight (IBW) is an estimate of healthy weight for a patient. A commonly used, empiric method for estimating IBW for adults in clinical settings is the Hamwi equation:[73]

> IBW in Males = 106 lb (48 kg) for first 60 inches of height + 6 lb (2.7 kg) per each additional inch

> IBW in Females = 100 lb (45 kg) for first 60 inches of height + 5 lb (2.3 kg) per each additional inch

Methods to estimate IBW in children include calculating the weight that would place the child at the 50th percentile curve for BMI for age; the McLaren-Read method, in which a child's stature is plotted on a weight-for-stature chart and then IBW is estimated to be the weight along the 50th percentile curve for that height; and the Moore method, which uses the weight along the same curve as height on a weight-for-stature chart.[74] However, there is no consensus on a standardized method, and the various methods provide a range of estimates.[74] Furthermore, anthropometric data for pediatric patients are frequently inaccurate, either because the information is out of date or because height and/or weight were measured imprecisely, which throws an IBW estimate based on such data into doubt.

Height/Length

Height (stature) can be measured directly or estimated using indirect methods such as knee height. Direct methods using a stadiometer or measuring rod require the patient to stand erect or lie flat. For those who cannot be moved and do not have musculoskeletal deformities, a recumbent bed length measurement can assist in determining height.

In pediatrics, recumbent lengths are measured with a length board for infants and toddlers. A stadiometer is used for children ages 2 years and older (if they can stand). With a stadiometer, heights are measured in stocking feet and with feet together, back straight, and arms hanging freely.

Head Circumference

Birth to age 36 months is a time of rapid brain growth. Head circumference should be routinely monitored during this time.[75] A flexible, narrow tape measure is used to measure the head circumference. Ideally, three measurements are done, and the results averaged. The CDC and WHO have published growth curves and z score data to use in assessing the measurements from 0–36 months and 0–24 months, respectively.[53,54] Arrested head growth (microcephaly) may indicate cranial defects or abnormal brain growth; accelerated growth may indicate catch-up growth or developmental defects (eg, hydrocephalus).

Interpretation of Weight Data

In adults, comparison of a patient's current and usual body weights can indicate the severity of malnutrition (see Tables 1-7 and 1-8, earlier in this chapter).[25] Recent involuntary weight changes can accurately predict nutrition risk.[25] When obtainable, the weight history of the individual is therefore more helpful than comparison of current weight to IBW. Caution is recommended when interpreting current weight as a percentage of IBW.[76] Body shape and weight tend to vary across age and population groups, which can skew interpretation of IBW vs current weight.[76]

Recent weight changes in children can indicate acute nutrition issues. A weight-for-age z score or percentile is not independently indicative of nutrition issues. Weight gain velocity based on the WHO growth velocity standards can be an indicator of undernutrition in children ages 0–24 months. Weight loss in patients older than 2 years can be used to assess malnutrition (see Table 1-9, earlier in this chapter).

Factors that influence interpretation of weight measurements include the following:

- Edema, ascites, hydrocephalus, diuretic therapy, and other fluid alterations can significantly alter body weight within short time periods.
- Fluid shifts from the intravascular space to the extravascular space and the intracellular space to the extracellular space with a concurrent decline in lean body mass occur in malnutrition. Therefore, loss of lean body mass may be masked, with little obvious change in weight, by fluid shifts.

Mid–Upper Arm Circumference and Triceps Skinfold Thickness

MUAC measures muscle, fat, and bone in the mid–upper arm, and TSF thickness measures subcutaneous fat stores in the upper arm. Both MUAC and TSF thickness can be used to estimate the fat-free and fat mass in a body. Clinicians require training to obtain reliable and reproducible measurements. Instructions for obtaining these measurements are described in the National Health and Examination Survey Anthropometry Manual.[77] These measurements are appropriate for assessing change over time in individual patients. Single measurements are less useful than serial measurements over time. A 2005 reference provides standards tables in the US population.[78]

MUAC should be used in nutrition assessment of pediatric patients as it can be an independent indicator of malnutrition in children ages 6–59 months.[45] TSF thickness is not used as an independent indicator of malnutrition, but this measurement can be used to monitor progress of a nutrition intervention as fat lost or fat gained.

Bioelectrical Impedance Analysis

Bioelectrical impedance analysis (BIA) is a body composition assessment technique based on the principle that lean tissue has higher electrical conduction and lower impedance than fat. Three types of BIA devices are available (single-frequency, multiple-frequency, and spectroscopy). Using a standardized protocol, imperceptible, low currents of electricity pass through electrodes attached to the extremities of an individual to measure resistance and reactance to estimate fat-free mass and fat mass.[79] BIA estimates of body composition are then calculated from the data with established modeling or predictive equations that are device-specific.[79,80]

BIA has been favored over other methods to analyze body composition because it is portable, safe, easy to use, and noninvasive, and because it obtains measures quickly and with relatively low associated costs. Various studies have validated the use of BIA in healthy, normal weight individuals under highly controlled situations, and research investigating the use of BIA to obtain raw bioimpedance values (eg, phase angle, impedance ratio, and fat-free mass index) to evaluate nutrition status and clinical outcomes has had some promising results.[79] However, other studies attempting to use BIA to estimate whole body lean tissue of clinical populations have produced mixed results regarding accuracy. Obese patients, and those with conditions that cause fluid overload, are particularly affected by errors in whole body estimations based on BIA.[79] Other factors affecting the precision or accuracy of BIA include the electrolyte status and skin temperature of the patient, room temperature, proximity to other electronic devices or metal, and variability in measurement protocols.[80] For these reasons, the use of BIA in clinical settings may not be appropriate. Further research on the use of BIA methods, especially in hospitalized patients, is needed.

Computed Tomography and Ultrasound

Within the last several years, computed tomography (CT) imaging and bedside ultrasound have emerged as valuable tools for assessment of body composition. CT scans at the level of the third lumbar vertebra (L3) are precise, accurate, and valid means to distinguish and quantify skeletal muscle and adipose tissue. These measures, obtained by a trained clinician with the assistance of computer software, can then be used to estimate muscle volume throughout the entire body. Repeated measures in certain patient populations also show that changes in lean tissue can be observed and monitored through CT scans. However, this monitoring method is not a realistic option for all patients because of its cost and the emission of high doses of radiation.[81] Therefore, CT scans should not be obtained for the sole purpose of nutrition assessment.

Bedside ultrasound has the ability to quantify muscle layer thickness and is generally regarded as safe, noninvasive, portable, cost effective, and relatively easy to perform.[82,83] It has been studied in a variety of hospitalized and critically ill patient populations to measure muscle thickness, a proxy for lean soft tissue.[81,82] Measurements taken at the quadriceps muscle have been shown to signify overall lean body mass.[82,83] Bedside ultrasound is less accurate than CT images, and the measurement can be subject to errors related to optimal positioning of the transducer, muscle compressibility, presence of edema, variances between clinicians' techniques, and reliable site selection.[81] However, given the benefits previously described, and the fact that an array of disciplines can use bedside ultrasound in practice, this tool shows promise as a quantifiable method to assess lean body mass.[81–83]

Functional Status

Malnutrition, especially when caused by disease, diminishes muscle strength, decreases muscle mass, and impairs functional capacity over time.[40,84] Both SGA and ASPEN/ AND criteria recognize that strength and functional status are important components of nutrition assessment in adults.[23,25,45] However, it is also important to understand that various factors unrelated to nutrition status can alter muscle function and strength, including acute and chronic diseases, inflammatory states, sensory loss caused by neuromuscular damage, and atrophy from inactivity.[84] Furthermore, impairment of muscle function has consequences regarding recovery from disease, morbidity, and mortality.[40] At this time, assessment of functional status is not routinely performed in the nutrition assessment of pediatric patients.[45]

Handgrip strength can be measured with a handgrip dynamometer, and such measurements can be used as a validated surrogate for upper body muscle strength in adults.[84] Handgrip strength is feasible for bedside care in non-critical-care situations and correlates well with other tests of muscle function, although it should be noted that age and gender influence results and studies with younger adult patients demonstrate better correlations with nutrition status than those with elderly patients.[40] Variations in measurement technique, imprecise cutoff values, and a lack of consensus on protocols are limitations of this method.[40,84] Furthermore, clinicians must be trained in the proper use of dynamometers, which may not be available in all facilities, and patients with certain diseases and conditions (eg, dementia, arthritis, heavy sedation) may not be able to grip the tool.[28,40,84] In addition to handgrip strength, other measures of functional status have been proposed and may become of value for assessing different patient populations as they become validated.[40,84]

Vitamin and Trace Mineral Abnormalities

The medical history, nutrition history, and NFPE are all used to assess patients for potential vitamin and trace mineral deficits. Patients with malnutrition generally exhibit signs and symptoms associated with multiple nutrient deficiencies rather than a single nutrient deficiency. Laboratory assessment is usually required to confirm clinically abnormal signs and symptoms. Clinicians should consult with their facility's laboratory regarding available tests, reference ranges, and results indicative of micronutrient deficiency or toxicity. See Tables 1-16 through 1-19 for guidance on assessment of vitamin and trace mineral status in adult and pediatric patients.[85–87]

TABLE 1–16. Possible Indicators of Vitamin Deficiency or Toxicity from the Physical Exam or Medical History

Vitamin	Indicators of Nutrient Imbalance
A	• **Deficiency**: Dermatitis, keratomalacia, infection (measles), night blindness, and xerophthalmia • **Toxicity**: Liver damage, vascular dilation, flushing, and irritation
Biotin	• **Deficiency**: Dermatitis, depression, alopecia, fatigue, muscle pain, somnolence, anorexia, and paresthesia • **Toxicity**: None known
Cyanocobalamin (B$_{12}$)	• **Deficiency**: Pernicious (megaloblastic) anemia, glossitis, spinal cord degeneration, and peripheral neuropathy • **Toxicity**: (Rare) irritability, headache, insomnia, and interference with B$_2$ and B$_6$
Folate (B$_9$)	• **Deficiency**: Macrocytic anemia, stomatitis, paresthesia, diarrhea, glossitis, lethargy, and neural tube defects of fetus • **Toxicity**: Diarrhea
Niacin (B$_5$)	• **Deficiency**: Pellagra: dementia (loss of memory), diarrhea, dermatitis, headaches, and glossitis • **Toxicity**: Osmotic diarrhea, oxalate kidney stones, interference with anticoagulation therapy, and rebound deficiency after high intake
Pantothenic acid (B$_3$)	• **Deficiency**: Fatigue, malaise, headache, insomnia, vomiting, and abdominal cramps • **Toxicity**: Acute: nausea, vomiting, headache, and dizziness

(continued)

TABLE 1-16. *(Continued)*

Vitamin	Indicators of Nutrient Imbalance
Pyridoxine (B_6)	• **Deficiency**: Dermatitis, neuritis, irritability, glossitis, cheilosis, depression, confusion, seizures, and microcytic anemia • **Toxicity**: Chronic: peeling/scaly skin, bone pain, pseudotumor cerebri, hepatomegaly, gingivitis, and alopecia
Riboflavin (B_2)	• **Deficiency**: Mucositis, glossitis, angular cheilitis or angular stomatitis (cold sores), dermatitis, vascularization of cornea, photophobia, lacrimation, decreased vision, impaired wound healing, and normocytic anemia • **Toxicity**: Excess bone and soft tissue calcification, kidney stones, constipation, myositis ossificans, and hypercalcemia
Thiamin (B_1)	• **Deficiency**: Beriberi: cardiomyopathy, peripheral neuropathy, encephalopathy (Wernicke-Korsakoff syndrome), and lactic acidosis • **Toxicity**: Prolonged clotting time
C	• **Deficiency**: Scurvy: capillary hemorrhage of gingiva, skin, and bone; poor wound healing, enlargement and keratosis of hair follicles, anemia, lethargy, and depression • **Toxicity**: None known
D	• **Deficiency**: Rickets, osteomalacia, tetany, hypophosphatemia, and muscle weakness • **Toxicity**: None known

(continued)

TABLE 1-16. (Continued)	
Vitamin	**Indicators of Nutrient Imbalance**
E	• **Deficiency**: Hemolysis (in preterm infant), anemia, peripheral neuropathy, and myopathy • **Toxicity**: Neuropathy
K	• **Deficiency**: Bleeding, purpura, and bruising • **Toxicity**: None known

Source: Information is from references 85 and 86.

Nutrition Support Care Plan

Increased morbidity and mortality are associated with malnutrition.[88,89] Malnutrition results in loss of lean body mass and subsequent loss of structure or function of body systems. Impaired respiratory function, reduced cardiac contractility, impaired renal function, altered immune function, and poor wound healing are known consequences of malnutrition.[90] Based on data gathered from the comprehensive nutrition assessment, clinicians make a nutrition diagnosis and set a plan of care. Decisions involved in a nutrition intervention include timing of the intervention, the route of therapy, and whether specialized nutrition formulations are needed.

Nutrition Diagnosis

A malnutrition diagnosis is associated with a longer hospital length of stay, increased comorbidities, higher medical costs, and more ongoing medical care needs for a patient after discharge.[90,91] The malnutrition criteria for adults

TABLE 1-17. Possible Indicators of Trace Mineral Deficiency or Toxicity from the Physical Exam or Medical History

Mineral	Indicators of Nutrient Imbalance
Ceruloplasmin	• **Deficiency**: Copper deficiency (90%–95% of plasma copper in ceruloplasmin) • **Toxicity**: None known
Copper	• **Deficiency**: Neutropenia, microcytic anemia, osteoporosis, decreased hair and skin pigmentation, dermatitis, hypotonia, zinc toxicity, growth failure, Wilson's disease, and neuropathy • **Toxicity**: Nausea, vomiting, epigastric pain, cirrhosis, Fanconi nephropathy, corneal pigmentation, and diarrhea
Iron (ferritin)	• **Deficiency**: Anemia and pica • **Toxicity**: Hemosiderosis
Selenium	• **Deficiency**: Muscle weakness and pain; anemia; cardiomyopathy; growth failure • **Toxicity**: Hair loss, dermatitis, garlic odor, brittle nails
Zinc	• **Deficiency**: Growth failure, dermatitis, hypogonadism, hypogeusia, diarrhea, apathy, depression, impaired wound healing, and immunosuppression • **Toxicity**: Nausea, vomiting, metallic taste, chills, and headache

Source: Information is from references 85 and 86.

and pediatrics described earlier in this chapter should be used to accurately and uniformly diagnose malnutrition. Documentation of the malnutrition diagnosis is important for timely interventions, reimbursement, and resource allocation.

TABLE 1–18. Selected Laboratory Tests to Assess Vitamin Status

Vitamin	Laboratory Assay
A	Serum retinol *or* serum retinol-binding protein
Biotin	Serum or urine
Cyanocobalamin (B_{12})	Serum
Folate (B_9)	Serum
Niacin (B_5)	Urinary metabolites
Pantothenic acid (B_3)	Urine
Pyridoxine (B_6)	Serum or plasma
Riboflavin (B_2)	Urine
Thiamin (B_1)	Urine
C	Serum or plasma; whole blood, leukocyte-platelet
D	Plasma 25-hydroxyvitamin D
E	Plasma alpha-tocopherol (whole blood)
K	PIVKA-II, INR, PT

Abbreviations: INR, international normalized ratio; PIVKA, protein induced by vitamin K absence; PT, prothrombin time.

Source: Information is from reference 87.

TABLE 1–19. Selected Laboratory Tests to Assess Trace Element Status

Trace Element	Laboratory Assay
Ceruloplasmin	Serum
Copper	Serum value
Iron (ferritin)	Serum
Selenium	Serum
Zinc	Serum value

Source: Information is from reference 87.

Nutrition Support Therapy

Integral to the process of nutrition care and the administration of nutrition support therapy is the decision regarding the route of administration. In most cases, enteral nutrition (EN) is recommended when a patient's nutrient requirements are not met by oral intake and there is a functional GI tract of sufficient length and condition to allow adequate nutrient absorption.[92,93] Parenteral nutrition should be used when the GI tract is not functional or cannot be accessed and in patients who cannot be adequately nourished by oral diets or EN.[94] Indications for EN are discussed in further detail in Chapter 2.

Timing of the Nutrition Intervention

Initiation of EN can be considered in well-nourished, stable adult patients unable to achieve 50% of their estimated nutrient requirements orally after 7 days.[92] For high-risk, hemodynamically stable, critically ill adults, it is recommended that EN be initiated within 24–48 hours of initial trauma or medical insult if it is not possible to maintain adequate volitional intakes and/or when patients are expected to require mechanical ventilation for at least 72 hours.[20] For adult patients deemed severely malnourished, those with moderate to severe pancreatitis, or individuals who just received a liver transplant, starting early EN within 24–48 hours is also recommended.

Advancement of nutrition support to goal protein and energy ranges depends on risk of refeeding, clinical status, and expected tolerance of therapy, but clinicians are encouraged to advance EN as quickly as the patient tolerates it. For non–critically ill adult patients, as well as some hemodynamically stable critically ill adult patients, aiming to achieve goal energy provisions within 24–48 hours of initiating EN will maximize nutrient delivery. Providing at least 80% of estimated energy and protein goals within 48–72 hours of initiation can impart clinical benefit.[20]

Pediatric patients with insufficient oral intake require nutrition support therapy. According to expert consensus, EN is the preferred route for delivery of nutrition for such patients, including those in an intensive care setting. Initiation of EN within the first 24–48 hours of admission to a pediatric intensive care unit and reaching at least two-thirds goal volume within the first week of critical illness have been associated with improved outcomes.[93]

Nutrition Monitoring and Evaluation

Once the nutrition assessment is complete and nutrition intervention begins, continuous reassessment (otherwise known as *monitoring*) is needed.[1] Many of the assessment parameters used initially are repeated serially to assess the efficacy of the intervention and any potential complications associated with the therapy. The data collected also determine the need to continue or cease nutrition care. See Chapter 8 for additional information.

Practice Resources

Malnutrition

- Jensen GL, Hsiao PY, D Wheeler. Adult nutrition assessment tutorial. *JPEN J Parenter Enteral Nutr*. 2012;36(3):267–274. doi:10.1177/014860711 2440284.
- American Society for Parenteral and Enteral Nutrition Malnutrition Committee. *Malnutrition Matters: A Call to Action for Providers Caring for Adult*

Patients (video). https://www.youtube.com/watch?v=JORLgsyri5U&list=PL-rWCu1T1wTKyItZtLZow_NLUJUeeM3JYU&index=5&t=0s. Published September 2018. Accessed November 21, 2018.

- American Society for Parenteral and Enteral Nutrition Malnutrition Committee. *Malnutrition Matters: A Call to Action for Providers Caring for Pediatric Patients* (video). https://www.youtube.com/watch?v=tjyCepbtDT0&list=PL-rWCuTTwTKyItZtLZow_NLUJUeeM3JYU&index=5. Published September 2018. Accessed November 21, 2018.
- American Society for Parenteral and Enteral Nutrition. Malnutrition Toolkit website. http://www.nutritioncare.org/MalToolkit. Accessed November 21, 2018.

Interpretation of Albumin and Prealbumin

- Chen Y, Henson S, Jackson AB, Richards JS. Obesity intervention in persons with spinal cord injury. *Spinal Cord*. 2006;44(2):82–91. doi:10.1038/sj.sc.3101818.
- Nova E, Lopez-Vidriero I, Varela P, et al. Indicators of nutritional status in restricting-type anorexia nervosa patients: a 1-year follow-up study. *Clin Nutr*. 2004;23(6):1353–1359. doi:10.1016/j.clnu.2004.05.004.
- Jensen GL. Inflammation as the key interface of the medical and nutrition universes: a provocative examination of the future of clinical nutrition and medicine. *JPEN J Parenter Enteral Nutr*. 2006;30(5):453–463.
- Davis CJ, Sowa D, Keim KS, Kinnare K, Peterson S. The use of prealbumin and C-reactive protein for monitoring nutrition support in adult patients receiving enteral nutrition in an urban medical center. *JPEN J Parenter Enteral Nutr*. 2012;36(2):197–204. doi:10.1177/0148607111413896.

Nutrition-Focused Physical Exam

- Hamilton C, ed. *Nutrition-Focused Physical Exam: An Illustrated Handbook.* Silver Spring, MD: American Society for Parenteral and Enteral Nutrition; 2016.
- DeTallo C, ed. *The Practitioner's Guide to Nutrition-Focused Physical Exam of Infants, Children, and Adolescents: An Illustrated Handbook.* Silver Spring, MD: American Society for Parenteral and Enteral Nutrition; 2019.

Anthropometrics

- National Center for Health Statistics. Growth charts. Centers for Disease Control and Prevention website. http://www.cdc.gov/growthcharts. Accessed November 21, 2018.
- World Health Organization child growth standards. World Health Organization website. http://who.int/childgrowth/standards/en. Accessed November 21, 2018.
- PediTools website (includes calculators for growth percentiles and z scores for WHO, CDC, Olsen, Down syndrome, and MUAC growth curves). http://www.peditools.org. Accessed November 21, 2018.
- National Health and Nutrition Examination Survey (NHANES). Anthropometry procedures manual. Centers for Disease Control and Prevention website. https://www.cdc.gov/nchs/data/nhanes/nhanes_07_08/manual_an.pdf. Accessed November 21, 2018.
- University of Vermont Department of Food and Nutrition Sciences. Bioelectric impedance analysis tutorial. University of Vermont website. http://nutrition.uvm.edu/bodycomp/bia/lesson1.html. Accessed November 21, 2018.

- Earthman CP. Body composition tools for assessment of adult malnutrition at the bedside: a tutorial on research considerations and clinical applications. *JPEN J Parenter Enteral Nutr.* 2015;39(7):787–822. doi:10.1177/0148607115595227.
- Gomez-Perez SL, Haus JM, Sheean P, et al. Measuring abdominal circumference and skeletal muscle from a single cross-sectional CT image: a step-by-step guide for clinicians using National Institutes of Health ImageJ. *JPEN J Parenter Enteral Nutr.* 2016;40(3):308–318. doi:10.1177/0148607115604149.
- Galindo Martín CA, Zepeda EM, Lescas Méndez OA. Bedside ultrasound measurement of rectus femoris: a tutorial for the nutrition support clinician. *J Nutr Metabol.* 2017;2017: 2767232. doi:10.1155/2017/2767232.

Functional Status

- Dietitians in Nutrition Support. *Handgrip Strength Assessment: A Skill to Enhance the Diagnosis of Disease-Related Malnutrition* (toolkit). 2017. Available for purchase at https://www.dnsdpg.org/store.cfm.

References

1. Lacey K, Pritchett E. Nutrition care process and model: ADA adopts road map to quality care and outcomes management. *J Am Diet Assoc.* 2003;103:1061–1072.
2. Field LB, Hand RK. Differentiating malnutrition screening and assessment: a nutrition care process perspective. *J Acad Nutr Diet.* 2015;115(5):824–828.
3. American Society for Parenteral and Enteral Nutrition. *Improve Patient Outcomes: A.S.P.E.N.'s Step-by-Step Guide to Addressing Malnutrition.* Silver Spring, MD: American Society for Parenteral and Enteral Nutrition; 2015.

4. A.S.P.E.N. pediatric nutrition care pathway (age 1 month–18 years) (infographic). Malnutrition solution center. American Society for Parenteral and Enteral Nutrition website. https://www.nutritioncare.org/Continuing_Education/Programs/Malnutrition_Awareness/Malnutrition. Accessed November 17, 2018.

5. Ukleja A, Freeman KL, Gilbert K, et al. Standards for nutrition support: adult hospitalized patients. *Nutr Clin Pract.* 2010;25(4):403–414.

6. Skipper A, Ferguson M, Thompson K, Castellanos VH, Porcari J. Nutrition screening tools: an analysis of the evidence. *JPEN J Parenter Enteral Nutr.* 2012;36(3):292–298.

7. Kruizenga HM, Van Tuldar MW, Seidell JC, et al. Effectiveness and cost-effectiveness of early screening and treatment of malnourished patients. *Am J Clin Nutr.* 2005;82:1082–1089.

8. van Bokhorst-de van der Schueren MA, Guaitoli PR, Jansma EP, de Vet HC. Nutrition screening tools: does one size fit all? A systematic review of screening tools for the hospital setting. *Clin Nutr.* 2014;33(1):39–58.

9. Academy of Nutrition and Dietetics. Nutrition screening adults: summary of all tools evaluated (2010). Evidence Analysis Library website. https://www.andeal.org/topic.cfm?cat=5437&conclusion_statement_id=251197&highlight=nutrition%20screen%20tool&home=1. Accessed November 21, 2018.

10. Heyland DK, Dhaliwal R, Jiang X, Day AG. Identifying critically ill patients who benefit the most from nutrition therapy: the development and initial validation of a novel risk assessment tool. *Crit Care.* 2011;15(6):R268.

11. Rahman A, Hasan RM, Agarwala R, Martin C, Day AG, Heyland DK. Identifying critically-ill patients who will benefit most from nutritional therapy: further validation of the "modified NUTRIC" nutritional risk assessment tool. *Clin Nutr.* 2016;35(1):158–162.

12. Lee YJ. Nutritional screening tools among hospitalized children: from past and to present. *Pediatr Gastroenterol Hepatol Nutr.* 2018;21(2):79–85.

13. Joosten KFM, Hulst JM. Nutritional screening tools for hospitalized children: methodological considerations. *Clin Nutr.* 2014;33:1–5.

14. Sermet-Gaudelus I, Poisson-Salomon AS, Colomb V, et al. Simple pediatric nutritional risk score to identify children at risk of malnutrition. *Am J Clin Nutr*. 2000;72:64–70.

15. McCarthy H, Dixon M, Crabtree I, et al. The development and evaluation of the Screening Tool for the Assessment of Malnutrition in Paediatrics (STAMP©) for use by healthcare staff. *J Hum Nutr Diet*. 2012; 25:311–318.

16. Huysentruyt K, Devreker T, Dejonckheere J, De Schepper J, Vandenplas Y, Cools F. Accuracy of nutritional screening tools in assessing the risk of undernutrition in hospitalized children. *J Pediatr Gastroenterol Nutr*. 2015;61(2):159–166.

17. Murphy AJ, White M, Viani K, Mosby TT. Evaluation of the nutrition screening tool for childhood cancer (SCAN). *Clin Nutr*. 2016;35(1):219–224.

18. Wonoputri N, Djais JT, Rosalina I. Validity of nutritional screening tools for hospitalized children. *J Nutr Metabol*. 2014;2014:143649.

19. Jensen GL, Compher C, Sullivan DH, Mullin GE. Recognizing malnutrition in adults: definitions and characteristics, screening, assessment, and team approach. *JPEN J Parenter Enteral Nutr*. 2013;37(6):802–807.

20. McClave SA, Taylor BE, Martindale RG, et al. Guidelines for the provision and assessment of nutrition support therapy in the adult critically ill patient: Society of Critical Care Medicine (SCCM) and American Society for Parenteral and Enteral Nutrition (A.S.P.E.N.). *JPEN J Parenter Enteral Nutr*. 2016;40(2):159–211.

21. Shronts EP, Cerra FB. The rational use of applied nutrition in the surgical setting. In: Paparella M, ed. *Otolaryngology*. Philadelphia, PA: WB Saunders; 1990.

22. Jeejeebhoy KN. Nutritional assessment. *Gastroenterol Clin North Am*. 1998;27(2):347–369.

23. Detsky AS, McLaughlin JR, Baker JP, et al. What is subjective global assessment of nutritional status? *JPEN J Parenter Enteral Nutr*. 1987;11:8–13.

24. Baker JP, Detsky AS, Wesson DL, et al. Nutritional assessment: a comparison of clinical judgment and objective measurements. *N Engl J Med*. 1988;306:969–973.

25. White JV, Guenter P, Jensen G, et al. Consensus statement: Academy of Nutrition and Dietetics and American Society for Parenteral and Enteral Nutrition: characteristics

recommended for the identification and documentation of adult malnutrition (undernutrition). *JPEN J Parenter Enteral Nutr.* 2012;36(3):275–283. doi:10.1177/0148607112440285.

26. Guenter P, Jensen G, Patel V, et al. Addressing disease-related malnutrition in hospitalized patients: a call for a national goal. *Jt Comm J Qual Patient Saf.* 2015;41(10):469–473.

27. JeVenn AK, Galang M, Hipskind P, Bury C. Malnutrition screening and assessment. In: Mueller CM, ed. *The ASPEN Adult Nutrition Support Core Curriculum.* 3rd ed. Silver Spring, MD: American Society for Parenteral and Enteral Nutrition; 2017:185–211.

28. Malone A, Hamilton C. The Academy of Nutrition and Dietetics/the American Society for Parenteral and Enteral Nutrition consensus malnutrition characteristics: application in practice. *Nutr Clin Pract.* 2013;28(6):639–650.

29. Jensen GL, Hsiao PY, Wheeler D. Adult nutrition assessment tutorial. *JPEN J Parenter Enteral Nutr.* 2012;36(3):267–274.

30. Riley LK, Rupert J. Evaluation of patients with leukocytosis. *Am Fam Physician.* 2015;92(11):1004–1011.

31. McDowell S. What is leukopenia? *Healthline.* June 1, 2017. https://www.healthline.com/health/leukopenia. Accessed June 15, 2018.

32. Marcin J. C-reactive protein test. *Healthline.* May 22, 2017. https://www.healthline.com/health/c-reactive-protein. Accessed June 15, 2018.

33. Ferritin, serum. Mayo Medical Laboratories website. https://www.mayomedicallaboratories.com/test-catalog/Clinical+and+Interpretive/88153. Accessed June 15, 2018.

34. Hypotension—what causes hypotension? National Heart, Lung, and Blood Institute website. https://www.nhlbi.nih.gov/node/3740. Accessed June 15, 2018.

35. Tachycardia. Mayo Clinic website. https://www.mayoclinic.org/diseases-conditions/tachycardia/symptoms-causes/syc-20355127. Accessed June 15, 2018.

36. Bradycardia. Mayo Clinic website. https://www.mayoclinic.org/diseases-conditions/bradycardia/symptoms-causes/syc-20355474. Accessed June 15, 2018.

37. McCullough L, Arora S. Diagnosis and treatment of hypothermia. *Am Fam Physician.* 2004;70(12):2325–2332.

38. Fever. Mayo Clinic website. https://www.mayoclinic.org/diseases-conditions/fever/symptoms-causes/syc-20352759. Accessed June 15, 2018.

39. Norman K, Stobaus N, Gonzalez MC, Schulzke JD, Pirlich M. Hand grip strength: outcome predictor and marker of nutritional status. *Clin Nutr.* 2011;30:135–142.

40. Jensen GL, Bistrian B, Roubenoff R, Heimburger DC. Malnutrition syndromes: a conundrum vs continuum. *JPEN J Parenter Enteral Nutr.* 2009;33(6):710–716.

41. Jensen GL, Mirtallo J, Compher C, et al. Adult starvation and disease-related malnutrition: a proposal for etiology-based diagnosis in the clinical practice setting from the International Consensus Guideline Committee. *JPEN J Parenter Enteral Nutr.* 2010;34(2):156–159. doi:10.1177/0148607110361910.

42. Hudson L, Chittams J, Griffith C, Compher C. Malnutrition identified by Academy of Nutrition and Dietetics/American Society for Parenteral and Enteral Nutrition is associated with more 30-day readmissions, greater hospital mortality, and longer hospital stays: a retrospective analysis of nutrition assessment data in a major medical center. *JPEN J Parenter Enteral Nutr.* 2018;42(5):892–897. doi:10.1002/jpen.1021.

43. Ceniccola GD, Holanda TP, Pequeno RSF, et al. Relevance of AND-ASPEN criteria of malnutrition to predict hospital mortality in critically ill patients: a prospective study. *J Crit Care.* 2018;44:398–403.

44. Mehta NM, Corkins MR, Lyman B, et al. Defining pediatric malnutrition: a paradigm shift toward etiology-related definitions. *JPEN J Parenter Enteral Nutr.* 2013;37(4):460–481. doi:10.1177/0148607113479972.

45. Becker P, Carney LN, Corkins M, et al. Consensus statement of the Academy of Nutrition and Dietetics/American Society of Parenteral and Enteral Nutrition: indicators recommended for the identification and documentation of pediatric malnutrition (undernutrition). *Nutr Clin Pract.* 2015; 30(1):147–161. doi:10.1177/0884533614557642.

46. Ireton-Jones CS, Hasse JM. Comprehensive nutritional assessment: the dietitians' contribution to the team effort. *Nutrition.* 1992;8(2):75–81.

47. Fischer M, JeVenn A, Hipskind P. Evaluation of muscle and fat loss as diagnostic criteria for malnutrition. *Nutr Clin Pract.* 2015;30(2):239–248.

48. Secker DJ, Jeejeebhoy KN. How to perform subjective global nutritional assessment in children. *J Acad Nutr Diet.* 2012;112(3):424–431.

49. DeTallo C, ed. *The Practitioner's Guide to Nutrition-Focused Physical Exam of Infants, Children, and Adolescents: An Illustrated Handbook.* Silver Spring, MD: American Society for Parenteral and Enteral Nutrition; 2019.

50. Tanner JM. *Growth in Adolescents.* 2nd ed. Boston, MA: Blackwell Scientific Publications; 1962.

51. Chumlea WC. Physical growth and maturation. In: Samour PM, Lang CE, eds. *Handbook of Pediatric Nutrition.* 3rd ed. Boston, MA: Jones & Bartlett; 2005:1–10.

52. Assessment of nutritional status. In: Kleinman RE, Greer FR, eds. *Pediatric Nutrition.* 7th ed. Elk Grove Village, IL: American Academy of Pediatrics. 2014:609–642.

53. Centers for Disease Control and Prevention. Growth charts. https://www.cdc.gov/growthcharts/index.htm. Accessed November 21, 2018.

54. World Health Organization child growth standards. World Health Organization website. http://who.int/childgrowth/standards/en. Accessed November 21, 2018.

55. Olsen IE, Groveman SA, Lawson L, Clark RH, Zemel BS. New intrauterine growth curves based on United States data. *Pediatrics.* 2010;125(2):e214–e224. doi:10.1542/peds.2009-0913.

56. Fenton TR, Kim JH. A systematic review and meta-analysis to revise the Fenton growth chart for preterm infants. *BMC Pediatr.* 2013;13:59. doi:10.1186/1471-2431-13-59.

57. Cronk C, Crocker AC, Pueschel SM, et al. Growth charts for children with Down syndrome. *Pediatrics.* 1988;81:102–110.

58. Lyon AJ, Preece MA, Grant DB. Growth curve for girls with Turner syndrome. *Arch Dis Child.* 1985;60:932–935.

59. Morris CA, Demsey MS, Leonard CL, et al. Height and weight of males and females with Williams syndrome. *Williams Syndr Assoc Newslett.* Summer 1991:29–30.

60. Butler MG, Meany FJ. Standards for selected anthropometric measurements in Prader-Willi syndrome. *Pediatrics.* 1991;88:853–858.

61. Krick J, Murphy-Miller P, Zeger S, et al. Pattern of growth in children with cerebral palsy. *J Am Diet Assoc.* 1996;96:680–685.

62. Brooks J, Day SM, Shavelle RM, Strauss DJ. Low weight, morbidity, and mortality in children with cerebral palsy: new

clinical growth charts. *Pediatrics.* 2011;128:e299. doi:10.1542/peds.2010-2801.

63. Cerebral palsy: new growth charts. Life Expectancy Project website. http://www.lifeexpectancy.org/articles/newgrowthcharts.shtml. Accessed November 21, 2018.

64. Maternal Child and Health Bureau. The CDC growth charts for children with special health care needs [training module]. http://depts.washington.edu/growth/cshcn/text/intro.htm. Accessed November 21, 2018.

65. Guenter PA, Smithgall JM, Williamson JM, Rombeau JL. Body weight. In: Rombeau JL, Caldwell MD, Forlaw L, Guenter PA, eds. *Atlas of Nutrition Support Techniques.* Boston, MA: Little, Brown; 1989:1–12.

66. Heymsfield SB, Baumgartner RN, Pan SF. Nutritional assessment of malnutrition by anthropometric methods. In: Shils M, Olson JA, Shike M, Ross AC. *Modern Nutrition in Health and Disease.* 9th ed. Baltimore, MD: Williams and Wilkins; 1999.

67. *Lippincott's Nursing Procedures.* 7th ed. Philadelphia, PA: Lippincott Williams & Wilkins; 2015.

68. National Heart, Lung, and Blood Institute. *Clinical Guidelines on the Identification, Evaluation, and Treatment of Overweight and Obesity in Adults: Executive Summary.* Washington, DC: National Institutes of Health; 2002.

69. World Health Organization. Obesity: preventing and managing the global epidemic. Report of a WHO Consultation presented at: the World Health Organization; June 3–5, 1997; Geneva, Switzerland. Publication WHO/NUT/NCD/98.1.

70. American Academy of Family Physicians, American Dietetic Association, and National Council on Aging. *Nutrition Interventions Manual for Professionals Caring for Older Americans.* Washington, DC: Nutrition Screening Initiative; 1992.

71. Barlow SE; Expert Committee. Expert Committee recommendations regarding the prevention, assessment, and treatment of child and adolescent overweight and obesity: summary report. *Pediatrics.* 2007;120(Suppl 4):S164–S192.

72. Freeman DS, Sherry B. The validity of BMI as an indicator of body fatness and risk among children. *Pediatrics.* 2009;124(Suppl 1):S23–S34. doi:10.1542/peds.2008-3586E.

73. Hamwi GJ. Changing dietary concepts. In: Danowski TS, ed. *Diabetes Mellitus: Diagnosis & Treatment.* Vol. 1. New York, NY: American Diabetes Association; 1964:73–78.

74. Phillips S, Edlbeck A, Kirby M, Goday P. Ideal body weight in children. *Nutr Clin Pract.* 2007;22(2):240–245. doi:10.1177/0115426507022002240.

75. Sentongo T. Growth assessment and monitoring. In: Corkins MR, Balint J, Bobo E, Plogsted E, Yaworski JA, eds. *The A.S.P.E.N. Pediatric Nutrition Support Core Curriculum.* 2nd ed. Silver Spring, MD: American Society for Parenteral and Enteral Nutrition; 2010:142.

76. Knapp TR. A methodological critique of the "ideal weight" concept. *JAMA.* 1983;250:506–510.

77. Centers for Disease Control and Prevention. National Health and Nutrition Examination Survey (NHANES). Anthropometry manual. https://wwwn.cdc.gov/nchs/data/nhanes/2013-2014/manuals/2013_Anthropometry.pdf. Published January 2013. Accessed June 18, 2018.

78. McDowell MA, Fryar CD, Hirsch R, Ogden CL. Anthropometric reference data for children and adults: U.S. population, 1999–2002. *Adv Data.* 2005;(361):1–5.

79. Mulasi U, Kuchnia AJ, Cole AJ, Earthman CP. Bioimpedance at the bedside: current applications, limitations, and opportunities. *Nutr Clin Pract.* 2015;30(2):180–193.

80. Earthman CP. Body composition tools for assessment of adult malnutrition at the bedside: a tutorial on research considerations and clinical applications. *JPEN J Parenter Enteral Nutr.* 2015;39(7):787–822.

81. Prado CM, Heymsfield SB. Lean tissue imaging: a new era for nutritional assessment and intervention. *JPEN J Parenter Enteral Nutr.* 2014;38(8):940–953.

82. Tillquist M, Kutsogiannis DJ, Wischmeyer PE, et al. Bedside ultrasound is a practical and reliable measurement tool for assessing quadriceps muscle layer thickness. *JPEN J Parenter Enteral Nutr.* 2014;38(7):886–890.

83. Gruther W, Benesch T, Zorn C, et al. Muscle wasting in intensive care patients: ultrasound observation of the M. quadriceps femoris muscle layer. *J Rehabil Med.* 2008; 40(3):185–189.

84. Russell MK. Functional assessment of nutrition status. *Nutr Clin Pract.* 2015;30(2):211–218.

85. Esper DH. Utilization of nutrition-focused physical assessment in identifying micronutrient deficiencies. *Nutr Clin Pract.* 2015;30(2):194–202. doi:10.1177/0884533615573054.

86. McKeever L. Vitamins and trace minerals. In: Mueller CM, ed. *The ASPEN Adult Nutrition Support Core Curriculum.* 3rd ed. Silver Spring, MD: American Society for Parenteral and Enteral Nutrition; 2017:139–182.

87. Russell MK. Laboratory monitoring. In: Matarese LE, Gottschlich MM, eds. *Contemporary Nutrition Support Practice.* Philadelphia, PA: WB Saunders; 2003:45–62.

88. Black DR, Sciacca JP, Coster DC. Extremes in body mass index: probability of health care expenditures. *Prev Med.* 1994;23:385–393.

89. Seres DS. Nutritional assessment: current concepts and guidelines for the busy physician. *Pract Gastroenterol.* 2003; 8:30–39.

90. Tignanelli CJ, Bukowiec JC. Hospital-based nutrition support: a review of the latest evidence. *J Clin Nutr Diet.* 2017; 3:22. doi:10.4172/2472-1921.100057.

91. Abdelhadi RA, Bouma S, Bairdain S. Characteristics of hospitalized children with a diagnosis of malnutrition: United States, 2010. *JPEN J Parenter Enteral Nutr.* 2016;40(5):623–635.

92. McClave SA, DiBaise JK, Mullin GE, Martindale RG. ACG clinical guideline: nutrition therapy in the adult hospitalized patient. *Am J Gastroenterol.* 2016;111(3):315–334.

93. Mehta NM, Skillman HE, Irving SY, et al. Guidelines for the provision and assessment of nutrition support therapy in the pediatric critically ill patient: Society of Critical Care Medicine and American Society for Parenteral and Enteral Nutrition. *JPEN J Parenter Enteral Nutr.* 2017;41(5):706–742.

94. Worthington P, Balint J, Bechtold M, et al. When is parenteral nutrition appropriate? *JPEN J Parenter Enteral Nutr.* 2017;41:324–377.

CHAPTER 2

Overview of Enteral Nutrition and Patient Selection

Introduction

When adequate oral intake is compromised or contraindicated, nutrition support may be warranted for survival. Enteral nutrition (EN), the provision of nutrients via the gastrointestinal (GI) tract through a feeding tube, is the preferred route for delivering nutrition in patients who cannot meet their nutrition needs through voluntary oral intake.[1] When access is available and the GI tract can be safely used, EN is associated with numerous physiological, metabolic, safety, and cost benefits over parenteral nutrition (PN).[1]

The physiological benefits of EN include using normal digestive and absorptive pathways. In contrast to PN, nutrients that are administered enterally undergo first-pass metabolism, which promotes the efficient utilization of nutrients. EN is also an important therapeutic tool that can diminish the adverse structural and functional consequences associated with gut disuse.[2] The presence of nutrients in the gut lumen, even in small amounts, helps maintain normal digestive and absorptive functions of the GI tract. EN also assists with maintenance of the gut-associated lymphoid tissue and mucosa-associated lymphoid tissue, both of which play an integral role in immunity.[2] In prospective, randomized clinical trials (RCTs), EN has been associated with reduced infectious complications, likely through the maintenance of GI integrity.[2–4] Alterations in gut integrity due to loss of villous height, reduction in secretory immunoglobulin A production, and increased gut permeability can lead to systemic infectious complications and multiorgan dysfunction syndrome.[3,4] By maintaining gut integrity through the use of EN, the stress and immune responses are modulated and disease severity may therefore be decreased.[5,6] Lastly, EN is also associated with fewer complications and is less expensive than PN. The time-tested adage "If the gut works, use it" has become the guiding principle when identifying patients for EN.

Technological advancements in enteral formulations and equipment have greatly expanded the number of patients who can receive EN. The EN use process (Figure 2-1) is the system within which EN is used.[7] It involves a number of major steps: initial patient assessment, recommendations for an EN regimen, selection of the enteral access device (EAD), the EN prescription, review of the EN order, product selection or preparation, product labeling and dispensing, administration of the EN to the patient, and patient monitoring and reassessment, with documentation at each step. This process requires a multidisciplinary team of competent clinicians working in concert to provide safe nutrition care.[7] This chapter briefly surveys the various aspects of the process; refer to the other chapters in this handbook for more detailed information.

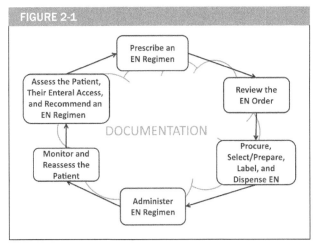

FIGURE 2-1

The enteral nutrition (EN) use process. Reprinted with permission from reference 7: Boullata J, Carrera AL, Harvey L, et al. ASPEN safe practices for enteral nutrition therapy. *JPEN J Parenter Enteral Nutr.* 2016;41(1):15–103. doi:10.1177/0148607116673053.

History of Enteral Nutrition

In ancient times, equipment such as wooden or glass tubes was used to administer various combinations of liquids to individuals who were unable or unwilling to consume adequate quantities of food.[8] Given the difficulty and danger involved in such attempts, enteral feeding was often viewed as an option of last resort. During the 18th and 19th centuries, equipment remained fairly primitive, and nutrition choices were limited to liquids such as broth, milk, eggs, and wine.[9] In the late 19th century—a time when efficient nutrient absorption was thought to take place in the colon—rectal feedings were commonly used to circumvent the challenges of achieving reliable access to the upper GI tract.[9]

With the advent of modern medicine, technological advances have led to the availability of a plethora of

EADs and formulas that have improved the safety and efficacy of EN. Additionally, a multitude of studies have demonstrated that improved outcomes are associated with EN.[2–6,10–12]

Indications for Enteral Nutrition and Patient Selection

A thorough nutrition assessment facilitates the identification of patients who may benefit from the initiation of nutrition support (see Chapter 1). Data collected in the assessment process guide decisions related to nutrition interventions by determining the most appropriate route for providing nutrition (see Figure 2-2), identifying the optimal timing for initiation of therapy, establishing nutrient requirements, detecting potential complications, and identifying any need for specialty formulations.[13]

The process of determining which patients actually should receive a feeding tube and EN can be quite challenging. Table 2-1 lists important factors to consider before placement of any type of EAD. Addressing these issues may take some time. Therefore, waiting a few days before placing a feeding tube may be appropriate for patients who are not critically ill or malnourished. For critically ill patients, the patient should be hemodynamically stable and fully resuscitated before EN support is initiated.[14]

Individuals who have a functional GI tract but have clinical conditions in which oral intake is impossible, inadequate, or unsafe are candidates for EN. EN should be considered for malnourished patients and those who are at high risk for becoming malnourished because they cannot maintain adequate nutrition status through oral intake alone. Other possible indications for EN include the following:

FIGURE 2-2

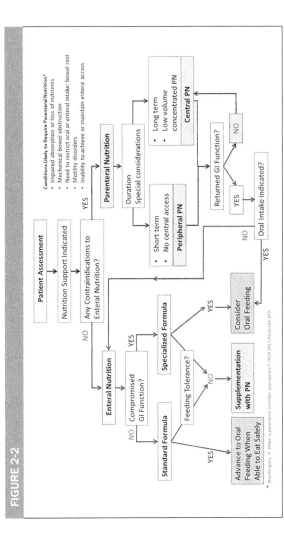

Selecting routes for delivery of nutrition in adults. Reprinted with permission from reference 13: Ukleja A, Gilbert K, Mogensen KM, et al. Standards for nutrition support: adult hospitalized patients. *Nutr Clin Pract.* 2018;33(6):906–920. doi:10.1002/ncp.10204.

TABLE 2-1. Factors to Consider Before Initiating Enteral Nutrition

- The patient's clinical and nutrition status, medical diagnosis, and prognosis
- Risks and benefits of therapy
- Discharge plans
- Quality of life
- Ethical issues
- The patient's or family's wishes
- Cost and reimbursement issues

- Poor appetite, which may be associated with a chronic medical condition or treatment
- Dysphagia, which may be related to neurological disease, oropharyngeal dysfunction, or another issue
- Major trauma, burns, wounds, and/or critical illness

Additionally, severely malnourished preoperative patients who have a functional GI tract may benefit from a course of EN prior to surgery.[15]

Infants and children have a higher rate of energy expenditure than adults; on a weight basis, energy requirements are 3 to 4 times higher for infants than for adults. Therefore, infants and children are at greater risk for nutrition compromise than adults.[16,17] The nutrition goals for the pediatric patient are to provide adequate nutrition for growth, development, and the preservation and proliferation of lean body mass.[5,18] Extended periods of malnutrition during childhood can manifest in growth failure and have adverse effects on cognitive and behavioral development. In hospitalized children, malnutrition is associated with longer length of stay, higher infection rates, and worse clinical outcomes (eg, longer times to wean off ventilator support).[19,20] For these reasons, identifying malnutrition and optimizing nutrition provision in children is vital.

Initiation of EN may be considered in infants and children who have a functioning GI tract in the following circumstances:

- Prolonged *nil per os* (NPO) status during hospitalization:
  - If the patient is age 1 year or older, consider EN if patient is NPO or is anticipated to remain NPO ≥5 days.[21]
  - If the patient is younger than age 1 year, consider EN if the patient is NPO or is anticipated to remain NPO ≥3 days.[21]
- Disorders of oral feeding (eg, abnormal sucking and swallowing, discoordination, aspiration, dysphagia, congenital abnormalities of upper GI tract, severe gastroesophageal reflux, esophagitis, feeding/oral aversion, anorexia nervosa)[21]
- Disorders of digestion and/or absorption (eg, congenital abnormalities of the GI tract, GI dysmotility, intractable diarrhea of infancy, autoimmune enteropathy, immunodeficiency, short bowel syndrome, organ transplantation, graft-versus-host disease, pancreatitis, cystic fibrosis)[21]
- Conditions with increased nutrient and/or metabolic requirements (eg, cystic fibrosis, burn, injury, recurrent infection, congenital heart defects, chronic renal or pulmonary disease)
- Poor growth velocity (weight decrease of more than 2 standard deviations based on z score)
- Inadequate growth, weight loss, or no weight change[21]
- Weight for height less than the fifth percentile or z score of less than −2
- Mid–upper arm circumference less than the fifth percentile for age
- Inability to consume at least 80% of estimated energy needs by mouth[22]

- Disorders where EN is a key component of disease treatment, such as the use of exclusive EN for Crohn's disease, the ketogenic diet for epilepsy, or specialty formulas for inborn errors of metabolism[21]

Contraindications to Enteral Nutrition

In certain situations, patients should not receive EN. Table 2-2 summarizes selected contraindications to EN.[14,21,23–25]

TABLE 2-2. Selected Contraindications to Enteral Nutrition Support
Potential contraindications for patients of all ages: • Nonoperative mechanical GI obstruction   • Hemodynamic instability (eg, mean arterial pressure <50 mmHg)   • Intractable vomiting/diarrhea refractory to medical management   • Severe short bowel syndrome (<100 cm small bowel remaining)   • Distal high-output fistulas   • Severe GI bleed   • Severe GI malabsorption[a]   • Inaccessible GI tract   • Aggressive intervention is not warranted or not desired by the patient
Relative contraindications in pediatric patients: • Intestinal dysmotility   • Necrotizing enterocolitis   • Toxic megacolon   • Diffuse peritonitis   • GI bleeding

Abbreviations: EN, enteral nutrition; GI, gastrointestinal.

[a]For example, EN failed as evidenced by progressive deterioration in the patient's nutrition status.

Source: Information is from references 14, 21, and 23–25.

To determine whether contraindications are relative or absolute, the patient's clinical status should be thoroughly assessed. In particular, a thorough and objective evaluation of GI function is needed to identify any obstacle to successful enteral feeding. Additionally, patients receiving EN should be monitored closely to detect any complications or signs of intolerance that may require a change in the EN regimen.

Often, potential barriers to EN can be circumvented with careful selection of the appropriate EAD, formula, and route of administration. For example, patients with minimally functional digestive and absorptive capabilities can often be fed using elemental or small-peptide formulations (see Chapters 4 and 5 for further discussion on EN formulas).

It was previously thought that paralytic ileus, defined as absence of bowel sounds or flatus, presented a contraindication to enteral feedings. However, it is now known that the absence of bowel sounds does not preclude safe EN.[14] Ileus has varied effects on different areas of the intestine. For example, postoperative ileus appears to affect colonic and gastric function to a greater extent than small intestinal function.[26] While similar conditions, such as partial small bowel obstruction and motility disorders, also present challenges to successful EN, these problems are not considered absolute barriers.

Vomiting and diarrhea are frequently identified as contraindications to EN. Vomiting presents challenges in maintaining nasal tube placement. However, successful enteral administration may be promoted by (a) the initiation of small bowel feedings with simultaneous gastric decompression and (b) the use of prokinetic agents. Patients with diarrhea should be evaluated to identify the cause (eg, *Clostridium difficile* infection or medications) and type of diarrhea (osmotic vs secretory).[14] The patient's nutrition status as well as the risk for a general overall deterioration in clinical status should also be considered (see Chapter 9 for further discussion of nausea and diarrhea).

In some situations, GI fistulas may preclude the initiation of EN. Enteral feedings are generally better tolerated by patients with more proximal or distal fistulas (rather than midgut), and low to moderate fistula output. High-output fistulas in the mid-jejunal area tend to be the most problematic. Patients should be monitored closely to ensure efficacy and tolerance of EN support. An increase in fistula output with enteral feeding suggests that other means of nutrition support, such as PN, may be indicated.

A mechanical obstruction of the GI tract, or pseudo-obstruction that does not resolve, is generally an absolute contraindication to enteral feedings. Patients with a partial obstruction may receive EN; however, careful monitoring is essential in order to ensure efficacy and tolerance of EN therapy.

The use of EN for patients with GI bleeding presents another clinical dilemma. GI bleeding was previously considered an absolute contraindication for enteral feedings since the literature in the past suggested that any GI bleeding was associated with adverse outcomes.[27] Etiology, location, and severity of the bleeding are all factors that should be evaluated before initiating enteral support. For most patients, lower GI bleeding does not affect the administration of EN.[28] Conversely, enteral feedings for patients who present with upper GI bleeding due to esophageal varices, portal hypertension, or cirrhosis should be delayed until risk of bleeding has diminished.[15]

While the Society of Critical Care Medicine (SCCM) and American Society for Parenteral and Enteral Nutrition (ASPEN) clinical practice guidelines for the provision of nutrition support for critically ill adults generally recommend early initiation of EN in critically ill patients (see Optimal Timing for Enteral Nutrition section later in this chapter), the guidelines also state that EN should be withheld for patients with hypotension (mean arterial pressure <50 mmHg), during initiation of catecholamine agents (ie, dopamine, epinephrine, norepinephrine, etc), and when doses of catecholamine agents are increased.[14] In the NUTRIREA-2 study, critically ill patients who were mechanically ventilated receiving vasopressor support and early EN experienced bowel ischemia to a greater degree than patients receiving PN (19 patients in EN group vs 5 patients in PN group; $P = 0.007$), supporting the importance of providing EN to stable patients.[29] Conversely, stable patients receiving low-dose vasopressor support had lower mortality rates for both intensive care unit (ICU) mortality and hospital mortality when EN was initiated early.[30]

During periods of hemodynamic instability in pediatric patients, clinicians may be reluctant to provide EN because of the risk of bowel ischemia. However, studies have shown that critically ill pediatric patients can tolerate full-strength, continuous EN while receiving extracorporeal membrane oxygenation and tolerate EN administered at the goal rate while receiving cardiovascular medication support (ie, vasopressors) that affect gut perfusion.[31,32]

Optimal Timing for Enteral Nutrition

The optimal times to initiate EN depend on the patient's clinical and nutrition status (eg, medically stable, critically ill, acutely ill, nourished, malnourished). Medical and nutrition assessment is required to determine the best timing for the individual patient.

Medically Stable Patients

The precise length of time that a patient can tolerate suboptimal nutrition intake is unknown. In a 2017 consensus document on the use of PN, PN support is recommended after 7 days in well-nourished, medically stable adult patients who are unable to achieve 50% of estimated nutrient requirements.[33] In this document, it is recommended that in patients "at risk" for malnutrition, PN intervention should begin within 3–5 days with inadequate oral or enteral intake. The principles underlying these recommendations can be applied to support the initiation of enteral feedings in the patient unable to achieve adequate oral intake.

Worse outcomes, including increased morbidity and longer hospital length of stay, have been reported for hospitalized adult patients who do not eat for 10 to 14 days following admission or surgery.[14] The optimal timing to promote positive clinical outcomes in general nonsurgical and non–critically ill patients requires further evaluation in large clinical trials.

Critically Ill Patients

In contrast to patients who are medically stable, critically ill patients seem to benefit from early initiation of EN. When EN initiation is delayed, patients are exposed to energy deficits, which are correlated with increased incidence of complications in critical illness.[34] Although the optimal timing for EN support in critically ill patients has not been clearly elucidated, the SCCM/ASPEN guidelines for critically ill adults recommend initiating EN within 24 to 48 hours postoperatively or following injury requiring admission to the ICU because evidence suggests that early initiation improves clinical outcomes.[14] In agreement with adult critical care guidelines, recommendations for patients in the pediatric intensive care unit (PICU) also support early EN initiation (ie, within 24–48 hours of PICU admission).[35]

Starting EN as trophic feeds in the first week of critical illness may be an option for patients who cannot initially tolerate full feedings. Several RCTs comparing EN therapy initiated with trophic feeding vs full feeding have found no differences in outcomes.[36–39]

Most of the more recent studies of trophic vs full feeds have focused on the delivery of EN within the first week of critical illness. No prospective RCTs have investigated whether delaying full feeds until the second week of critical illness would be more beneficial than advancing more quickly to full feeds. Some researchers have theorized that minimal feeding during the first week or "initial phase" of critical illness may be beneficial for critically ill adults to promote autophagy during the height of critical illness; others advocate for the goal of providing full nutrition support, if possible, at this critical time period.[14,40,41] In published studies comparing underfeeding to full feeding, 8 out of 9 studies report more favorable outcomes with underfeeding.[42–50] After removing the studies with methodological flaws, 4 observational studies and 1 RCT found worse outcomes were associated with full feeds.[42–45,47] In RCTs, investigators have found no difference in outcomes between the feeding strategies.[36,38,39,46]

The initial feeding goal for critically ill pediatric patients is to provide up to two-thirds of the estimated nutrient needs in the first week of critical illness. Optimizing protein intake is also crucial to the recovery of PICU patients.[35,51,52] Efficient advancement of EN to achieve goal feeds is best supported by protocols or algorithms in the PICU.[53,54] Each medical center has different protocols or algorithms for feeding advancement in pediatric patients, but the rates for initiation and advancement of tube feeds typically depend on the child's body weight and overall clinical status. See the Administration Methods section of this chapter for additional information.

Critically ill patients are a heterogeneous group. Clinicians must always monitor patients closely to avoid the potential deleterious effects (eg, bowel ischemia, aspiration) of early EN.

Acutely Ill Patients

Several reviews comparing early EN versus early PN in acutely ill patients have been published. A criticism commonly voiced regarding the results of these reviews is that the studies include heterogeneous populations, making it difficult to determine what advantages are conveyed to specific populations. The results of several early meta-analyses of RCTs of hospitalized patients clearly support recommendations to use early EN over early PN to achieve positive clinical outcomes; however, more recent trials have found no difference in outcomes when comparing early EN with early PN.[29,55–58]

Lack of consistency in the definition of "early" intervention is a limitation when comparing studies of early nutrition support interventions. Protocols for early EN typically begin EN within 24 to 36 hours of admission, but the initiation of feedings ranges from within 3 hours of injury to as late as 96 hours following hospitalization.[14] Some evidence suggests that the time of initiation of feeding can make a difference in outcomes. When EN was initiated less than 72 hours postadmission, it was associated with a 2-day reduction in length of stay, compared with EN initiated more than 72 hours following admission.[14] Given the inconsistent results and methodological flaws in studies of early nutrition support interventions, further research is clearly needed to delineate more precisely the optimal timing and amount delivered for nutrition intervention in acutely ill patients.

Enteral Access Device Selection

The selection of the correct EAD is critical to the successful delivery of EN. Factors influencing the selection include the following:

- Clinical status and patient history
- Functional status of the GI tract (eg, gastric emptying, absorptive capacity)
- Anatomy of the GI tract
- Expected duration of EN: short term (eg, <4 weeks) vs long term (eg, >4 weeks)
- Aspiration risk
- Patient wishes
- Quality of life

Refer to Chapter 3 for additional information on the various feeding routes and EAD types available for administering EN formulations, including their benefits, limitations, and potential complications.

Formula Selection and Preparation

Many types of EN formulas are available in the marketplace. Most medical institutions have an established EN formulary that reflects the needs of their patient populations, and outpatients can either receive formula from an infusion or durable medical equipment company or purchase standard EN formulas over the counter. Before selecting an EN formula, the clinician should complete a comprehensive assessment of the patient's nutrition needs, clinical status, and possible benefits that may be derived from the formula.

Standard adult formulas, ranging from 1 kcal/mL to 2 kcal/mL with varying amounts of protein, are readily available and are recommended for most adult patient populations (see Chapter 4). Standard pediatric formulas are indicated for patients ages 1 to 13 years. These products typically provide 1 kcal/mL (30 kcal/oz). Most pediatric formulations are available as ready-to-feed products and some are available in the retail setting (see Chapter 5). Homemade or commercially prepared blenderized tube feedings (BTFs) derived from whole food may also be used in EN therapy for adults and children. However, these types of formulas may increase the risk for microbial contamination and clogging of the feeding tube.[38] Refer to Chapters 4, 5, 7, 8, and 11 for additional information on BTFs.

Human milk (HM) is typically the first choice for neonates; however, the optimal choice for a specific infant depends on the family's feeding goals. HM is assumed to be between 19 and 20 kcal/oz, although the energy density can vary. Standard infant formulas are available over the counter. To match the energy provided by HM, standard dilution of infant formula ranges from 19 to 20 kcal/oz. See Chapter 5 for additional information on the selection of HM and infant formulas.

The concentration of energy provided by powdered formulas may be adjusted by altering the amount of fluid mixed with the powder. See Chapter 7 for guidance on the preparation of powdered formulas.

Nutrient levels in both liquid and powdered products can be adjusted with the addition of a variety of modular components that augment energy, protein, fiber, and micronutrients. For example, modulars may be used to increase the energy density of feeds for pediatric patients while avoiding the high renal solute load of excessively concentrated formula. The osmolarity of the final formula must be considered to avoid hyperosmolar formula, which may not be well tolerated in some infants and children.[59]

See Chapters 4 and 5 for additional information on modular products.

Pediatric and adult enteral formulas do not generally meet the patient's fluid requirements. Additional fluid is therefore needed to maintain normal fluid status. Infants should rarely be offered free water because of the possible risk for oral water intoxication, which can cause hyponatremia, convulsions, and even death.[60] See Chapter 1 for information on assessing fluid status, Chapter 6 for information on the fluid requirements in the nutrition prescription, and Chapter 9 for guidance on dehydration prevention.

Regardless of the type of tube feeding used, clinicians must follow best-practice recommendations for the safe storage, preparation, labeling, and dispensing of EN products. These recommendations are reviewed in Chapter 7.

Administration Methods

Bolus, intermittent, continuous, and cyclic methods are options for administering EN. The following should be considered when choosing an administration method:

- The patient's clinical status and GI function
- Location of feeding tube tip location
- The patient's functional status, quality of life, and treatment preferences

When initiating feedings, clinicians should select the infusion method that promotes the best initial tolerance of EN and is most likely to meet the patient's nutrition needs. The infusion method may be changed, if necessary or desirable, once feedings are established with good tolerance.

The following reviews the various infusion methods. Refer to Chapter 8 for additional information on administration methods. **Note**: Before initiating any type of enteral feeding, tube placement should be confirmed with imaging or by checking the medical record for documentation of what type of tube was placed and precisely where the tip of the feeding tube is located.

Bolus Infusion

Bolus feedings use a syringe or gravity drip via a feeding container to infuse a specific volume of enteral formula over a short period of time (eg, ≤30 minutes), several times throughout the day. For example, a bolus feeding regimen might be to infuse 1 can (237 mL) of formula over 10–15 minutes every 3 to 4 hours, 4 or more times per day during the daytime. The volume infused per feeding can range widely depending on the patient's tolerance. The rate at which the volume is infused can also be adjusted depending on the patient's tolerance.

The advantages of bolus feedings are that they reflect typical eating patterns, allow for greater ambulation than other administration methods, and are inexpensive.[61] For some patients, providing feedings only during the day may improve their quality of life and support their autonomy. In infants, bolus feedings can be helpful when the goal is to increase the amount of oral intake because patients can drink part of the feeding and then the remaining amount can be provided as a bolus through a feeding tube. Bolus feedings are generally only used when feeding into the stomach.

Intermittent Infusion

Like the bolus method, the intermittent method infuses a specific volume of enteral formula over a specific amount of time, several times per day. However, the intermittent method infuses the volume of feeding over a longer period of time (eg, 20–60 minutes in adults; 120–180 minutes in pediatrics); typically intermittent feedings are administered 4 or more times per day every 3 to 4 hours. The volumes infused can be similar to those used with bolus feedings. An infusion pump or the gravity-drip method can be used to infuse the intermittent feeding.

Intermittent feedings are typically used for patients receiving gastric feedings. They may be used prior to trying bolus feedings or tried when bolus feedings are poorly tolerated.

Continuous Infusion

Continuous infusions run 24 hours a day at a steady rate (mL/h) that provides adequate total volume to meet the patient's nutrition prescription. The volume infused can range widely (eg, from less than 50 mL/h to more than 150 mL/hour in adults), depending on the patient's nutrition prescription and feeding tolerance. Continuous infusion is most often administered using an enteral infusion pump or can be delivered via the gravity-drip method.[62]

Continuous infusions can be used when the feeding tube tip is in any location (gastric or postpyloric) because the formula is administered in a slow and steady fashion. This administration method is most often used for critically ill patients or when administering feedings into the small bowel.[62] A variety of EN infusion pumps are available on the market, including small, lightweight pumps for home use. See Chapter 11 for additional information on EN in the home setting.

Cyclic Feedings

Cyclic feedings are similar to continuous feedings, except the daily volume of EN formula is infused in less than

24 hours. Like continuous feedings, cyclic feedings can be administered via an EN infusion pump or gravity drip.

With cyclic feedings, the rate (mL/h) of administration may be increased while the feeding times are condensed. For example, if a patient has been receiving EN at a rate of 100 mL/h over 24 hours, the EN volume may be increased to 135 mL/h and infused over 18 hours to provide a similar volume per day. As long as the patient is tolerating the EN, the rate of EN administration could be continually increased while the time span for infusing the formula is decreased to as little as 8 hours per day.

Compared with continuous feedings, the primary advantage of cyclic feedings is that time off the pump may give the patient more autonomy and improved quality of life. Cyclic feedings are also an option when nocturnal feedings are desired. For example, a patient may consume a normal diet during the day with nightly EN feedings supplementing oral intake. Sometimes, infants will be allowed to work on oral feeding with oral/nasogastric boluses during the day while catching up on energy and/or volume with overnight continuous feeds. This technique is especially helpful in children who are already sleeping through the night and may enhance quality of life for both the patient and family if the patient is receiving EN at home.

Volume-Based Administration

Volume-based feedings can be used to achieve established nutrient goals in some patients. Rather than using a fixed rate of infusion, clinicians using this method can adjust the rate of feeding throughout the day based on the volume needed per day to achieve the patient's nutrient goals. This approach to EN administration is discussed in greater detail in Chapter 8.

Advancing Enteral Nutrition

The SCCM/ASPEN clinical practice guidelines for critically ill adults recommend that EN should be advanced to goal within 48–72 hours or provide at least 80% of nutrient needs in the first week of ICU admission in patients who are stable and have been adequately resuscitated.[14] Patients should be monitored closely for refeeding syndrome and be reevaluated for feeding tolerance until stable.

The SCCM/ASPEN recommendation reflects evidence showing that the administration of trophic feeds—which are usually begun in the critically ill adult at a rate from 10 to 20 mL/h—for up to 6 days is associated with positive clinical outcomes such as less GI intolerance (ie, diarrhea), more ventilator- and ICU-free days, fewer infectious complications, and reduced 60-day mortality when compared to full feeds.[30,36] Trophic feeds may be sufficient to maintain GI physiology and immune-enhancing benefits in patients who are at low to moderate nutrition risk and adequately nourished upon admission.[14] However, in many relevant studies, patients in the full-feeding groups never achieved their prescribed nutrient needs, which complicates the comparison of trophic and full-feeding strategies.[46,63] In 2 observational studies, when greater amounts of energy and protein were provided to critically ill patients at high nutrition risk, feedings administered for at least 12 days were associated with better outcomes such as reduced mortality.[64,65] More specifically, these investigators suggest that providing sufficient protein is important to improve ICU outcomes; meeting the energy goal seems less crucial. These findings are supported by others.[66–68]

Non–critically ill adult patients may begin EN at their goal rate when continuous infusions are used. Feedings are started at full strength. When patients cannot start at their goal rate, feedings can begin at a rate of 25–30 mL/h and be advanced as tolerated in increments of 20–30 mL/h every 4–8 hours until the goal rate is achieved.

In adults, bolus feedings are typically begun at 120–237 mL for the first feeding, with subsequent feedings increased by similar volumes every 3–4 hours as tolerated. Patients should also be monitored for refeeding syndrome.

In pediatrics, the volumes for initiating and advancing EN are tailored to reflect the size and age of the infant or child. It is rare to start EN at the goal rate for non–critically ill pediatric patients. Full-strength feedings are preferred. Laboratory values should be monitored for refeeding syndrome during the initiation and advancement of nutrition support in children who are malnourished or taking in minimal energy.

Challenges Associated with Enteral Nutrition

Many of the common challenges associated with EN may be prevented if patients are assessed thoroughly and monitored closely.[7,14,69] See Chapter 1 for information on nutrition assessment, Chapter 8 for further discussion of monitoring patients receiving EN, and Chapter 9 for a review of complications associated with EN.

The establishment of institutional policies and procedures can promote the safe delivery of optimal EN and reduce costs such as those associated with hospital admissions. Protocols addressing the following are recommended:[7]

- EAD assessment and care (Chapter 3)
- Formula and modular handling, preparation, labeling, and storage (Chapter 7)

- EN hang-time requirements (Chapter 8)
- Administration of medications (Chapter 10)
- Standardization of EN delivery and advancement (Chapter 8)
- Clarification of EN orders
- Review of EN errors
- Establishment of competency measurements for EN providers

Ethical Considerations

Artificial nutrition, including EN, is not associated with improved outcomes during advanced dementia and other terminal illnesses, and it may result in increased burdens.[14,70] When patients have advanced dementia or another terminal illness, decisions to initiate, continue, or withdraw nutrition support can be ethically challenging and may generate considerable distress among patients, family members, clinicians, and other caregivers. Careful consideration and respect must be given to the patient and family's wishes regarding the placement of a feeding tube or the cessation of aggressive therapies, including EN. In such circumstances, the healthcare team should review the risks and benefits with all involved in the patient's care. Factors such as the patient's religious and cultural beliefs as well as the patient's wishes should also be considered.

Guidelines are available from a variety of professional organizations to help guide decision-making related to ethical decisions involved in whether to initiate, withhold, or withdraw support.[14,70–73] Table 2-3 summarizes selected legal and ethical recommendations from ASPEN.[14,70–73]

TABLE 2-3. Selected Legal and Ethical Recommendations Regarding Nutrition Support Therapy

- Legally and ethically, nutrition support therapy should be considered a medical therapy.
- The decision to receive or refuse nutrition support therapy should reflect the autonomy and wishes of the patient. Clinicians should consider the benefits and burdens of nutrition support therapy, and the interventions required to deliver it, before offering this therapy.
- The healthcare team should strive for clear communication with the patient and his or her caregivers, family, and/or surrogate decision-makers.
- Clinicians should be familiar with current evidence of the benefits and burdens of nutrition support therapy.
- Adult patients should be encouraged to have living wills and/or advance directives and to discuss with their loved ones their wishes in the event of a serious or terminal accident or disease. These directives should address the use of nutrition support therapy.
- Competent patients or the legal surrogate of incompetent patients shall be involved in decisions regarding the withholding or withdrawal of treatment. Incompetent patients' wishes (as documented in advance directives) shall be considered in making decisions to withhold or withdraw nutrition support therapy.
- Nutrition support therapy should be modified or discontinued when there are disproportionate burdens for the patient or when benefit to the patient can no longer be demonstrated.
- Institutions should develop clear policies regarding the withdrawal or withholding of nutrition support therapy and communicate these policies to patients in accordance with the Patient Self-Determination Act.

Source: Information is from references 14 and 70–73.

References

1. A.S.P.E.N. Board of Directors and the Clinical Guidelines Task Force. Guidelines for the use of parenteral and enteral nutrition in adult and pediatric patients. *JPEN J Parenter Enteral Nutr.* 2002;26(suppl):1SA–138SA. (Errata *JPEN J Parenter Enteral Nutr.* 2002;26:144.)

2. Jabbar A, Chang WK, Dryden GW, McClave SA. Gut immunology and the differential response to feeding and starvation. *Nutr Clin Pract.* 2003;18(6):461–482.

3. Kudsk KA. Current aspects of mucosal immunology and its influence by nutrition. *Am J Surg.* 2002;183(4):390–398.

4. Kang W, Kudsk KA. Is there evidence that the gut contributes to mucosal immunity in humans? *JPEN J Parenter Enteral Nutr.* 2007;31(3):246–258.

5. Windsor AC, Kanwar S, Li AG, et al. Compared with parenteral nutrition, enteral feeding attenuates the acute phase response and improves disease severity in acute pancreatitis. *Gut.* 1998;42(3):431–435.

6. Ammori BJ. Importance of the early increase in intestinal permeability in critically ill patients. *Eur J Surg.* 2002; 168(11):660–661.

7. Boullata J, Carrera AL, Harvey L, et al. ASPEN safe practices for enteral nutrition therapy. *JPEN J Parenter Enteral Nutr.* 2016;41(1):15–103. doi:10.1177/0148607116673053.

8. Randall JT. The history of enteral nutrition. In: Rombeau JL, Caldwell MD, eds. *Clinical Nutrition: Enteral and Tube Feeding.* 2nd ed. Philadelphia, PA: WB Saunders; 1990.

9. Harkness L. The history of enteral nutrition therapy: from raw eggs and nasal tubes to purified amino acids and early postoperative jejunal delivery. *J Am Diet Assoc.* 2002;102(3): 399–404.

10. Heyland DK, Dhaliwal R, Drover JW, Gramlich L, Dodek P; Canadian Critical Care Clinical Practice Guidelines Committee. Canadian clinical practice guidelines for nutrition support in mechanically ventilated, critically ill adult patients. *JPEN J Parenter Enteral Nutr.* 2003;27(5):355–373.

11. Doig GS, Heighes PT, Simpson F, Sweetman EA, Davies AR. Early enteral nutrition, provided within 24 h of injury or intensive care unit admission, significantly reduces mortality

in critically ill patients: a meta-analysis of randomised controlled trials. *Intensive Care Med.* 2009;35(12):2018–2027.

12. Tian F, Heighes P, Allingstrup MJ, Doig GS. Early enteral nutrition provided within 24 hours of ICU admission: a meta-analysis of randomized controlled trials. *Crit Care Med.* 2018;46(7):1049–1056. doi:10.1097/CCM.0000000000003152.

13. Ukleja A, Gilbert K, Mogensen KM, et al. Standards for nutrition support: adult hospitalized patients. *Nutr Clin Pract.* 2018;33(6):906–920. doi:10.1002/ncp.10204.

14. McClave SA, Taylor BE, Martindale RG, et al. Guidelines for the provision and assessment of nutrition support therapy in the adult critically ill patient: Society of Critical Care Medicine (SCCM) and American Society for Parenteral and Enteral Nutrition (A.S.P.E.N.). *JPEN J Parenter Enteral Nutr.* 2016;40(2):159–211.

15. Weimann A, Braga M, Carli F, et al. ESPEN guideline: clinical nutrition in surgery. *Clin Nutr.* 2017;36:623–650.

16. Chwals WJ. Energy metabolism and appropriate energy repletion in children. In: Baker S, Baker R, Davis A, eds. *Pediatric Nutrition Support.* Boston, MA: Jones and Bartlett Publishers; 2007:66.

17. Institute of Medicine. *Recommended Dietary Allowances.* 10th ed. Washington DC: National Academies Press; 1989.

18. Sentongo T. Assessment of nutrition status by age and determining nutrient needs. In: Corkins M, ed. *The A.S.P.E.N. Pediatric Nutrition Support Core Curriculum.* 2nd ed. Silver Spring, MD: American Society for Parenteral and Enteral Nutrition; 2015:531–565.

19. Carvalho-Salemi J, Salemi J, Wong-Vera M, et al. Malnutrition among hospitalized children in the United States: changing prevalence, clinical correlates, and practice patterns between 2002 and 2011. *J Acad Nutr Diet.* 2018;118(1):40–51.

20. Becker P, Carney L, Corkins M, et al. Consensus statement of the Academy of Nutrition and Dietetics/American Society for Parenteral and Enteral Nutrition: indicators recommended for the identification and documentation of pediatric malnutrition (undernutrition). *Nutr Clin Pract.* 2015;30(1):147–161.

21. Yi DY. Enteral nutrition in pediatric patients. *Pediatr Gastroenterol Hepatol Nutr.* 2018;21(1):12–19.

22. Axelrod D, Kazmerski K, Iyer K. Pediatric enteral nutrition. *JPEN J Parenter Enteral Nutr.* 2006;30(1 Suppl):S21–S26.

23. Bankhead R, Boullata J, Brantley S, Corkins M, et al. Enteral nutrition practice recommendations. *JPEN J Parenter Enteral Nutr.* 2009;33(2):122–167.

24. DiBaise J, Parrish CR. Short bowel syndrome in adults— part 5: trophic agents in the treatment of short bowel syndrome. *Pract Gastroenterol.* 2015;39(5):10–18.

25. Corkins M, ed. *The A.S.P.E.N. Pediatric Nutrition Support Core Curriculum.* 2nd ed. Silver Spring, MD: American Society for Parenteral and Enteral Nutrition; 2015.

26. Lord L, Harrington M. Enteral nutrition implementation and management. In: Merritt R, ed. *The A.S.P.E.N. Nutrition Support Practice Manual.* 2nd ed. Silver Spring, MD: American Society for Parenteral and Enteral Nutrition; 2005:76–89.

27. MacLaren R, Jarvis CL, Fish DN. Use of enteral nutrition for stress ulcer prophylaxis. *Ann Pharmacother.* 2001;35: 1614–1623.

28. McClave SA, Change WK. When to feed the patient with gastrointestinal bleeding. *Nutr Clin Pract.* 2005;20:544–550.

29. Reignier J, Boisramé-Helms J, Brisard L, et al. Enteral versus parenteral early nutrition in ventilated adults with shock: a randomized, controlled, multicenter, open-label, parallel-group study (NUTRIREA-2). *Lancet.* 2018;391:133–143.

30. Khalid I, Doshi P, DiGiovine B. Early enteral nutrition and outcomes of critically ill patients treated with vasopressors and mechanical ventilation. *Am J Crit Care.* 2010;19(3): 261–268.

31. Greathouse K, Sakellaris K, Tumin D, et al. Impact of early initiation of enteral nutrition on survival during pediatric extracorporeal membrane oxygenation. *JPEN J Parenter Enteral Nutr.* 2018;42(1):205–211.

32. King W, Petrillo T, Pettignano R. Enteral nutrition and cardiovascular medications in the pediatric intensive care unit. *JPEN J Parenter Enteral Nutr.* 2004;28:334–338.

33. Worthington P, Balint J, Bechtold M, et al. When is parenteral nutrition appropriate? *JPEN J Parenter Enteral Nutr.* 2017;41(3):324–377. doi:10.1177/0148607117695251.

34. Villlet S, Chiolero RL, Bollmann MD, et al. Negative impact of hypocaloric feeding and energy balance on clinical outcome in ICU patients. *Clin Nutr.* 2005;24(4):502–509.

35. Mehta N, Skillman H, Irving S, et al. Guidelines for the provision and assessment of nutrition support therapy in the pediatric critically ill patient: Society of Critical Care Medicine and American Society for Parenteral and Enteral Nutrition. *JPEN J Parenter Enteral Nutr.* 2017;18(7):675–715.

36. National Heart, Lung, and Blood Institute Acute Respiratory Distress Syndrome (ARDS) Clinical Trials Network, Rice TW, Wheeler AP, et al. Initial trophic vs full enteral feeding in patients with acute lung injury: the EDEN randomized trial. *JAMA.* 2012;307(8):795–803.

37. Arabi YM, Aldawood AS, Haddad SH, et al. Permissive underfeeding or standard enteral feeding in critically ill adults. *N Engl J Med.* 2015;372(25):2398–2408.

38. Rice TW, Mogan S, Hays MA, Bernard GR, Jensen GL, Wheeler AP. Randomized trial of initial trophic versus full-energy enteral nutrition in mechanically ventilated patients with acute respiratory failure. *Crit Care Med.* 2011;39(5):967–974.

39. Charles EJ, Petroze RT, Metzger R, et al. Hypocaloric compared with eucaloric nutritional support and its effect on infection rates in a surgical intensive care unit: a randomized controlled trial. *Am J Clin Nutr.* 2014;100(5):1337–1343.

40. Marik PE. Is early starvation beneficial for the critically ill patient? *Curr Opin Clin Nutr Metab Care.* 2016;19(2):155–160.

41. Patel JJ, Martindale RG, McClave SA. Controversies surrounding critical care nutrition: an appraisal of permissive underfeeding, protein, and outcomes. *JPEN J Parenter Enteral Nutr.* 2018;42:508–515.

42. Krishnan JA, Parce PB, Martinez A, Diette GB, Brower RG. Caloric intake in medical ICU patients: consistency of care with guidelines and relationship to clinical outcomes. *Chest.* 2003;124(1):297–305.

43. Ash J, Gervasio JM, Zaloga GP. Does the quantity of enteral nutrition affect outcomes in critically ill trauma patients? *JPEN J Parenter Enteral Nutr.* 2005;29(suppl):S10.

44. Arabi YM, Haddad SH, Tamim HM, et al. Near-target caloric intake in critically ill medical-surgical patients is associated with adverse outcomes. *JPEN J Parenter Enteral Nutr.* 2010;34(3):280–288.

45. Crosara IC, Melot C, Preiser JC. A J-shaped relationship between caloric intake and survival in critically ill patients. *Ann Intensive Care.* 2015;5(1):37.

46. Arabi YM, Aldawood AS, Haddad SH, et al. Permissive underfeeding or standard enteral feeding in critically ill adults. *N Engl J Med*. 2015;372(25):2398–2408.

47. Braunschweig CA, Sheean PM, Peterson SJ, et al. Intensive nutrition in acute lung injury: a clinical trial (INTACT). *JPEN J Parenter Enteral Nutr*. 2015;39(1):13–20.

48. Heyland DK, Cahill N, Day AG. Optimal amount of calories for critically ill patients: depends on how you slice the cake! *Crit Care Med*. 2011;39(12):2619–2626.

49. Ibrahim EH, Mehringer L, Prentice D, et al. Early versus late enteral feeding of mechanically ventilated patients: results of a clinical trial. *JPEN J Parenter Enteral Nutr*. 2002;26(3):174–181.

50. Casaer MP, Wilmer A, Hermans G, Wouters PJ, Mesotten D, Van den Berghe G. Role of disease and macronutrient dose in the randomized controlled EPaNIC trial: a post hoc analysis. *Am J Respir Crit Care Med*. 2013;187(3):247–255.

51. Mehta N, Bechard L, Cahill N, et al. Nutritional practices and their relationship to clinical outcomes in critically ill children—an international multicenter cohort study. *Crit Care Med*. 2012;40(7):2204–2211.

52. Joffe A, Anton N, Lequier L, et al. Nutritional support for critically ill children. *Cochrane Database Syst Rev*. 2016;(5): CD005144.

53. Wong J, Ong, C, Han W, et al. Protocol-driven enteral nutrition in critically ill children: a systematic review. *JPEN J Parenter Enteral Nutr*. 2014;38(1):29–39.

54. Martinez E, Bechard L, Mehta N. Nutrition algorithms and bedside nutrient delivery practices in pediatric intensive care units: an international multicenter cohort study. *Nutr Clin Pract*. 2014; 29(3):360–367.

55. Braunschweig CL, Levy P, Sheean PM, et al. Enteral compared with parenteral nutrition: a meta-analysis. *Am J Clin Nutr*. 2001; 74:534–542.

56. Peter JV, Moran JL, Phillips-Hughes J. A meta-analysis of treatment outcomes of early enteral versus early parenteral nutrition in hospitalized patients. *Crit Care Med*. 2005;33:213–220.

57. Windsor AC, Kanwar S, Li AG, et al. Compared with parenteral nutrition, enteral feeding attenuates the acute phase response and improves disease severity in acute pancreatitis. *Gut*. 1998;42:431–435.

58. Harvey SE, Parrott F, Harrison DA, et al. Trial of the route of early nutritional support in critically ill adults. *N Engl J Med*. 2014;371(18):1673–1684.

59. Alpers DH, Stenson WF, Bier DM, eds. *Manual of Nutritional Therapeutics*. 3rd ed. Boston, MA: Little Brown and Company; 1995:281–320.

60. Keating JP, Schears GJ, Dodge PR. Oral water intoxication in infants: an American epidemic. *Am J Dis Child*. 1991;145(9):985–990. doi:10.1001/archpedi.1991.02160090037018.

61. Seron-Arbeloa C, Zamora-Elson M, Labarta-Monzon L, Mallor-Bonet T. Enteral nutrition in critical care. *J Clin Med Res*. 2013;5(1):1–11.

62. Read J, Guenter P. *ASPEN Enteral Nutrition by the Numbers: EN Data Across the Healthcare Continuum*. Silver Spring, MD: American Society for Parenteral and Enteral Nutrition; 2017.

63. Rice TW, Wheeler AP, Thompson BT, et al. Initial trophic vs full enteral feeding in patients with acute lung injury: the EDEN randomized trial. *JAMA*. 2012;307(8):795–803.

64. Compher C, Chittams J, Sammarco T, Nicolo M, Heyland D. Greater protein and energy intake may be associated with improved mortality in higher risk critically ill patients: a multicenter, multinational observational study. *Crit Care Med*. 2017;45(2):156–163.

65. Yeh DD, Cropano C, Quraishi SA, et al. Implementation of an aggressive enteral nutrition protocol and the effect on clinical outcomes. *Nutr Clin Pract*. 2017;32(2):175–181.

66. Wijs PJ, Stapel SN, de Groot SD, et al. Optimal protein and energy nutrition decreases mortality in mechanically ventilated, critically ill patients: a prospective observational cohort study. *JPEN J Parenter Enteral Nutr*. 2012;36(1):60–68.

67. Nicolo M, Heyland DK, Chittams J, Sammarco T, Compher C. Clinical outcomes related to protein delivery in a critically ill population: a multicenter, multinational observation study. *JPEN J Parenter Enteral Nutr*. 2016;40(1):45–51.

68. Zusman O, Theilla M, Cohen J, Kagan I, Bendavid I, Singer P. Resting energy expenditure, calorie and protein consumption in critically ill patients: a retrospective cohort study. *Crit Care*. 2016;20(1):367.

69. Drake R, Ozols A, Nadeau WJ, Braid-Forbes MJ. Hospital inpatient admissions with dehydration and/or malnutrition

in Medicare beneficiaries receiving enteral nutrition: a cohort study. *JPEN J Parenter Enteral Nutr.* 2018;42(4):730–738. doi:10.1177/0148607117713479.

70. A.S.P.E.N. Ethics Position Paper Task Force, Barrocas A, Geppert C, Durfee SM, et al. A.S.P.E.N. ethics position paper. *Nutr Clin Pract.* 2010;25(6):672–679.

71. O'Sullivan Maillet J, Baird Schwartz D, Posthauer ME; Academy of Nutrition and Dietetics. Position of the Academy of Nutrition and Dietetics: ethical and legal issues in feeding and hydration. *J Acad Nutr Diet.* 2013;113:828–833.

72. American Medical Association *Code of Medical Ethics'* opinions on care at the end of life. *Virtual Mentor.* 2013;15(12): 1038–1040.

73. American Nurses Association. Position statement. Nutrition and hydration at the end of life. 2017. https://www.nursingworld.org/~4af0ed/globalassets/docs/ana/ethics/ps_nutrition-and-hydration-at-the-end-of-life_2017june7.pdf. Accessed December 14, 2018.

CHAPTER 3

Enteral Access Devices

Introduction

The selection of an enteral access device (EAD) requires an evaluation of the patient's disease state, upper gastrointestinal (GI) anatomy (including past surgeries), GI motility and function, and the estimated length of therapy. Determination of the appropriate type and location of the feeding tube is critical to the success of enteral feeding. The clinician must weigh the overall risks vs benefits to the patient whenever a feeding tube is considered. Advance directives and religious, cultural, and ethical issues must also be considerations, especially in end-stage or terminal disease states. See Chapter 2 for additional information on ethical issues related to enteral nutrition (EN) therapy.

Selection of Enteral Access Devices

Once the decision has been made to administer EN, the next decision is to select the type of EAD. Primary factors to consider in this decision include how long EN therapy will likely be required, where the EN should be delivered (ie, at what level—gastric or small bowel), patient preferences, risk factors associated with the type of EAD, and tube characteristics. The specific type of feeding tube a patient receives may also depend on the expertise and availability of nutrition support clinicians at the particular institution. See Figure 3-1 for a decision algorithm for tube selection based on anticipated duration of need and patient preferences, goals, and aspiration risk.

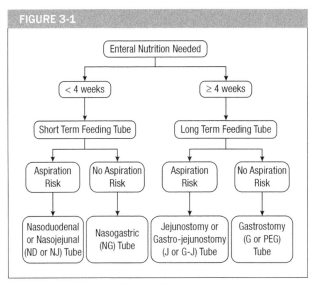

FIGURE 3-1

Enteral access device selection algorithm. PEG, percutaneous endoscopic gastrostomy.

Anticipated Duration of Enteral Nutrition Therapy

Clinicians should consider the estimated duration of enteral therapy when determining whether to place (a) an orogastric (OG), nasogastric (NG), or nasoenteric (NE) tube or (b) an enterostomy (gastrostomy, gastrojejunostomy, or jejunostomy) tube. EADs inserted via the nasal and oral routes (Figure 3-2) are usually placed for short-term use (<4–6

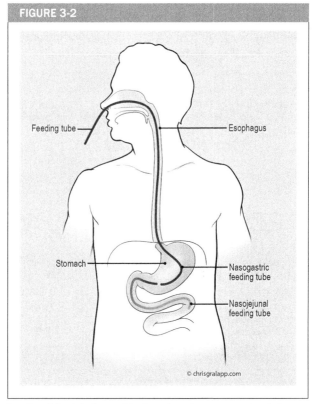

FIGURE 3-2

Feeding tube

Esophagus

Stomach

Nasogastric feeding tube

Nasojejunal feeding tube

© chrisgralapp.com

Location of distal tip for nasal feeding tubes. Illustration copyright © Christine Gralapp. Reprinted with permission of the artist.

weeks) in the hospitalized patient. They can also provide an opportunity to assess tolerance of enteral feedings prior to placement of enterostomy tubes when longer-term access is required. Additionally, there are many situations when NG and NE feeding tubes are appropriate for use in the outpatient setting, especially in the pediatric population.[1] (NE tubes include nasoduodenal and nasojejunal tubes.)

OG and NG feeding tubes can be placed at the bedside (either blindly or using electromagnetic guidance), endoscopically, or under fluoroscopic guidance.[2] Some patients or caregivers are able to self-place OG or NG tubes. However, the placement of an NE feeding tube should only be performed by clinicians who have been properly trained to insert the device. Insertion techniques are described in greater detail later in this chapter.

Decisions regarding the selection of an EAD for long-term EN (>4–6 weeks) involve the anticipated length of EN therapy, the patient's disposition, and the special needs of the patient and caregivers. For long-term EN, enterostomy tubes are placed into the stomach or small bowel using a variety of techniques (ie, endoscopic, fluoroscopic, laparoscopic, and open surgical laparotomy routes). Placing a long-term EAD with local anesthesia of the abdominal wall with or without intravenous (IV) sedation by fluoroscopic and endoscopic routes is often a better option than placement under general anesthesia, especially in patients with extensive comorbidities. See the section on insertion of long-term EADs later in this chapter for additional information.

To clarify the terminology, enterostomy tubes placed via endoscopy are called *percutaneous endoscopic gastrostomy* (PEG) or *percutaneous endoscopic jejunostomy* (PEJ) tubes; when enterostomy tubes are placed radiologically or surgically, they are simply called *gastrostomy* tubes (which may be further classified as balloon or nonballoon gastrostomy tubes), *gastrojejunostomy* tubes, or *jejunostomy* tubes. When a gastrostomy tube is placed at the bedside, it should not be referred to as a PEG tube.

Gastrostomy tubes are generally the preferred EAD for medium-term and long-term EN therapy, unless the use of gastrostomy tubes is medically contraindicated.[3] Two studies of adult patients with persistent dysphagia due to neurologic diseases randomly assigned patients to be fed via an NG tube or a PEG tube.[4,5] These studies found that the patients fed with a PEG tube had greater weight gain and fewer missed feedings, whereas the patients fed by NG received significantly less formula because of tube difficulties. In 1 of the studies, patients with NG tubes were switched to a PEG tube if they experienced difficulties (usually displacement) with the NG tube; at the end of 4 weeks, only 1 of 19 patients had an NG tube in place.[5]

When long-term enteral access is needed, the condition of the external abdominal wall, the ability to correct coagulopathies, and the patient's tolerance to sedation and general anesthesia must be assessed. Other factors to evaluate are the presence of open wounds or fistulas on the exterior abdominal wall, the presence of ostomies or future requirements for ostomies, the patient's need for other percutaneous or intra-abdominal infusion devices and peritoneal dialysis catheters, the patient's history of previous abdominal surgeries, and the condition of the upper GI anatomy.

Level of Delivery

EN can be delivered either into the stomach or into the small bowel. Gastric access relies on a functional stomach free of delayed gastric emptying, aspiration from gastric contents, obstruction, or fistulas. In patients who have had previous gastric bypass surgery, the EAD can be placed into the gastric remnant, which is typically accessed through laparoscopic surgery.[6,7] Small bowel placement and feedings are more appropriate than gastric for patients with gastric outlet obstruction, gastroparesis, reflux with aspiration of gastric contents, or superior mesenteric artery syndrome, and when patients have failed gastric feeds (including patients with pancreatitis).[2,8] Gastrojejunal access with a single combined gastrojejunostomy tube or with separate gastrostomy and jejunostomy tubes allows for simultaneous gastric decompression and small bowel feedings.[9,10]

In most cases, including in some patients with previous gastric surgery, gastric access is chosen first. The largest multicenter randomized controlled trial (RCT) comparing gastric vs small bowel feeding in critically ill patients found no difference in the most important outcomes, including length of stay, mortality, nutrient delivery, and incidence of pneumonia. Two meta-analyses have found that gastric feedings were initiated sooner than small bowel feedings because gastric feedings avoided the delay from difficulties in obtaining postpyloric placement.[11,12] The most recent guidelines from the Society of Critical Care Medicine (SCCM) and American Society for Parenteral and Enteral Nutrition (ASPEN) on nutrition support in critically ill adults aggregated data from relevant RCTs and found that small bowel feeding decreases the risk of pneumonia; however, there are no differences in length of stay or mortality between small bowel and gastric feeding.[13] The ASPEN/SCCM guidelines recommended that if timely obtainment of small bowel enteral access is not feasible, early EN via the gastric route may provide more benefit than delaying feeding initiation while awaiting small bowel access.[13]

Existing data are insufficient to make universal recommendations regarding the optimal site to deliver EN to critically ill children. On the basis of observational studies, SCCM and ASPEN suggest that the gastric route is the preferred site for EN in critically ill pediatric patients.[14] The postpyloric or small intestinal site for EN may be used for pediatric patients unable to tolerate gastric feeding or for those at high risk for aspiration.[11]

Device-Related Risk Assessment

When selecting an EAD, the risk factors associated with the type of device must be considered. For example, a concern with NG feedings in critically ill patients has been the risk of reflux associated with bronchopulmonary aspiration and pneumonia. Multiple studies and meta-analyses have attempted to address this issue.[11,12,15] Complications that may occur with gastrojejunostomy tubes include a gastric lumen that is too small to decompress adequately; a tendency to clog, leading to frequent replacements; and the jejunal extension tube migrating back into the stomach. In a 2016 case report of jejunal perforation in 3 low–birth weight infants due to gastrojejunostomy tube placement, the authors recommended caution when infants with a clinical indication for gastrojejunostomy tube weigh <10 kg.[16] Reported complications related to jejunostomies in pediatric patients have included dislodgement, bowel obstruction, tube leakage, and wound dehiscence in one-third of the patients studied, with most complications occurring within 4 weeks of surgery.[17] Complications related to EADs are discussed in greater detail later in this chapter.

Tube Characteristics

Physical Characteristics

Patient comfort, tube performance, and available commercial options are important considerations when choosing a feeding tube. Most commercially manufactured feeding tubes are made of polyurethane or silicone, each with its specific advantages and disadvantages (Table 3-1).[18]

	Polyurethane	**Silicone**
Comfort	Lower	Higher
Stiffness	Higher	Lower
Wall width	Thinner	Thicker
Fungal degradation	More resistant	Less resistant
Common use	Nasoenteric feeding tubes	Percutaneous abdominal feeding tubes

TABLE 3-1. Comparison of Polyurethane and Silicone Tube Characteristics

Source: Reprinted with permission from reference 18: Fang JC, Kinikini M. Enteral access devices. In: Mueller CM, ed. *The ASPEN Adult Nutrition Support Core Curriculum.* 3rd ed. Silver Spring, MD: American Society for Parenteral and Enteral Nutrition; 2017:251–264.

Most short-term feeding tubes are constructed of polyurethane, which can provide a relatively larger inner tube diameter for a given outer diameter size, thereby decreasing the risk of clogging. Most percutaneous tubes are constructed from silicone because of its inherent material compliance and comfort.

Rubber- and latex-based tubes (eg, Foley-type catheters and red rubber tubes) are *not* indicated for feeding. These are inferior tubes because (a) they degrade rapidly; (b) they lack internal (red rubber tubes) or external (red rubber tubes and Foley-type catheters) retention devices; and (c) their use puts the patient at risk for enteral misconnections with nonenteral devices. Tube connections and misconnections are discussed in greater detail later in this chapter.

Tube Configurations

As shown in Table 3-2, NE and enterostomy tubes are measured by their external diameter in French size

TABLE 3-2. Nasoenteric and Enterostomy Tube Types, Sizes, and Lengths

Tube Type	Size, Fr	Length, cm
Nasogastric (for adults)	8–16	38–91
Nasogastric (for pediatrics)	3.5–16	15–170
Nasoenteric (for adults)	8–12	91–240
Nasoenteric (for pediatrics)	3.5–16	15–170
Gastrostomy	12–30	n/a
Gastrojejunostomy	6–14	n/a
Jejunal extension through existing gastrostomy	8–12	15–95
Dual-lumen (gastric and jejunal)	16–30	n/a
Single lumen (jejunal only)	12–24	15–58
Low-profile gastrostomy (replacement)	12–24	0.8–6.0
Low-profile gastrojejunostomy	14–22	15–45

1 Fr = 0.33 mm; n/a, not applicable.

Source: Adapted with permission from reference 18: Fang JC, Kinikini M. Enteral access devices. In: Mueller CM, ed. *The ASPEN Adult Nutrition Support Core Curriculum.* 3rd ed. Silver Spring, MD: American Society for Parenteral and Enteral Nutrition; 2017:251–264. Pediatric data are from reference 19.

(1 Fr = 0.33 mm).[18,19] However, flow through the tube and a tube's susceptibility to clogging depend on the inner diameter, which may vary depending on the specific material used to construct the tube. In general, a polyurethane tube will have a larger internal diameter than a silicone tube of the same outer diameter.

NE feeding tubes come in a wide array of diameters and lengths, with a variety of options such as stylets, feeding and medication ports, and distal weighted and unweighted tips. A stylet or guidewire is included with most NE feeding tubes to provide tube structure and/or guidance while inserting these relatively floppy tubes. Stylets and guidewires are designed to be shorter than the length of the tube and have a flexible distal tip to avoid perforation of the GI mucosa/wall when placing the tube. A water-activated lubricant coats the tube's internal lumen to allow for easier removal of the stylet or guidewire after the tube is in place. Commercially available NE feeding tubes have a single lumen with either 1 port for feeding or 2 ports in a Y configuration, 1 for feeding and 1 for medication administration and/or irrigation. These ports can accommodate either a feeding set or a syringe or both. Dual ports can allow for concomitant feeding and medication administration and/or irrigation. However, to minimize the risk of tube clogging, medications should be administered separately through the tube only after enteral feedings are held and the feeding tube is flushed with water. (See Chapter 10 for further information on administration of medication via the feeding tube.)

Weighted tube tips were once thought to facilitate transpyloric passage. However, critical analysis of the literature has not demonstrated a clear advantage of either weighted or unweighted tips.[20] In fact, a study showed that weighted tips were less likely to migrate into the small bowel, and there have been reports that the weighted tip can separate from the tube and become a foreign body.[20,21]

Feeding tube tips come in a wide variety of shapes and sizes, and the number, size, and location of distal end openings can also vary. There are no data to demonstrate that any particular design is preferable. Therefore, the choice of feeding tube tip is determined by the personal preference of the individual clinician, the patient's preference, and available stock from the institution.

The internal retention bolster of the percutaneous enterostomy tube is constructed of either solid material (silicone

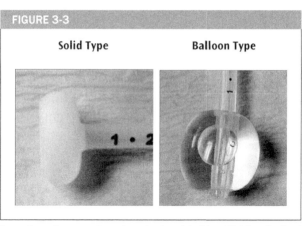

FIGURE 3-3

| Solid Type | Balloon Type |

Types of percutaneous endoscopic gastrostomy tube internal bolsters. Reprinted with permission from reference 18: Fang JC, Kinikini M. Enteral access devices. In: Mueller CM, ed. *The ASPEN Adult Nutrition Support Core Curriculum.* 3rd ed. Silver Spring, MD: American Society for Parenteral and Enteral Nutrition; 2017:251–264.

or polyurethane) or silicone balloons (Figure 3-3).[18] Solid internal bolsters are commonly used in initial percutaneous enterostomy tube placement. Balloon-type internal bolsters (or encapsulated internal bolsters) are commonly inserted when a tube is fluoroscopically or surgically placed or when a tube is replaced. The balloons generally have a lifespan of only 3–6 months, whereas solid internal bolsters typically last 1 year or longer.[22] Enterostomy feeding tubes typically have 2 ports: 1 for feeding and 1 for medication and/ or irrigation. If the internal bolster is of the balloon type, an additional third port is present for balloon inflation or deflation.

Traditionally, 2-piece gastrojejunostomy feeding tubes are placed by passing a smaller-bore jejunal extension tube through an existing gastrostomy tube through the pylorus, beyond the duodenum, and into the jejunum. There are also single-piece gastrojejunostomy tubes manufactured with designated gastric and jejunal lumens to allow for both jejunal feeding and gastric decompression.

Direct jejunostomy tubes are placed directly into the jejunum without passage through the stomach. There are no enterostomy tubes commercially available for this specific use; clinicians usually use smaller-bore percutaneous gastrostomy tubes but place them directly into the jejunum.

Low-profile tubes are skin-level devices. They can be placed as the initial feeding tube, but they are typically used as replacement devices for gastrostomies and gastrojejunostomies. The length of the existing stoma tract is measured before the most appropriately sized low-profile device is chosen and placed. Commercially available low-profile devices have either balloon or solid internal bolsters (Figure 3-4).[18] Balloon-type internal bolsters are used more commonly because they can be easily replaced by simply deflating the balloon and sliding the tube, without trauma, in or out of the existing stoma tract.

In pediatric patients, it is common practice to use a low-profile balloon gastrostomy tube as the initial gastrostomy tube. Caregivers are taught to replace the low-profile balloon gastrostomy tube at home.

FIGURE 3-4

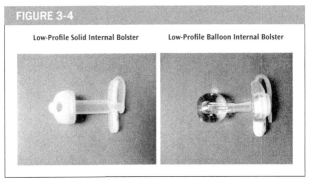

Low-Profile Solid Internal Bolster   Low-Profile Balloon Internal Bolster

Bolsters for low-profile replacement percutaneous gastrostomies. Reprinted with permission from reference 18: Fang JC, Kinikini M. Enteral access devices. In: Mueller CM, ed. *The ASPEN Adult Nutrition Support Core Curriculum*. 3rd ed. Silver Spring, MD: American Society for Parenteral and Enteral Nutrition; 2017:251–264.

Solid internal bolster replacement tubes require an obturator to deform the internal bolster to allow it to be inserted through the stoma tract. There is also a unique solid internal bolster tube that is constrained in a capsule such that it can be placed like a balloon-type tube, with minimal trauma; once placed, the capsule is split and the bolster deployed.

Insertion of Short-Term Enteral Access Devices

As noted previously, OG, NG, and NE feeding tubes are inserted when short-term access (<4–6 weeks) is indicated. Short-term EADs can be passed transorally or transnasally, although the nasal approach is better tolerated in the conscious patient. During the first 4 to 6 months of life, the infant is an obligate nose breather; therefore, an OG feeding tube may be the best option in these patients. However, in a study with a crossover design, 32 infants showed no significant difference in apnea or bradycardia using either the OG or NG tube.[23]

NG or NE feeding tube placement is contraindicated if the patient has an obstructing head, neck, and esophageal pathology or injury that would make insertion unsafe. Once placed, NG or NE feeding tubes should not be used until proper position of the EAD is confirmed.[24,25] It is imperative that clinicians use *only* evidence-based methods to verify OG, NG, or NE tube placement, such as measuring the pH of aspirate, evaluating a radiograph, or using specific technology that is proven to accurately determine placement.

NG tubes are the easiest feeding tubes to insert. Placement may be performed by a clinician with the appropriate training, competencies, and privileges to do so. When possible, larger, stiffer tubes used for gastric decompression should be converted to a smaller-bore feeding tube (6–12 Fr) for patient comfort and to decrease the risk of associated complications.

The most reliable method for measuring the length of NG tube necessary for gastric placement is known as NEMU (which is shorthand for "direct distance from *n*ose to *e*arlobe to *mid*umbilicus"), although many clinicians use a NEX (nose-to-earlobe-to-xiphoid process) measurement in adult patients.[26] For either an NEMU or NEX measurement, the patient is positioned as upright as possible and an NG tube is passed through a patent naris. If the patient is alert, he or she can help guide the tube appropriately through the esophagus by dry-swallowing or taking sips of water through a straw while the tube is being inserted and advanced.

Once the tube is in position at the predetermined length, attempted aspiration of gastric contents and auscultation of insufflated air over the stomach using a 30- to 60-mL syringe may be attempted. The volume, color, and pH level of the aspirate can be assessed. (To measure pH, place a drop of aspirate on a colorimetric pH strip.) Fasting gastric fluid typically is clear and colorless (pH <3) or grassy green (pH <5) and is of larger volume. In contrast, gastric fluid from a tube that has perforated into the pleural space is small in volume and has a pale-yellow serous appearance with pH of >7. Clinicians should *not* assess the position of a placed tube by the visual appearance of aspirated gastric contents; auscultation of insufflated air; or the absence of coughing, choking, or respiratory distress.[27–29]

Correct initial position of an NG tube should be confirmed by first checking the pH of gastric aspirate, with the desired result being ≤5.5 for all patients from neonates to older adults.[30–33] Although many institutions use abdominal radiograph as their gold standard for assessing the initial placement of a feeding tube, the National Health Service

(NHS) in the United Kingdom has reported multiple problems with inaccurate interpretation of radiographs.[32,34] Furthermore, a study conducted in a neonatal intensive care unit in Korea compared the interpretation of radiographs for OG tube placement by pediatric residents with interpretation by staff with expertise in interpreting radiographs and found that the residents correctly marked the position of the OG tube tip only 85.7% of the time.[35]

Both the American Association of Critical-Care Nurses and NHS recommend that the pH of aspirate be evaluated to assess placement of NG feeding tubes inserted at the bedside.[31,34] The NHS does not recommend radiographic confirmation of an NG tube as the first-line placement verification method.[31] Continuous feedings can skew the pH measurement, and it is recommended the feeds be held for 10–20 minutes (longer for patients receiving high administration rates).[30] The use of an acid-suppressing medication does not necessarily mean the pH will be ≥5.5 and is not a contraindication for checking pH.[36]

An abdominal radiograph should be obtained to confirm tube position in certain situations, such as cases with a pH measurement of ≥6 or when aspirate cannot be collected from the NG tube even after the patient is repositioned. Radiographic confirmation may also be warranted if the patient has a high-risk condition, such as critical illness with intubation; decreased or absent gag or cough reflex; neurologic impairment with decreased level of consciousness; sedation and/or chemical paralysis; or clinical status that warrants use of an X-ray even though pH is less than 5 or 5.5. ASPEN's New Opportunities for Verification of Enteral Tube Location (NOVEL) Project has published additional information and an algorithm to help clinicians place NG tubes in pediatric patients.[30] To learn more about the NOVEL Project or download the

algorithm, visit the NOVEL web page (www.nutritioncare
.org/NOVEL).

When a radiograph is necessary, it should be done in
such a way that the tube can be traced from the pharynx
to the stomach with the tip within the frame of the radiograph.[36] The report needs to specifically state that the tube
placement is appropriate to use for feeding or medication
administration.[36] Use of abdominal radiograph to assess
NG tube placement is not common in pediatric care settings, but many adult centers continue to consider radiographic assessment to be the "gold standard" method.[3,19]

Nursing documentation of the NG tube insertion procedure must include the centimeter mark that is visible
at the naris. Once the NG tube is in place, nurses should
recheck the centimeter mark to determine whether it has
changed, which would indicate tube migration. Currently,
there is no evidence to guide practice regarding how often
to routinely reconfirm placement. If there are indicators
that the tube has migrated while in place, such as vomiting
or deep coughing, the pH of an aspirate sample should
be checked and the patient's respiratory status should be
thoroughly assessed.

Carbon dioxide (CO_2) monitoring can help clinicians
determine when an NG or NE tube has taken an inadvertent course into the trachea during the insertion process.[37–40] Use of capnography or a colorimetric CO_2
detector (Medtronic, Minneapolis, MN) assumes that a
tube misplaced into the respiratory tract will reveal (a) a
characteristic exhaled CO_2 waveform when attached to
CO_2 monitoring equipment or (b) a color change when
using the calorimetric CO_2 detector. However, CO_2 detection cannot determine whether the depth of insertion
into the GI tract is proper; therefore, radiography and/or
pH testing should be used to verify that the tip position

is appropriate before enteral feeding is initiated or whenever dislodgement is suspected. Tube migration is further discussed in the Tube Maintenance Considerations section later in this chapter.

NE feeding tubes are placed anywhere distal to the pylorus, with NJ tubes positioned distal to the ligament of Treitz. NE tubes, which are more difficult to place than NG tubes, can be placed blindly at the bedside, endoscopically, or fluoroscopically.

Bedside placement usually requires specialized training and should be done by an experienced clinician. A number of methods have been described for bedside blind placements,[41] including a method described by Zaloga.[42] In this technique, the patient lies on his or her right side, and a feeding tube with bent tip is passed through a naris into the stomach. The tip of the tube is bent by removing the stylet and bending it 30° about 2 cm from the distal end and reinserting it into the feeding tube. A 60-mL syringe is used to pump air into the stomach. The bend allows for the tip of the tube to cover a greater surface area during rotation and helps the tip to "hook" the pyloric outlet during tube advancement. After air insufflation, the feeding tube is slowly rotated and advanced in short (4- to 5-cm) bursts until it is inserted the appropriate length (ie, compatible with a small bowel location). The tube is allowed to slowly advance and is not forced forward. Prokinetic agents (erythromycin or metoclopramide) may be used as adjuvants to bedside placement techniques and may increase success rates.[43] A meta-analysis recently showed the most effective maneuvers to assist with postpyloric tube placement are air insufflation and the use of prokinetic agents in adult patients.[44] The authors of that review did not recommend use of prokinetic agents in children when placing a postpyloric feeding tube.[44] Finally, compared with feeding tubes with weighted tips, feeding tubes with unweighted tips have been shown to increase the likelihood of trans-pyloric passage.[20]

NE feeding tube placement is reliably achieved with endoscopic or fluoroscopic techniques. However, these methods are costlier and require advanced training, and endoscopy is more invasive than the bedside method. Radiographic confirmation of placement is not required for these methods.

When inserting NE tubes in pediatric patients, it is most important to swaddle the child and slowly advance the tube 5–10 cm past the measured number obtained using the NEMU method at the umbilicus. Older children will require advancement of the tube up to 20 cm past that number.

Infants with increased work of breathing can pose a challenge for NG or NE tube placement. Blowing in the patient's face to elicit a startle reflex will cause the infant to swallow, which facilitates proper tube passage. It is typical to slowly instill a small volume of sterile water (3–10 mL) to help "float" the tube postpylorically and to check for a "snap back" of an empty syringe when attempting to aspirate. When water is slowly instilled during tube advancement, kinking of the tube is readily identified and remedied; a kinked tube will result in a false-positive "snap back." NG or NE tubes are secured to the cheek with a skin-protectant base and transparent tape. An abdominal radiograph is required to confirm placement for any patient who has a blindly placed NE tube. It is uncommon in pediatrics to change the position of the child during tube placement unless placement is difficult. Prokinetic agents are not often used when placing feeding tubes in pediatric patients.

Efforts are being made to improve technological aids for tube insertion. An electromagnetic placement device system has been developed to assist with NG and NE tube placement. An electromagnetic signal is sent by a transmitter at the distal end of the feeding tube stylet to a receiver unit, which is positioned on the patient's chest at the xiphoid process (corresponding to the base of the diaphragm). The triangulated signal from the tip of the feeding tube stylet is tracked on a portable monitor as the tube is advanced through the esophagus and into the stomach and small intestine.[45] The most recent version of this system provides both anterior and lateral positioning screens, allowing 2-dimensional tracking of the tube tip. This technology has reported success rates of 70%–90% when physicians or nurses pass the feeding tube into the small intestine.[46–48] Before using this technology, clinicians should be trained with a combination of didactic and clinical observation, and periodic competency assessment after initial training is recommended. The electromagnetic placement device system has been approved by the US Food and Drug Administration (FDA) for confirmation of the final tip position by qualified operators, without the need for radiographic confirmation. However, tracheobronchial misplacements have been reported with the device, and radiographic confirmation is suggested if there is any concern for incorrect tube position.[49]

Another technological innovation is a single-use, small-bore NG feeding tube with a miniature camera embedded in the distal end to aid in tube placement. This system allows clinicians to visually identify anatomical markers during the placement procedure. Preliminary studies have demonstrated correct identification of gastric mucosa in ≥90% of patients.[50,51]

When placing NG or NE tubes, clinicians must be aware that malpositioning may occur without any apparent symptoms, particularly in patients with decreased level of consciousness.[24,52,53] Also, the auscultatory method or bubbling of air from the proximal end of the tube placed in water cannot reliably differentiate placement in the esophagus, stomach, or small bowel from tracheobronchial placement and therefore should not be used to assess tube tip location.[30,31,36,52] Pulmonary aspiration, pneumonia, and pneumothorax have been reported with all tube insertion methods, including use of the electromagnetic signal device technology.[54]

The overall success rate for NG or NE tube placement is high (90%–100%), but the success rate for placement in the distal duodenum is lower (84%–90%), and the success rate is just 25%–50% for placement past the ligament of Treitz, no matter which insertion method is employed.[55] Table 3-3 summarizes the ASPEN practice recommendations for short-term feeding tube placement.[3]

TABLE 3-3. Practice Recommendations for Short-Term Feeding Tube Placement

1. For all blindly placed tubes, obtain evidence-based confirmation of proper tube positioning in the GI tract prior to initial use.

2. Do not rely on the auscultation method to differentiate between gastric and respiratory placement or to differentiate between gastric and small bowel placement.

3. Mark the exit site of a feeding tube at the time of the initial radiograph; observe for a change in the external tube length during feedings. If a significant increase in the external length is observed, use other bedside tests to help determine whether the tube has become dislocated. If in doubt, obtain a radiograph to determine tube location.

4. In pediatric and neonatal patients, the first-line method to verify NG tube placement is pH measurement of aspirate, with a cutoff level of ≤5.5. When pH is greater than this number, pH is unattainable, or a radiograph is clinically indicated, radiographic assessment is the best practice. The use of radiography in children should be judicious given the cumulative effect of radiation exposure. It is also noted that several cases have been identified where the X-ray has been misinterpreted by a physician who is not trained in radiology.

(continued)

TABLE 3-3. *(Continued)*

5. Consider pH measurement of aspirate as the first-line method for NG tube placement in adult patients. A radiograph would be the first- or second-line method to confirm that any blindly placed tube (small-bore or large-bore) is properly positioned in the GI tract prior to the tube's initial use for administering feedings and medications in adult patients.

6. When attempting to insert a feeding tube into the stomach of an adult patient, it may be helpful to use capnography to detect inadvertent entry of the tube into the trachea. Be aware that radiographic confirmation is needed before the tube is used for feedings.

7. When attempting to insert a feeding tube into the small bowel, observe for a change in the pH and appearance of aspirates as the tube progresses from the stomach into the small bowel; use the findings to determine when a radiograph should be done to confirm small bowel placement.

Abbreviations: GI, gastrointestinal; NG, nasogastric.

Source: Adapted with permission from reference 3: Boullata JI, Carrera AL, Harvey L, et al. ASPEN safe practices for enteral nutrition therapy. *JPEN J Parenter Enteral Nutr.* 2016;41(1):15–103. doi:10.1177/0148607116673053.

Insertion of Long-Term Enteral Access Devices

As discussed earlier in this chapter, enterostomy tubes are placed when long-term enteral access (>4–6 weeks) is anticipated. These tubes may be placed by endoscopic, radiologic, or surgical (laparoscopic or open) methods. All of these methods have similar success rates; however, endoscopic or fluoroscopic techniques have less morbidity and cost less than surgical methods; therefore, endoscopic and fluoroscopic methods are more commonly employed.[56–60] The choice of procedure depends on local resources and expertise, anatomical considerations (eg, contraindications to endoscopic or radiologic placement), and whether the patient is undergoing surgery for another reason where operative gastrostomy can be performed in combination with the primary surgical procedure. See Table 3-4 for practice recommendations for long-term EAD placement.[61]

TABLE 3-4. Practice Recommendations for Long-Term Enteral Access Device Placement
1. Long-term feeding devices should be considered in adults, children, and infants, including neonates after term age, when the need for enteral feeding exceeds at least 4–6 weeks.
2. In premature infants with the ability to eat by mouth at the normal time for development of oral feeding skills, a long-term feeding device should not be considered before the usual age of development of independent oral feeding.
3. Evaluation by a multidisciplinary team is indicated prior to insertion of a long-term feeding device to establish whether (a) benefit outweighs the risk of access placement; (b) insertion of a feeding tube near the end of life is warranted; or (c) insertion of a feeding tube is indicated in the situation where patients are close to achieving oral feeding.
4. Abdominal imaging should be performed prior to long-term feeding device placement if a possible anatomical difficulty exists.
5. Gastrostomy tube placement does not mandate fundoplication. The possible exception is children with neurologic impairment who also have abnormal pH probe findings.
6. Direct placement of a jejunostomy tube is indicated in patients requiring long-term small bowel feeding. For patients who require gastric venting or decompression, consideration of a gastrojejunostomy tube is appropriate. In the pediatric population, gastrojejunostomy tubes are not typically the first enterostomy tube placed.

(continued)

TABLE 3-4. *(Continued)*

7. Low-profile devices require periodic resizing to increase the length of the stem of the device. Resizing should occur with any significant growth or weight change and, in the pediatric population, twice a year for patients under the age of 5 years and annually for patients after the age of 5 years.

8. Document tube type, tip location, and external markings in the medical record and in follow-up examinations.

9. Avoid placement of catheters or tubes not intended for use as enteral feeding devices, such as urinary or GI drainage tubes, which usually do not have an external anchoring device. Use of such tubes leads to enteral misconnection as well as tube migration, which can potentially cause obstruction of the gastric pylorus or small bowel and aspiration. In the rare instances that a non–enteral feeding tube is placed, use an anchoring device to keep the tube from migrating.

Abbreviation: GI, gastrointestinal.

Source: Adapted with permission from reference 61: Bankhead R, Boullata J, Brantley S, et al. Enteral nutrition practice recommendations. *JPEN J Parenter Enteral Nutr.* 2009;33(2):122–167.

Gastrostomy Tubes

Commercially available percutaneous gastrostomy tubes with balloon-type or solid distensible internal bolsters can be placed initially or for replacement by endoscopic or radiologic methods. Solid internal bolsters are not susceptible to balloon deflation and may be less susceptible to inadvertent dislodgement than balloon internal bolster gastrostomy tubes.

Percutaneous Endoscopic Placement

PEG is the most commonly used technique for obtaining long-term gastric access. It is generally performed under moderate IV sedation.[62] Absolute contraindications for endoscopic placement of a gastrostomy tube include obstruction of the GI tract proximal to the stomach and the inability to transilluminate the abdominal wall for identification of a safe abdominal access site.[63] Additional relative contraindications include ascites, coagulopathy, gastric varices, morbid obesity, and neoplastic, infiltrative, or inflammatory disease of the gastric or abdominal wall.[64] If a patient is not already receiving a broad-spectrum antibiotic, a single dose of an appropriate antibiotic administered prophylactically before tube placement has been shown to decrease peristomal infection rates.[65-67] PEG placement offers several advantages over other methods. For example, clinicians can perform it at the bedside; it does not expose the patient to radiation; and clinicians can perform diagnostic and therapeutic endoscopic procedures simultaneously.

Routine preprocedural testing of coagulation parameters and platelets is no longer recommended for patients undergoing endoscopic tube placement; however, these tests should be considered if the patient is at risk for abnormal coagulation due to anticoagulant medication, medical history of excessive bleeding, or recent antibiotic use. American Society for Gastrointestinal Endoscopy guidelines consider placement of a percutaneous feeding tube to be a high-bleeding-risk procedure.[68] Thienopyridines (eg, clopidogrel) should be held, whenever possible, for 5 to 7 days before PEG placement. If holding the thienopyridine is not possible, some institutions will add epinephrine to the lidocaine for local anesthesia (vasoconstriction), avoid vessels on the skin and mucosa, and make sure the bolsters are relatively firm (not tight) for 3 to 4 days before loosening them.[68,69] Aspirin regimens should be continued in patients with high thromboembolic risk.[68] Warfarin should be held 5 days before PEG placement, and patients at high risk for clots may be bridged with short-acting heparin. The new, direct-acting oral anticoagulants should be held for at least 48 hours before high-risk procedures and restarted up to 48 hours after the procedure, depending on renal function.[69]

The most common method of PEG insertion is the "pull" technique first described by Ponsky.[70] Air is insufflated into the stomach, and the optimal site for placement is determined through simultaneous endoscopic transillumination noted on the abdominal wall and finger indentation at the site visualized endoscopically. A sounding needle is inserted initially to confirm a safe track. A small incision is then made at this site, and a larger-bore (14- to 18-Fr) needle/trocar is inserted through the abdominal wall and into the stomach. A guidewire is passed through the needle/trocar, snared endoscopically, and withdrawn through the mouth. A gastrostomy tube is affixed to the guidewire and pulled through the esophagus into the stomach and out the abdominal wall. The gastrostomy tube is held in place by a solid distensible internal bolster as well as an external bumper (see Figure 3-5).[71]

Percutaneous Radiologic Placement

Two common methods for placing percutaneous gastrostomy tubes fluoroscopically are the antegrade (transoral) and the retrograde (transabdominal) techniques. With either method, identification of a safe window can be aided by using oral barium administered the day before the procedure to opacify the colon; more commonly, an abdominal computed tomography (CT) scan or ultrasound examination can be performed and/or reviewed prior to the procedure. If patients are not already receiving a broad-spectrum antibiotic, a single dose of an appropriate antibiotic is administered prophylactically for fluoroscopic placement using the antegrade method; prophylactic antibiotic administration is optional for the retrograde method.

FIGURE 3-5

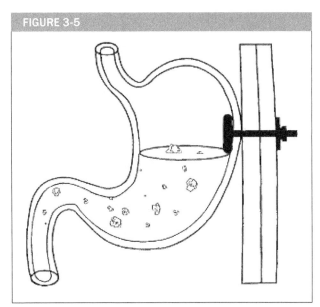

Properly placed percutaneous endoscopic gastrostomy. Reprinted with permission from reference 71: Heximer B. Pressure necrosis: implications and interventions for PEG tubes. *Nutr Clin Pract.* 1997;12:256–258.

Advantages of fluoroscopic gastrostomy placement include the following: Some patients will not need sedation; placement can be done in patients with severe stenosis/ trauma of the upper GI tract; and the risk of tumor seeding from active upper aerodigestive tract cancers may potentially be decreased when the retrograde approach is used.[72] Society of Interventional Radiology guidelines designate these procedures as category 2, implying a moderate risk of bleeding. Those guidelines recommend the following:[72]

1. Correct international normalized ratio to ≤1.5.
2. Verify that platelet count is >50,000.
3. Withhold clopidogrel for 5 days before the procedure.
4. Do not withhold aspirin.

5. Withhold 1 dose of low-molecular-weight heparin before the procedure.

6. Measurement of partial thromboplastin time is recommended only for patients receiving unfractionated heparin.

However, some institutions do not routinely check coagulation status when there is no reason to suspect coagulopathy before tube placement.

In the retrograde method, an NG tube is placed to insufflate the stomach, a safe window is identified under fluoroscopy, and 1–4 T-fasteners are used to perform a gastropexy to secure the stomach wall to the abdominal wall. The stomach is then punctured, usually with an 18-gauge needle directed toward the pylorus, to facilitate future conversion of the gastrostomy tube to a gastrojejunostomy tube if the latter type of tube is needed later. A guidewire is advanced through the needle, and the tract is dilated sequentially until it is a large enough for the gastrostomy tube. The gastrostomy tube is placed through the tract using a peel-away sheath, and contrast material is injected to confirm correct tube placement.[63]

In the antegrade technique, 2 tubes are usually advanced into the stomach—an NG tube is used to inflate the stomach with air, and an OG tube is used to insert and advance a snare. However, it is possible to use only 1 OG catheter, which can be used to inflate the stomach and then introduce the snare. The stomach is punctured percutaneously with a needle under fluoroscopic guidance, and a wire is introduced. The OG snare is then used to grasp the wire and pull it out of the mouth, giving wire access from the mouth, down the esophagus, and out of the gastric puncture. The percutaneous gastrostomy tube is introduced over this wire, and the tube is pulled out of the anterior abdominal wall (similar to the endoscopic pull method), which allows for placement of a standard PEG-type gastrostomy tube with a solid distensible internal bolster.[73]

Surgical Placement

Gastrostomy tube insertion using the laparoscopic or open method is performed in the operating room using general anesthesia. Placement of these tubes may take place during other operative procedures, including tracheostomy, or when endoscopic or fluoroscopic methods fail.

Laparoscopic techniques access the peritoneal cavity by way of small ports that enter through the abdominal wall. A pneumoperitoneum is created by way of a port inserted through the umbilicus, and a camera is passed through this site. A second port enters the left upper quadrant of the abdomen and is used to access the stomach. T-fasteners are placed to approximate the stomach to the abdominal wall. A gastrostomy tube is then placed over a guidewire into the stomach. A third port may be placed in the right upper quadrant so atraumatic graspers can be inserted to hold the stomach in place.[74]

The Stamm technique is the most commonly used open surgery technique for placement of a gastrostomy tube.[75,76] It requires a small laparotomy in the upper midline of the abdomen. The gastrostomy tube is brought into the stomach through a small incision in the upper abdominal wall. Another small incision is then made into the stomach through which the feeding tube enters and around which a purse-string suture is placed to secure the stomach around the gastrostomy tube. The stomach is then sutured to the anterior abdominal wall. This tube is held in place with an inflated balloon.

Percutaneous Gastrojejunostomy Tubes

With a gastrojejunostomy tube, 1 lumen opens to the stomach and the distal opening is in the jejunum, so the patient can benefit from gastric decompression while receiving enteral feeds into the small bowel (see Figure 3-6).[77] A gastrojejunostomy tube should be placed any time that enteral feeding into the small bowel with simultaneous stomach decompression is required. It may be indicated in patients with gastric feeding intolerance, impaired gastric motility, a previous gastric surgery, or pancreatitis, and in those undergoing pancreatic surgery.[78,79]

Percutaneous endoscopic gastrojejunostomy (PEGJ) may be performed initially or at any time after gastrostomy tube placement. In this procedure, a guidewire is placed

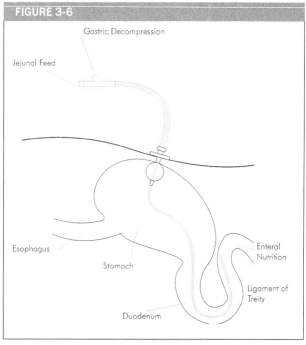

FIGURE 3-6

Gastric Decompression

Jejunal Feed

Esophagus

Stomach

Enteral Nutrition

Ligament of Treity

Duodenum

Gastrojejunostomy feeding and decompression tube. Reprinted from reference 77: Vanek VW. Ins and outs of enteral access. Part 3: long-term access—jejunostomy. *Nutr Clin Pract.* 2003;18:201–220.

through the existing gastrostomy and then grasped endoscopically and carried into the jejunum. The endoscope is then withdrawn, leaving the guidewire in place. The jejunal extension tube is threaded over the guidewire and placed within the small bowel.[64,80]

A more recently described PEGJ technique uses reclosable clips. The jejunostomy feeding tube with a suture on its tip is inserted through the PEG or existing gastrostomy stoma into the stomach lumen. A clip is passed through the working channel of an endoscope and used to grasp the suture and drag the tube into the jejunum as the endoscope is advanced. The suture is then clipped to the jejunal mucosa, securing the feeding tube to the small bowel.[81]

Another PEGJ technique uses an ultrathin endoscope (5–6 mm in diameter) or pediatric bronchoscope (3–4 mm) passed through a large-diameter gastrostomy tube or mature gastrostomy tract into the small intestine. A guidewire is fed through the endoscope deep into the small bowel, and the endoscope is removed. The gastrojejunostomy tube is then passed over the wire into position, and the wire is removed.[82]

Fluoroscopy may be used as an adjunct with any method of endoscopic placement. However, it is not absolutely required.

Fluoroscopic techniques to provide gastrojejunal access are becoming much more common for both initial and replacement gastrojejunostomy feeding tubes. Initial steps are similar to the previously described fluoroscopic gastrostomy placement. For initial placement, the stomach is punctured in the direction of the pylorus to facilitate placement of the gastrojejunostomy. A guiding catheter and/or wire is advanced through the gastrostomy to or beyond the ligament of Treitz, and the jejunal extension tube is advanced over the wire into the jejunum.[83,84]

Fluoroscopic techniques can be used when the patient cannot undergo endoscopy. However, fluoroscopic placement cannot be done at the bedside; it requires transport of the patient to the radiology suite.

Gastrojejunostomy tubes can be placed during laparotomy or by laparoscopic technique using any of the previously described laparoscopic gastrostomy methods. Using manual and/or endoscopic methods, the jejunostomy tube is positioned into the small bowel through the gastrostomy.

Percutaneous Direct Jejunostomy Tubes

Direct percutaneous jejunostomy using either endoscopic or fluoroscopic guidance is technically much more difficult than percutaneous gastrostomy and therefore is not available in all institutions. Success rates range from 68% to 100% for endoscopic jejunostomy and from 87% to 100% for fluoroscopic jejunostomy.[72] Endoscopic jejunostomy tubes may be more stable than fluoroscopically placed tubes because the endoscopic tubes have solid, mushroom-type internal bolsters and larger tube diameters (14- to 20-Fr tubes are used in endoscopic placement; 10- to 14-Fr tubes are placed fluoroscopically). Because endoscopic and radiologic methods for jejunostomies are more complex, surgical jejunostomies are usually more commonly performed, although this depends on local expertise and availability.

Direct PEJ is a modification of the PEG technique. A colonoscope or enteroscope is advanced through the stomach into the small bowel. Transillumination and finger palpation are performed over the jejunum instead of the stomach. A sounding needle and/or trocar is passed through the anterior abdominal wall into the jejunum. An insertion wire is advanced through the trocar and grasped. The procedure is then completed in the same manner as the "pull-type" PEG.[85] Higher rates of successful endoscopic placement have been reported when balloon enteroscopy and general anesthesia are used.[86,87]

Interventional radiologists have a variety of methods to place direct jejunostomy tubes. The initial step in all methods is to identify a target bowel loop. Historically, this has been done by advancing an angiographic catheter into the proximal jejunum and insufflating it with air and contrast or by placing an angioplasty balloon or snare loop in the desired location to serve as a target.[88,89] More recently introduced methods to identify the proximal jejunal loop include (a) ultrasound guidance following injection of the saline solution and contrast agent, and (b) use of cone fluoroscopy CT.[90] Once the jejunal loop is identified by any method, it is accessed with a needle, and a T-fastener device is used to secure the jejunal loop against the abdominal wall. A guidewire is then advanced through the needle, the tract is dilated, and the jejunostomy tube is placed and injected with contrast to confirm the position.

The technique of laparoscopic jejunostomy is similar to laparoscopic gastrostomy. Ports are placed in the left upper quadrant and lower abdominal midline. The jejunum is manipulated to affix it to the abdominal wall with T-fasteners. A guidewire is then placed into the lumen of the jejunum, and a jejunostomy tube is advanced into the small bowel through a peel-away sheath. An advantage with this approach is that a larger-diameter tube (18–20 Fr) with a solid bolster can be placed.

An open jejunostomy is placed using the Witzel technique (Figure 3-7).[77] In this procedure, a submucosal tunnel is created in the small bowel through which the jejunostomy tube is threaded. This method helps prevents leakage of small bowel contents onto the abdominal wall.[77,91]

Placing a needle-catheter jejunostomy by laparotomy or laparoscopy is a less common procedure.[77] In this

FIGURE 3-7

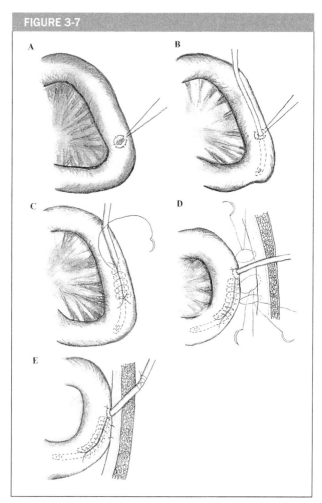

Witzel jejunostomy. Reprinted with permission from reference 77: Vanek VW. Ins and outs of enteral access. Part 3: long-term access—jejunostomy. *Nutr Clin Pract.* 2003;18(3):201–220.

procedure, a needle is threaded into the small bowel and a guidewire is passed into the jejunum. A small jejunostomy catheter (5–8 Fr) is passed over the guidewire into the jejunum. The small-bore size of needle-catheter jejunostomies makes them prone to occlusion.

Low-Profile Devices

Low-profile (skin-level) devices are excellent options for the patient who is concerned about cosmetic appearance and does not wish to have a feeding tube concealed or exposed through clothing. These devices may also be more comfortable for the patient who is active, sleeps in the prone position, only needs intermittent therapy, or is at risk for pulling out a standard-profile tube. Low-profile EADs are the preferred option for pediatric patients because these devices are easier to secure and less likely to be inadvertently dislodged. Balloon low-profile devices allow caregivers to manage and replace in the home setting. To attach a feeding connector to the skin-level device, reasonable manual dexterity or caregiver assistance is needed.

In adult patients, skin-level devices are usually placed as an exchange or replacement tube for a preexisting gastrostomy tube; however, they can also be placed at the time of initial tube placement.[92] In pediatric patients, they are typically placed as the initial EAD.[93] The devices are held in place with an inflated internal balloon or a distensible internal retention bolster that requires an obturator for placement. Low-profile, 1-piece gastrojejunostomy tubes are also available for jejunal feeding with or without gastric decompression.

Tube Maintenance Considerations

Maintaining Proper Placement

Once the feeding tube tip is properly positioned, it is necessary to verify that the tube has remained in the desired location (either the stomach or small bowel). Unfortunately, a nasally placed or transgastric small bowel tube may migrate upward into the stomach, or a nasally placed gastric tube may migrate downward into the small bowel; the worst-case scenario is when a tube tip displaces upward into the esophagus.[94] Obviously, X-rays cannot be obtained multiple times a day to confirm tube location; thus, clinicians may employ bedside methods for this purpose. These methods include the following:[95]

- Determining whether the external length of the tubing has changed since the time of the confirmatory radiograph
- Detecting any change in the measurement marking on the tube at the naris
- Observing for negative pressure when attempting to withdraw fluid from the feeding tube
- Observing for unexpected changes in gastric residual volumes (GRVs)
- Measuring the pH of the feeding tube aspirates

In a prospective study, observing for changes in external tube length was helpful in identifying outward migration of feeding tubes into the esophagus, as well as proximal migration from the small bowel into the stomach.[95] To allow for assessment of tube length, the measurement marking where a confirmed properly placed OG or NG tube exits the mouth or nares should be recorded in documentation accessible to all clinicians. Negative pressure is more likely to be felt during attempts to aspirate fluid from a small bowel tube than from a gastric tube.[96] A sharp increase in GRV may indicate displacement of a small bowel tube into the stomach.[97] Testing the pH of feeding tube aspirates is most likely to be helpful prior to an intermittent or bolus feeding, when less of the tube feeding formula is present (formula can alter the pH). For tubes placed using electromagnetic guidance, the stylet with transmitter can be reinserted to check the distal location of the tip.

As noted previously, the auscultatory method cannot distinguish between gastric and small bowel placement, and it cannot detect when the tube tip is in the esophagus. This method should not be used to evaluate tube placement.[53,98]

Tube Securement and Connections

There is nothing inherent to the design of available nasally placed tubes to prevent migration inward or outward. Therefore, an additional mechanism is needed to secure the tube to the nose or face. Nasal tubes are typically secured near the nares with tape, adhesive strips, a transparent physiologic dressing, or a nasal bridle. Securement is frequently done with adhesive tape that is split part way and wrapped around the tube and then attached to the nose, or it may be done with semipermeable transparent dressing, adhesive skin-closure strips, or manufactured fixation devices. After providing some slack so as not to exert pressure on the nares, the remaining tube length can then be brought to the side of the face and secured to the cheek with tape, adhesive strips, or a transparent physiologic dressing. For infants, it is important to watch the pacifier and make sure it does not catch in securement products.

Nasal bridles are typically reserved for patients who are at risk for pulling at their tubes or those with facial burns, but they can be used in any patient. Use of a nasal bridle involves a technique that results in small-bore tubing or twill tape entering 1 naris, looping around the nasal septum, and exiting the other naris. The 2 ends are then secured together, forming the bridle, and the feeding tube is clipped or tied to it. When the feeding tube is pulled or tugged, the bridle is also tugged and the patient feels nasal septal discomfort. There is a commercially manufactured nasal bridle that uses a magnetic retrieval technique to facilitate the movement of the blue polymer hypoallergenic, latex-free tubing (bridle) around the nasal septum (Applied Medical Technology, Brecksville, OH).

A meta-analysis found that nasal bridles were more effective for tube securement and preventing tube dislodgement when compared to adhesive tape.[99] This technique should be avoided in those patients with nasal airway obstructions and abnormalities and with facial or anterior cranial fractures. Excessive traction on a nasal bridle may cause serious nasal injury, and it is recommended to further secure the tube by other means.

As noted previously, percutaneous feeding tubes have an internal securement device or bolster to prevent external displacement, and most have an external securement device preventing internal displacement. Those that do not have the external retention device should be secured with tape, adhesive strips, sutures, or commercial tube-attachment devices. For patients who tend to pull at their percutaneous feeding tube, the tube should either be tucked away under clothing, covered with an abdominal binder, cut down to an external length of 6 to 8 cm, and/or transitioned to a low-profile feeding tube. Placing the patient's hands in mittens is another option to deter pulling. The use of medications or physical restraints is discouraged because those methods can increase the risk of agitation and delirium.

To administer formula, medication, or water to the patient, the EAD must be connected to a syringe or feeding bag. Misconnections between EADs and unrelated delivery systems such as IV lines, respiratory tubing, or urinary devices can lead to deleterious outcomes, including serious injury or death. The FDA has received reports of 2 deaths and 24 serious injuries related to enteral misconnections just since 2011. Furthermore, it is thought that many enteral misconnections do not get reported to the FDA. In response to such safety issues, the FDA published safety considerations regarding the risk of enteral feed misconnections with non-enteral small-bore connectors in 2015.[100] Healthcare facilities are encouraged to implement procedures and policies to reduce enteral misconnection risk.[3,101] See Table 3-5 for recommendations to prevent enteral misconnections.

To address the risk of enteral misconnections, the International Organization for Standardization (ISO) has published design standard ISO 80369-3 (commonly known as ENFit®). Enteral device manufacturers produce EADs with this connection to comply with the standard and improve patient safety (see Figure 3-8). Use of the ENFit connection is considered an effective method to reduce enteral misconnection risk because the ENFit connection is not physically compatible with non-enteral devices. The FDA released a letter on September 7, 2018, encouraging healthcare facilities to adopt the ISO 80369-3 connection.[102] The Global Enteral Device Supplier Association (GEDSA) is a nonprofit group created to promote the global adoption of ENFit connectors.[103,104] At the time of publication of this handbook, US healthcare facilities, manufacturers, and distributors are undergoing the transition from legacy to ENFit devices.[104] More information on ENFit may be found on GEDSA's website (www.stayconnected.org).

TABLE 3-5. Practice Recommendations for Enteral Misconnection Prevention

1. Review currently used systems to assess practices that include the potential for misconnection, including nonstandard, rigged work-arounds (Luer adapters, etc).

2. Train nonclinical staff and visitors not to reconnect lines but to seek clinical assistance instead. Only clinicians or users knowledgeable about the use of the device should make a reconnection, and they should do so under proper lighting.

3. Do not modify or adapt IV or feeding devices because doing so may compromise the safety features incorporated into their design.

4. When making a reconnection, practitioners should routinely trace lines back to their origins and then verify that they are secure.

5. Route tubes and catheters that have different purposes in unique and standardized directions (eg, IV lines should be routed toward the patient's head, and enteric lines should be routed toward the feet).

6. When arriving at a new setting or as part of a hand-off process, staff should recheck connections and trace all tubes.

7. Label or color-code feeding tubes and connectors, and educate staff about the labeling or color-coding process in the institution's enteral feeding system.

8. Identify and confirm the EN label, because a 3-in-1 PN admixture can appear similar to an EN formulation bag. Label the EN bags with large, bold statements such as "WARNING! For Enteral Use Only—NOT for IV Use."

9. Transition to enteral-specific connectors such as ENFit®.

10. Purchase an adequate number of enteral pumps so that IV pumps are not used for enteral delivery for adult patients. When syringe pumps are used in neonatal ICUs for human milk or other feedings, they should be clearly distinct from syringe pumps used for IV or other medical purposes. Ideally, enteral feeding pumps should be a different model, a different color, or as different in appearance from IV pumps as possible. Enteral feeding pumps should be clearly labeled as enteral feeding pumps.

(continued)

TABLE 3-5. *(Continued)*

11. Avoid buying prefilled enteral feeding containers, except for those with design technology labeled non-IV-compatible. In all cases, verify that the enteral administration set is packaged with the enteral feeding bag or container before it is sent to the patient care unit. (The set should be secured to the bag, perhaps with a rubber band, or preattached sets should be requested from the manufacturer.) In either case, the objective is to prevent bags or containers from being spiked with IV administration sets.

12. Purchase and use enteral syringes with ENFit connectors instead of Luer-lock syringes to draw up and deliver medications into the enteral feeding system. Include pharmacy department recommendations to verify the correct syringe type, along with dispensing and proper labeling protocols.

Abbreviations: EN, enteral nutrition; GI, gastrointestinal; ICU, intensive care unit; IV, intravenous; PN, parenteral nutrition.

Source: Adapted with permission from reference 3: Boullata JI, Carrera AL, Harvey L, et al. ASPEN safe practices for enteral nutrition therapy. *JPEN J Parenter Enteral Nutr.* 2017;41(1):15–103. doi:10.1177/0148607116673053.

FIGURE 3-8

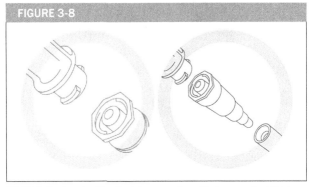

ENFit® design for enteral feeding tube connections. The image on the right shows a transition set to use with existing legacy devices. Reprinted with permission from Global Enteral Device Supplier Association (http://gedsa.org). For more information, visit: www.stayconnected.org.

Nasal, Oral, and Skin Care

Regardless of the feeding tube type or insertion technique, all patients receiving EN require appropriate oral hygiene. Oral care is especially important for preventing aspiration pneumonia in ventilator-dependent patients or in those with a depressed level of consciousness.[105]

Patients with nasal feeding tubes benefit from skin care to the nasal area to prevent or address harm caused by prolonged exposure to tape and adhesive products. Periodic repositioning of the nasal tube and efforts to avoid pressure on the nares are necessary to prevent pressure necrosis.

In patients with enterostomy feeding tubes, the area around the tube's exit site should be cleaned with mild soap and water daily. The area should then be rinsed and dried thoroughly, including underneath the external retention device. Routine use of antibiotic ointments or hydrogen peroxide at the tube site is not recommended. Hydrogen peroxide can impede wound healing and cause skin irritation. Antibiotic ointments are not routinely necessary and can promote yeast overgrowth with chronic use. Dressings are not needed at the tube site unless there is concern about drainage (some drainage is common).

Patients with enterostomies are at risk for skin breakdown with redness or excoriation at the exit site. Zinc-based products, such as diaper rash creams or absorptive powders, can be applied and the site covered with a semipermeable/breathable drainage sponge. If there is excessive site leakage, a dressing that is manufactured to wick away moisture is preferable to gauze. Alcohol-free, skin-barrier films or skin-barrier wafers can be used. Scattered, reddened and raised papules spreading from the stoma outward may indicate a candidal infection. This type of fungal infection can be treated by directly applying a topical antifungal, such as nystatin powder or cream, and a zinc oxide cream coating twice daily and then covering the area with a split-gauze dressing. Clinicians should consult with a wound or stoma nurse if these first-line treatments are ineffective.

Hypertrophic granulation tissue growth may develop at the stoma site, manifesting as reddened, lumpy, moist, shiny tissue growth protruding from the site. The presence of this excess tissue may, but does not always, lead to increased site drainage as the seal around the tube is compromised. The treatment involves dissolution of the granulated tissue, most commonly with silver nitrate applicators. If that fails, topical corticosteroid can be applied with a cotton tip applicator as needed. Other treatment options include mometasone furoate 0.1% once daily or triamcinolone acetonide 0.1% 3 times daily. Care must be taken not to apply the corticosteroid on healthy skin because it will cause tissue thinning of the skin over time. As a last resort, surgical excision of granulation tissue can be undertaken. A skilled clinician must perform the surgical intervention because the tissue can bleed easily, and a thorough assessment is needed to rule out malignancy.

To minimize the risk for granulation tissue, the site must be kept as dry as possible, the tube should be secured to prevent movement, and the movable external attachment device or low-profile tube should be positioned about a dime's width from the skin.

Exchange and Removal of Enterostomy Feeding Tubes

Depending on the tube type and provider's discretion, enterostomy tubes may be safely removed after the tract has matured, which usually happens 4–8 weeks after insertion in adults. In patients who are slow to heal or receiving steroids or immunosuppressive agents, longer wait times (up to 3 months) are advised. In pediatric patients, waiting 4–12 weeks may be advised.[106] Early dislodgement or removal of newly placed enterostomy tubes may result in the stomach falling away from the abdominal wall, allowing gastric contents to leak into the peritoneum. Inadvertent tube dislodgement before tract maturation requires tube replacement with the assistance of endoscopy, interventional radiology, or surgical intervention.

Removal of enterostomy tubes should be performed only by those trained and/or credentialed to do so. Removal of a percutaneous gastrostomy tube with an internal solid bolster is accomplished at the bedside using the traction pull method. The patient is placed in the supine position with knees bent to relax the abdominal muscles. The exposed gastric tube is firmly grasped and pulled using constant traction while the abdomen is held down around the stoma site for countertraction. The internal bolster deconforms through the stomal tract. Some clinicians cut the percutaneous gastrostomy tube close to the site, which allows the internal bolster to fall inside the stomach; however, the severed bolster could potentially cause a subsequent bowel obstruction. For devices held in place with an inflated balloon, the balloon is deflated and the tube is gently removed.

To insert replacement percutaneous feeding tubes with balloon internal bolsters, the deflated replacement tube is lubricated with water-soluble gel and inserted into the stoma tract and then the balloon is inflated with distilled or sterile water. Generally, 5–20 mL of sterile or distilled water should be used for gastric tubes and 2–3 mL should be used for small bowel tubes; follow the manufacturer's recommendations to determine the water volume to use. Clinicians can use stoma-measuring devices to select the appropriate replacement tube length when replacing a standard-profile tube with a low-profile tube or when there is uncertainty about the length of the low-profile replacement tube needed.

Complications of Enteral Access Devices

Nasal Tube Complications

Complications of nasally placed feeding tubes can be divided into those that occur during the insertion procedure and those that occur postprocedure. Procedure-related complications include epistaxis, aspiration, tube misplacement, esophageal perforation, and circulatory or respiratory compromise. The most-dreaded procedure-related complication is initial misplacement of the nasal tube into the bronchopulmonary tree. This complication has been reported to occur in 1.2%–2.3% of blind tube placements and may lead to pneumothorax, hemopneumothorax, empyema, or pneumonia.[107] Death has been reported to occur in 0.1%–0.5% of all blind tube placements, and the estimated mortality rate is 15% when a tube is misplaced into the bronchopulmonary tree.[108,109] Patients at the highest risk for feeding tube malposition include those who are critically ill, sedated, or intubated; patients with altered mental status; and those who have poor cough reflex.[107] Patients who require repeated tube placements or experience difficult tube placements are also at increased risk. Best practices for confirming tube position are reviewed earlier in this chapter.

Postprocedural complications include tube malfunction, tube displacement or dislodgement, tube clogging, pressure-related skin breakdown, sinusitis, aspiration, and intestinal ischemia. Malfunction of the tube, which includes breaking, cracking, or kinking, occurs 11% to 20% of the time.[110,111]

Tube dislodgement seems to be a fairly frequent occurrence. In a study of 49 intensive care units (ICUs), 28.9% of NG tubes were reported to have dislodged.[112] As noted earlier in the chapter, once a feeding tube is placed and the tube tip is determined to be in the proper position, the tube must be secured to prevent inward or outward migration. A tube can displace inward or outward by slipping through the external securement device. Tube dislodgement has been associated with patients who are agitated, confused, or restless, as well as those who have infections, untoward medication side effects, or a Glasgow coma scale score <9.[112,113] For these high-risk patients and patients with facial wounds or burns, a nasal bridle may be a good securement option. See the Tube Securement and Connections section earlier in this chapter for cautions regarding the use of nasal bridles.

In patients with nasally placed tubes, the incidence of sinusitis is approximately 12%.[114] Sinusitis is believed to be secondary to obstruction of physiological sinus drainage by the nasal tube; therefore, it may be prudent to avoid larger-diameter or stiffer tubes. Although the overall incidence of sinusitis is relatively low, incidence increases in patients who have both a nasoenteric tube and an endotracheal tube.[115]

Enterostomy Tube Complications

Complications of enterostomy tubes can be divided into major complications and those that tend to have less clinical significance. Major complications include aspiration, hemorrhage, peritonitis/necrotizing fasciitis, and death. Complications that are usually less serious include peristomal infection, peristomal leakage, buried bumper syndrome, inadvertent removal, and fistulous tracts.[18]

Another way to classify enterostomy-related complications is as procedural vs postprocedural events. Incidence of procedure-related complications (eg, intraprocedural aspiration, hemorrhage, perforation of the GI lumen, and prolonged ileus) has been estimated to be 1.5%–4%; procedure-related mortality occurs in less than 2% of cases.[116] Risk factors for aspiration include the supine position, advanced age, need for sedation, and neurologic impairment.[117] Pneumoperitoneum as a result of the percutaneous procedure is common, and, in the absence of peritoneal signs, it is of no clinical consequence.[118] Infusion of water-soluble contrast with fluoroscopic or CT imaging is the test of choice if perforation and peritonitis are suspected.

Peristomal infection is the most common complication of gastrostomy tube placement.[65,119] Most of these infections are mild, presenting with a painful area surrounding the tube with marked redness and induration. Early evaluation and management of peristomal wound infection and treatment with oral antibiotics are usually sufficient interventions. However, signs of systemic toxicity (ie, fever, tachycardia, hypotension) require hospital admission and IV antibiotics. Local wound care and incision and drainage of any significant fluid collections are the keys to successful management.[66,120] In rare cases, necrotizing fasciitis with high risks for morbidity and mortality can develop from peristomal infection. Necrotizing fasciitis is an emergent condition requiring surgical debridement, broad-spectrum antibiotics, and ICU admission.

Significant leakage around the gastrostomy site should be addressed promptly (see Table 3-6).[121] Of note, the color of the drainage around a gastrostomy tube does not necessarily signify infection—even green or cloudy yellow drainage, which may otherwise appear purulent, may be normal for gastric fluid. Prolonged exposure of the skin to gastrostomy secretions can lead to pain, skin breakdown, cellulitis, or a yeast infection. Risk factors include infection, excessive cleansing with irritant solutions (eg, hydrogen peroxide, povidone-iodine), an external bumper that

TABLE 3-6. Management of Drainage at an Enterostomy Tube Site

Type of Drainage	Management Recommendations
Thin clear (serous)	• Monitor for skin irritation and breakdown. • Clean site with mild soap and water. • Check water in the balloon/external bolster position if appropriate. • Confirm size of the tube is appropriate. • Use a skin-barrier product to protect the skin (cream, powder) or a moisture-wicking dressing.
Pink/bleeding serosanguineous	• Assess gastrostomy site for skin breakdown. • Assess whether a traumatic event occurred. • Identify where drainage is originating. • Clean site with mild soap and water. • Check water in the balloon if appropriate. • Confirm size is appropriate. • If skin breakdown is present, use a moisture-wicking dressing. • Consider using a silver-impregnated dressing.
Mucous—thick/clear white/cloudy	• Monitor site for skin breakdown. • Clean site with mild soap and water. • Use a skin-barrier product to protect the skin (cream, powder) or a moisture-wicking dressing.
Purulent yellow/ green thick	• Monitor site for signs and symptoms of infection and for skin breakdown. • Clean site with mild soap and water. • Check water in the balloon/external bolster position if appropriate.

(continued)

TABLE 3-6. *(Continued)*

Type of Drainage	Management Recommendations
	• Confirm size is appropriate. • Use a moisture-wicking dressing. • If skin breakdown is present, consider using a silver-impregnated dressing.
Thin, bright-yellow	• Protect skin from drainage, and monitor the site for skin breakdown. • Clean site with mild soap and water. • Check water in the balloon/external bolster position, if appropriate. • Confirm size of the tube is appropriate. • Use a skin-barrier product to protect the skin (cream, powder) or a moisture-wicking dressing.
Formula/food intake	• Protect skin from drainage, and monitor site for skin breakdown. • Monitor bowel movements and feeding tolerance. • Clean site with mild soap and water. • Check water in the balloon/external bolster position, if appropriate. • Confirm size of the tube, if appropriate. • Vent gastric port to release any air in the stomach. • Use a skin-barrier product to protect the skin (cream, powder) or a moisture-wicking dressing.
Dark-brown/black	• This is an indication that an injury has occurred to the gastric mucosa. Patient should be seen by a medical provider, and close follow-up is needed.

(continued)

TABLE 3-6. *(Continued)*	
Type of Drainage	**Management Recommendations**
	• Monitor site for skin breakdown.
	• Monitor site for signs and symptoms of infections.
	• Monitor site for signs and symptoms of buried bumper syndrome or other injury to stomach mucosa.
	• Confirm size is appropriate.
	• Protect skin from drainage with moisture-wicking dressing or skin-barrier products.
	• Consider whether patient needs a proton pump inhibitor to decrease the acidic environment and promote healing of the gastric mucosa.

Source: Adapted with permission from reference 121: Abdelhadi RA, Rahe K, Lyman B. Pediatric enteral access device management. *Nutr Clin Pract.* 2016;31: 748–761.

is either too loose or too tight, internal balloon deflation or rupture, and excessive tension and side torsion on the external portion of the feeding tube. Prompt treatment of infection, good ostomy skin care, adjustment of the outer bumper, checking for appropriate balloon volume, and stabilizing the gastrostomy tube to prevent torsion on the tube will address these issues.[122] Converting a gastrostomy to a gastrojejunostomy tube may be indicated to decrease leakage of formula. With a gastrojejunostomy, the gastric port can be used for drainage while feeding is infused through the jejunal port.

Buried bumper syndrome (Figure 3-9) is the embedding of the internal retention device into the gastric mucosa.[71] It can cause pain, tube obstruction, and stoma site drainage and may lead to GI bleeding, perforation, peritonitis,

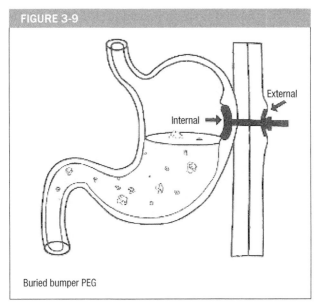

FIGURE 3-9

Buried bumper PEG

Buried bumper syndrome involving a gastrostomy tube. Reprinted with permission from reference 71: Heximer B. Pressure necrosis: implications and interventions for PEG tubes. *Nutr Clin Pract.* 1997;12:256–258.

abdominal abscesses, or phlegmon.[123] Risk factors include excessive tension between the internal and external bumpers, poor wound healing, and significant weight gain or abdominal distention that causes progressive tightness of the external bumper.[124–126] Buried bumper syndrome is highly suspected when a gastrostomy tube cannot be easily rotated or moved inward. Treatment is based on maintaining the existing stoma tract while restoring the internal bumper entirely within the stomach lumen; if that approach fails, tube removal and replacement may be warranted.[127,128] To prevent this complication, it is important to not place the external bumper too tightly and to loosen it if the patient gains a substantial amount of weight or has a distended abdomen.

A rare but serious complication is tumor implantation and metastasis at the gastrostomy tube site in patients with upper aerodigestive cancers. This complication may result from direct shearing of cancer cells during gastrostomy tube placement and subsequent tumor seeding at the tube site or from hematogenous spread of circulating tumor cells to a wound site. In a report of 218 patients with head and neck cancer with viable tumor at the time of PEG placement, 2 patients (0.92%) experienced PEG-site metastasis.[129] This may have been caused by cancer cells adhering to the endoscope and then seeding at the gastrostomy site. Gastrostomy-site tumors can be treated with palliative radiation or resection, but overall prognosis is poor. Because this complication has for the most part been reported with endoscopically placed gastrostomy tubes using the transoral approach, alternate tube placement methods, such as radiologic techniques using the transabdominal approach, can be considered in patients with active aerodigestive cancers.

Peritonitis can result from the premature removal of the percutaneous enterostomy tube before the stoma tract has matured (ie, within the first few days to weeks after insertion). If the stomach or small bowel falls away from the abdominal wall when the EAD is prematurely removed, gastric or small bowel contents can leak into the peritoneum. Gastrostomy tract maturation begins to take place in the first 7 to 10 days following initial gastrostomy tube placement, but it is recommended to wait at least 30 days for fusion between the stomach and peritoneum to occur.[3,116] Peritonitis can also occur during either initial placement or replacement if the tip of the tube is malpositioned into the peritoneum and enteral formula infuses into the peritoneal cavity.

Given the risk for peritonitis, unintended gastrostomy tube removal should be addressed urgently. If a gastrostomy tube is removed or dislodged prior to stoma tract maturation, the tube should be immediately replaced with endoscopic or fluoroscopic guidance. After stoma tract maturation has occurred, a replacement tube can be placed at the bedside or in an outpatient setting without endoscopy or fluoroscopy. If a standard replacement tube is not promptly available, a suitably sized Foley-type or urological red rubber catheter might be used to keep the tract open until a standard replacement tube can be placed. However, this intervention should be temporary and done only as a last resort. As noted earlier, these types of tubes are not indicated for enteral use and are not compatible with ENFit connections on feeding sets and syringes. Alternatively, tape may be used to hold the damaged tube in place until replacement can be achieved. Some patients are provided with a backup gastrostomy tube to be used for replacement in an emergency. If there is any concern about improper replacement, the tube position should be checked either radiographically with injection of contrast or by direct endoscopic visualization.

A cohort study published in 2015 sheds light on gastrostomy-related complications in pediatric patients.[130] The authors reviewed charts of 591 infants and children with PEG tubes, and the data collected indicated that mortality in the pediatric population was relatively low compared to the adult population cohort. Mortality in the pediatric patients was linked to comorbidities. In this review, infection at the stoma site was the most common complication with PEG placement. The presence of a ventriculoperitoneal shunt was a greater risk factor than other neurologic abnormalities. From the data reviewed, the authors predicted that 1 in 4 pediatric patients would have a complication, an extended hospital stay, or an additional procedure requiring anesthesia after the placement of a PEG. Laparoscopic techniques to place PEG tubes may have lower complication rates.[130]

Other studies involving pediatric patients have investigated the risk for gastroesophageal reflux disease (GERD) following PEG tube placement.[131,132] That risk seems to be minimal even when predicted based on preplacement studies. However, pediatric patients with a neurologic impairment are at increased risk for GERD after PEG tube placement.[131,132]

Patients with gastrojejunostomy tubes and jejunostomy tubes are at risk for many of the complications associated with gastrostomy tubes. Compared with gastrostomy feeding tubes, gastrojejunostomy feeding tubes are associated with higher risks of tube occlusion and kinking because the jejunostomy tube has a smaller diameter and longer length. To help prevent tube clogging, medications should be administered through the much-larger-diameter gastrostomy port of the gastrojejunostomy tube when possible (tube clogging is discussed in greater detail in the next section of this chapter).

A unique complication of transgastric GI and transgastric jejunal tubes is the retrograde migration of the jejunostomy tube tip back into the stomach.[72] Further complications may occur when the type of ostomy tube is incorrectly identified (eg, a balloon gastrostomy tube is confused with a gastrojejunostomy tube). This risk can be prevented when clinicians clearly understand and carefully inspect the labeling of the various ports (gastric, jejunal, or balloon). In addition, there should be clear documentation regarding which port is used for enteral formula delivery, which is used for water administration, and which is for medication administration (see Chapter 10).

A pediatric study described outcomes for patients requiring primary gastrojejunostomy tube placement.[133] The primary indications for gastrojejunostomy tube placement in this study were GERD, aspiration, and growth failure; secondary comorbidities included complex cardiac disease, prematurity, respiratory disease, and neurologic conditions. Of the 90 patients in the study, 16 had a complication of tube occlusion, tube migration, or jejunal perforation. The 30-day complication rate was 6.7%, and the mortality rate at 30 days was 4.4%.[133]

Complications specific to direct jejunostomy tubes include jejunal volvulus, small bowel perforation, and persistent enterocutaneous fistulas after the tube is removed.[72] However, jejunostomy tubes have the advantage of a more stable jejunal tip placement because they are inserted directly into the jejunum. Jejunal volvulus is a rare but potentially devastating complication of direct jejunostomy placement.[134] A retrospective study that compared outcomes of primary placement of jejunostomy tube and gastrojejunostomy tubes found comparable complication rates except that more pericatheter leakage was seen with the jejunostomy tubes.[135]

Gastrojejunostomy or direct jejunostomy intermittent feeding into the small bowel can result in dumping syndrome. The rapid infusion of tube feeding directly into the small bowel causes a release of gut hormones that shifts the fluid from the bloodstream into the bowel. The bowel becomes distended, and patients can experience diarrhea, abdominal discomfort and bloating, lightheadedness, and potential fainting.

Tube Clogging

Tube clogging is a frequent problem across all types of tubes, with incidence reported to be as high as 23%–35%; when tubes become clogged, they often must be replaced.[136] Risk factors for tube clogging include longer tube lengths, smaller internal tube calibers, inadequate water flushing, contaminated formula, improper medication delivery, and use of the tube to measure GRVs.[137]

The first strategy to unclog a feeding tube usually involves attaching a 60-mL syringe of warm water to the tube, using the syringe plunger to push the water into the tubing, massaging the tubing to loosen the clog, and then pulling back on the plunger to dislodge the clog. If this technique is ineffective, water penetration may be tried. Remove all fluid from the tube, instill the tube with warm water, and clamp the tube for 20–60 minutes, periodically moving the plunger back and forth to help loosen the clog.[138–140]

If water penetration fails, a declogging solution can be tried. A prospective study demonstrated that pancreatic enzyme activated with bicarbonate was more effective than traditional measures for resolving feeding tube clogs.[141] This declogging solution is made by first dissolving ¼ teaspoon of baking soda or a crushed 650-mg non-enteric-coated sodium bicarbonate tablet in 10 mL of warm water and then adding the contents of an opened 12,000-U pancrelipase capsule (Creon) or a crushed 10,440 U pancrelipase tablet (Viokace) to the solution; the solution is ready for use when all ingredients are fully dissolved.[29] To use the solution, all the fluid from the feeding tube should be withdrawn, the declogging solution instilled, and the tube clamped for up to 60 minutes. Afterward, the solution should be withdrawn to see whether the clog releases. The declogging technique with activated pancreatic enzyme can be repeated once. Once a clog is successfully withdrawn, a water flush should be administered to clear the tube.

An intermittent activated pancreatic enzyme lock has been suggested once weekly to prevent clogging in tubes prone to clogging.[29] A commercially available pancreatic enzyme cocktail (Clog Zapper, Avanos, Alpharetta, GA) is available in a preloaded syringe that is activated with water and gains close proximity to the clog through a smaller-bore tube placed inside the feeding tube. A 100% declogging success rate was reported with up to 2 attempts in feeding tubes with formula clogs.[142]

Another option is mechanical dislodgement of tube occlusion. This may be achieved using a cytology brush, an endoscopic retrograde cholangiopancreatography catheter, corrugated plastic rods (Bionix, Toledo, OH), or a machine-operated wire encased in a sheath that mechanically breaks up clogs with a back and forth motion (Tube-Clear, Actuated Medical, Bellefonte, PA).

Regular flushing of the tube is critical to maintain tube patency, with water as the fluid of choice. If medication is administered via the feeding tube, a water flush should be administered before and after each medication.[143] A pharmacist should be consulted if any medications are to be administered via the feeding tube. For example, some medications require activation in the stomach and should not be administered via a postpyloric route. See Chapter 10 for additional information on medication administration. Table 3-7 summarizes practice recommendations related to tube patency.[3,29]

TABLE 3-7. Practice Recommendations to Maintain Tube Patency
1. Use the largest-bore enteral tube possible that will be comfortable for the patient.
2. Follow best practices for enteral medication administration.[a]
3. Flush the tube with water every 4–8 hours during continuous feedings.
4. Flush the tube with water before and after all bolus enteral feeds.
5. Consult treating provider for the appropriate amount of water flushes.

[a]See Chapter 10.

References

1. Northington L, Lyman B, Guenter P, Irving SY, Duesing L. Current practices in home management of nasogastric tube placement in pediatric patients: a survey of parents and homecare providers. *J Pediatr Nurs*. 2017;33:46–53.

2. Vanek VW. Ins and outs of enteral access. Part 1: short-term enteral access. *Nutr Clin Pract*. 2002;17(5):275–283.

3. Boullata JI, Carrera AL, Harvey L, et al. ASPEN safe practices for enteral nutrition therapy. *JPEN J Parenter Enteral Nutr*. 2016;41(1):15–103. doi:10.1177/0148607116673053.

4. Norton B, Homer-Ward M, Donnelly MT, Long RG, Holmes GK. A randomised prospective comparison of percutaneous endoscopic gastrostomy and nasogastric tube feeding after acute dysphagic stroke. *BMJ*. 1996;312(7022):13–16.

5. Park RH, Allison MC, Lang J, et al. Randomised comparison of percutaneous endoscopic gastrostomy and nasogastric tube feeding in patients with persisting neurological dysphagia. *BMJ*. 1992;304(6839):1406–1409.

6. Attam R, Leslie D, Freeman M, Ikramuddin F, Andrade R. EUS-assisted, fluoroscopically guided gastrostomy tube placement in patients with Roux-en-Y gastric bypass: a novel technique for access to the gastric remnant. *Gastrointest Endosc*. 2011;74(3):677–682. doi:10.1016/j.gie.2011.05.01.

7. Moon R, Teixeira A, Potenza K, Jawad M. Routine gastrostomy tube placement in gastric bypass patients: impact on length of stay and 30-day readmission rate. *Obes Surg*. 2013;23(2):216–221. doi:10.1007/s11695-012-0835-5.

8. Levy H. Nasogastric and nasoenteric feeding tubes. *Gastrointest Endosc Clin N Am*. 1998;8(3):529–549.

9. Albrecht H, Hagel AF, Schlechtweg P, Foertsch T, Neurath MF, Mudter J. Computed tomography-guided percutaneous gastrostomy/jejunostomy for feeding and decompression. *Nutr Clin Pract*. 2017;32(2):212–218.

10. Haskins IN, Strong AT, Baginsky M, et al. Comparison of laparoscopic jejunostomy tube to percutaneous endoscopic gastrostomy tube with jejunal extension: long-term durability and nutritional outcomes. *Surg Endosc*. 2018;32(5):2496–2504.

11. Ho KM, Dobb GJ, Webb SA. A comparison of early gastric and post-pyloric feeding in critically ill patients: a meta-analysis. *Intensive Care Med*. 2006;32(5):639–649.

12. Marik PE, Zaloga GP. Gastric versus post-pyloric feeding: a systematic review. *Crit Care.* 2003;7(3):R46–R51.

13. McClave SA, Taylor BE, Martindale RG, et al. Guidelines for the provision and assessment of nutrition support therapy in the adult critically ill patient: Society of Critical Care Medicine (SCCM) and American Society for Parenteral and Enteral Nutrition (A.S.P.E.N.). *JPEN J Parenter Enteral Nutr.* 2016;40(2):159–211.

14. Mehta NM, Skillman HE, Irving SY, et al. Guidelines for the provision and assessment of nutrition support therapy in the pediatric critically ill patient: Society of Critical Care Medicine and American Society for Parenteral and Enteral Nutrition. *JPEN J Parenter Enteral Nutr.* 2017;41(5): 706–741.

15. Heyland DK, Drover JW, Dhaliwal R, Greenwood J. Optimizing the benefits and minimizing the risks of enteral nutrition in the critically ill: role of small bowel feeding. *JPEN J Parenter Enteral Nutr.* 2002;26(6 Suppl):S51–S55.

16. Massoumi R, Akdelhafeez HA, Christensen MA, Vo NJ. *JPEN J Parenter Enteral Nutr.* 2016;40(8):1177–1182.

17. Egnell C, Eclborg S. Grahnquist L. Jejunostomy enteral feeding in children: outcome and safety. *JPEN J Parenter Enteral Nutr.* 2014;38(5):631–636.

18. Fang JC, Kinikini M. Enteral access devices. In: Mueller CM, ed. *The ASPEN Adult Nutrition Support Core Curriculum.* 3rd ed. Silver Spring, MD: American Society for Parenteral and Enteral Nutrition; 2017:251–264.

19. Lyman B, Kemper CA, Northington L, et al. Use of temporary enteral access devices in hospitalized neonatal and pediatric patients in the United States. *JPEN J Parenter Enteral Nutr.* 2016;40(4):574–580.

20. Lord LM, Weiser-Maimone A, Pulhamus M, Sax HC. Comparison of weighted vs unweighted enteral feeding tubes for efficacy of transpyloric intubation. *JPEN J Parenter Enteral Nutr.* 1993;17(3):271–273.

21. Meyer TE, Verbrugge JK, Neutze JA. Ruptured, weighted, enteral feeding tube tip presenting as enteric foreign objects. *Radiol Case Rep.* 2010;5:429.

22. Heiser M, Malaty H. Balloon-type versus non-balloon-type replacement percutaneous endoscopic gastrostomy: which is better? *Gastroenterol Nurs.* 2001;24(2):58–63.

23. Bonhorst B, Cech K, Peter C, Doerdelmann M. Oral versus nasal route for placing feeding tubes: no effect on hypoxemia and bradycardia in infants with apnea of prematurity. *Neonatology.* 2010;98(2):143–149.

24. Rassias AJ, Ball PA, Corwin HL. A prospective study of tracheopulmonary complications associated with the placement of narrow-bore enteral feeding tubes. *Crit Care.* 1998;2(1): 25–28.

25. Marderstein EL, Simmons RL, Ochoa JB. Patient safety: effect of institutional protocols on adverse events related to feeding tube placement in the critically ill. *J Am Coll Surg.* 2004;199(1):39–50.

26. Ellett ML, Beckstrand J, Flueckiger J, Perkins SM, Johnson CS. Predicting the insertion distance for placing gastric tubes. *Clin Nurs Res.* 2005;14(1):11–31.

27. Metheny N, Reed L, Berglund B, Wehrle MA. Visual characteristics of aspirates from feeding tubes as a method for predicting tube location. *Nurs Res.* 1994;43(5):282–287.

28. Metheny NA. Preventing respiratory complications of tube feedings: evidence-based practice. *Am J Crit Care.* 2006;15(4): 360–369.

29. Lord LM. Enteral access devices: types, function, care, and challenges. *Nutr Clin Pract.* 2018;33(1):16–38.

30. Irving SY, Lyman B, Northington L, Bartlett JA, Kemper C. Nasogastric tube placement and verification in children: review of the current literature. *Crit Care Nurs.* 2014;34(3):67–78.

31. American Association of Critical-Care Nurses. *AACN Practice Alert: Verification of Feeding Tube Placement (Blindly Inserted).* Aliso Viejo, CA: American Association of Critical-Care Nurses; 2010.

32. National Health Service. Nasogastric tube misplacement: continuing risk of death and severe harm. Patient safety alert. https://improvement.nhs.uk/resources/patient-safety -alerts. Published July 2016. Accessed August 9, 2018.

33. Meert KL, Calverly M, Kelm LM, Metheny NA. The pH of feeding tube aspirates from critically ill infants. *Am J Crit Care.* 2015;24(5):72–77.

34. National Health Service. Resource set: initial placement checks for nasogastric and orogastric tubes. https:// improvement.nhs.uk/documents/193/Resource_set_

_Initial_placement_checks_for_NG_tubes_1.pdf. Published July 2016. Accessed August 9, 2018.

35. Lee KH, Cho HJ, Kim EY, Son DW, et al. Variation between residents and attending staff interpreting radiographs to verify placement of nutrition access devices in the neonatal intensive care unit. *Nutr Clin Pract*. 2015;30(3):389–401.

36. Patient Safety Movement Foundation. APSS—actionable patient safety solutions: challenge 15. Nasogastric feeding and drainage tube placement and verification. https:// patientsafetymovement.org/actionable-solutions/challenge -solutions/nasogastric-feeding-and-drainage-tube-placement -and-verification. Accessed December 23, 2018.

37. Asai T. Use of a capnograph during feeding tube insertion. *Crit Care Med*. 2002;30(7):1674.

38. Araujo-Preza CE, Melhado ME, Gutierrez FJ, Maniatis T, Castellano MA. Use of capnometry to verify feeding tube placement. *Crit Care Med*. 2002;30(10):2255–2259.

39. Kindopp AS, Drover JW, Heyland DK. Capnography confirms correct feeding tube placement in intensive care unit patients. *Can J Anaesth*. 2001;48(7):705–710.

40. Burns SM, Carpenter R, Truwit JD. Report on the development of a procedure to prevent placement of feeding tubes into the lungs using end-tidal CO_2 measurements. *Crit Care Med*. 2001;29(5):936–939.

41. DeLegge MH. Enteral access and associated complications. *Gastroenterol Clin North Am*. 2018;47(1):23–37.

42. Zaloga GP. Bedside method for placing small bowel feeding tubes in critically ill patients. A prospective study. *Chest*. 1991;100(6):1643–1646.

43. Booth CM, Heyland DK, Paterson WG. Gastrointestinal promotility drugs in the critical care setting: a systematic review of the evidence. *Crit Care Med*. 2002;30(7):1429–1435.

44. Tiancha H, Jiyong J, Min Y. How to promote bedside placement of postpyloric feeding tubes: a network meta-analysis of randomized controlled trials. *JPEN Parenteral Enteral Nutr*. 2015;39(5):521–530.

45. Powers J, Luebbehusen M, Spitzer T, et al. Verification of an electromagnetic placement device compared with abdominal radiograph to predict accuracy of feeding tube placement. *JPEN J Parenter Enteral Nutr*. 2011;35(4):535–539.

46. Akers AS, Pinsky M. Placement of a magnetic small bowel feeding tube at the bedside. *JPEN J Parenter Enteral Nutr.* 2017; 41(3):496–499.

47. Smithard D, Barrett NA, Hargroves D, Elliot S. Electromagnetic sensor-guided enteral access systems: a literature review. *Dysphagia.* 2015;30(3):275–285.

48. Gerritsen A, van der Poel MJ, de Rooij T, et al. Systematic review on bedside electromagnetic-guided, endoscopic, and fluoroscopic placement of nasoenteral feeding tubes. *Gastrointest Endosc.* 2015;81(4):836–847e2.

49. Bourgault AM, Aguirre L, Ibrahim J. Cortrak-assisted feeding tube insertion: a comprehensive review of adverse events in the MAUDE database. *Am J Crit Care.* 2017;26(2):149–156.

50. Wischmeyer PE, McMoon MM, Waldron NH, Dye EJ. Successful identification of anatomical markers and placement of feeding tubes in critically ill patients via camera-assisted technology with real-time video guidance. *JPEN J Parenter Enteral Nutr.* 2019;43(1):118–125. doi:10.1002/jpen.1313.

51. Mizzi A, Cozzi S, Beretta L, Greco M, Braga M. Real-time image-guided nasogastric feeding tube placement: a case series using Kangaroo with IRIS technology in an ICU. *Nutrition.* 2017;37:48–52.

52. Metheny N, Dettenmeier P, Hampton K, Wiersema L, Williams P. Detection of inadvertent respiratory placement of small-bore feeding tubes: a report of 10 cases. *Heart Lung.* 1990;19(6):631–638.

53. Metheny N, McSweeney M, Wehrle MA, Wiersema L. Effectiveness of the auscultatory method in predicting feeding tube location. *Nurs Res.* 1990;39(5):262–267.

54. US Food and Drug Administration. Feeding tube placement systems—letter to health care providers. https://www.fda.gov/MedicalDevices/Safety/LetterstoHealthCareProviders/ucm591838.htm. Published January 16, 2018. Accessed December 29, 2018.

55. McClave SA, Chang WK. Complications of enteral access. *Gastrointest Endosc.* 2003;58(5):739–751.

56. Cosentini EP, Sautner T, Gnant M, Winkelbauer F, Teleky B, Jakesz R. Outcomes of surgical, percutaneous endoscopic, and percutaneous radiologic gastrostomies. *Arch Surg.* 1998; 133(10):1076–1083.

57. Moller P, Lindberg CG, Zilling T. Gastrostomy by various techniques: evaluation of indications, outcome, and complications. *Scand J Gastroenterol.* 1999;34(10):1050–1054.

58. Laasch HU, Wilbraham L, Bullen K, et al. Gastrostomy insertion: comparing the options—PEG, RIG or PIG? *Clin Radiol.* 2003;58(5):398–405.

59. Stiegmann GV, Goff JS, Silas D, Pearlman N, Sun J, Norton L. Endoscopic versus operative gastrostomy: final results of a prospective randomized trial. *Gastrointest Endosc.* 1990;36(1):1–5.

60. Scott JS, de la Torre RA, Unger SW. Comparison of operative versus percutaneous endoscopic gastrostomy tube placement in the elderly. *Am Surg.* 1991;57(5):338–340.

61. Bankhead R, Boullata J, Brantley S, et al. Enteral nutrition practice recommendations. *JPEN J Parenter Enteral Nutr.* 2009;33(2):122–167.

62. Duszak R Jr, Mabry MR. National trends in gastrointestinal access procedures: an analysis of Medicare services provided by radiologists and other specialists. *J Vasc Interv Radiol.* 2003;14(8):1031–1036.

63. Lorentzen T, Skjoldbye B, Nolsoe C, Torp-Pedersen S, Mygind T. Percutaneous gastrostomy guided by ultrasound and fluoroscopy. *Acta Radiol.* 1995;36(2):159–162.

64. DiSario JA, Baskin WN, Brown RD, et al. Endoscopic approaches to enteral nutritional support. *Gastrointest Endosc.* 2002;55(7):901–908.

65. Gossner L, Keymling J, Hahn EG, Ell C. Antibiotic prophylaxis in percutaneous endoscopic gastrostomy (PEG): a prospective randomized clinical trial. *Endoscopy.* 1999;31(2):119–124.

66. Jain NK, Larson DE, Schroeder KW, et al. Antibiotic prophylaxis for percutaneous endoscopic gastrostomy. A prospective, randomized, double-blind clinical trial. *Ann Intern Med.* 1987;107(6):824–828.

67. Allison MC, Sandoe JA, Tighe R, et al. Antibiotic prophylaxis in gastrointestinal endoscopy. *Gut.* 2009;58(6):869–880.

68. Acosta RD, Abraham NS, Chandrasekhara V, et al. The management of antithrombotic agents for patients undergoing GI endoscopy. *Gastrointest Endosc.* 2016;83(1):3–16.

69. Veitch AM, Vanbiervliet G, Gershlick AH, et al. Endoscopy in patients on antiplatelet or anticoagulant therapy, including

direct oral anticoagulants: British Society of Gastroenterology (BSG) and European Society of Gastrointestinal Endoscopy (ESGE) guidelines. *Endoscopy.* 2016;48(4):385–402.

70. Ponsky JL, Gauderer MW. Percutaneous endoscopic gastrostomy: a nonoperative technique for feeding gastrostomy. *Gastrointest Endosc.* 1981;27(1):9–11.

71. Heximer B. Pressure necrosis: implications and interventions for PEG tubes. *Nutr Clin Pract.* 1997;12:256–258.

72. Itkin M, DeLegge MH, Fang JC, et al. Multidisciplinary practical guidelines for gastrointestinal access for enteral nutrition and decompression from the Society of Interventional Radiology and American Gastroenterological Association (AGA) Institute, with endorsement by Canadian Interventional Radiological Association (CIRA) and Cardiovascular and Interventional Radiological Society of Europe (CIRSE). *Gastroenterology.* 2011;141(2):742–765.

73. Crowley JJ, Hogan MJ, Towbin RB, et al. Quality improvement guidelines for pediatric gastrostomy and gastrojejunostomy tube placement. *J Vasc Interv Radiol.* 2014;25(12): 1983–1991.

74. Peitgen K, von Ostau C, Walz MK. Laparoscopic gastrostomy: results of 121 patients over 7 years. *Surg Laparosc Endosc Percutan Tech.* 2001;11(2):76–82.

75. Grant JP. Comparison of percutaneous endoscopic gastrostomy with Stamm gastrostomy. *Ann Surg.* 1988;207(5):598–603.

76. Vanek VW. Ins and outs of enteral access: part 2—long-term access—esophagostomy and gastrostomy. *Nutr Clin Pract.* 2003;18(1):50–74.

77. Vanek VW. Ins and outs of enteral access. Part 3: long-term access—jejunostomy. *Nutr Clin Pract.* 2003;18(3):201–220.

78. Rombeau JL, Twomey PL, McLean GK, Forlaw L, Del Rio D, Caldwell MD. Experience with a new gastrostomy-jejunal feeding tube. *Surgery.* 1983;93(4):574–578.

79. Mack LA, Kaklamanos IG, Livingstone AS, et al. Gastric decompression and enteral feeding through a double-lumen gastrojejunostomy tube improves outcomes after pancreaticoduodenectomy. *Ann Surg.* 2004;240(5):845–851.

80. DeLegge MH, Duckworth PF, McHenry L, Foxx-Orenstein A, Craig RM, Kirby DF. Percutaneous endoscopic gastrojejunostomy: a dual center safety and efficacy trial. *JPEN J Parenter Enteral Nutr.* 1995;19(3):239–243.

81. Udorah MO, Fleischman MW, Bala V, Cai Q. Endoscopic clips prevent displacement of intestinal feeding tubes: a long-term follow-up study. *Dig Dis Sci.* 2010;55(2):371–374.

82. Adler DG, Gostout CJ, Baron TH. Percutaneous transgastric placement of jejunal feeding tubes with an ultrathin endoscope. *Gastrointest Endosc.* 2002;55(1):106–110.

83. Ho CS. Radiologic placement of gastrostomy/jejunostomy tubes in high-risk patients. *Nutr Clin Pract.* 1997;12(1 Suppl): S17–S19.

84. Ho CS, Yeung EY. Percutaneous gastrostomy and transgastric jejunostomy. *AJR Am J Roentgenol.* 1992;158(2):251–257.

85. Shike M, Latkany L, Gerdes H, Bloch AS. Direct percutaneous endoscopic jejunostomies for enteral feeding. *Gastrointest Endosc.* 1996;44(5):536–540.

86. Al-Bawardy B, Gorospe EC, Alexander JA, et al. Outcomes of double-balloon enteroscopy-assisted direct percutaneous endoscopic jejunostomy tube placement. *Endoscopy.* 2016; 48(6):552–556.

87. Velazquez-Avina J, Beyer R, Diaz-Tobar CP, et al. New method of direct percutaneous endoscopic jejunostomy tube placement using balloon-assisted enteroscopy with fluoroscopy. *Dig Endosc.* 2015;27(3):317–322.

88. Richard HM, Widlus DM, Malloy PC. Percutaneous fluoroscopically guided jejunostomy placement. *J Trauma.* 2008; 65(5):1072–1077.

89. Yang ZQ, Shin JH, Song HY, et al. Fluoroscopically guided percutaneous jejunostomy: outcomes in 25 consecutive patients. *Clin Radiol.* 2007;62(11):1061–1068.

90. Sparrow P, David E, Pugash R. Direct percutaneous jejunostomy—an underutilized interventional technique? *Cardiovasc Intervent Radiol.* 2008;31:336–341.

91. Skandalakis LJ, Skandalakis JE. Small intestine. In: Skandalakis LJ, Skandalakis JE, eds. *Surgical Anatomy and Technique: A Pocket Manual.* 4th ed. New York, NY: Springer; 2014: 405–414.

92. Yarze JC, Herlihy KJ, Fritz HP, et al. Prospective trial evaluating early initiation of feeding in patients with newly placed one-step button gastrostomy devices. *Dig Dis Sci.* 2001;46(4):854–858.

93. Gothberg, G, Bjornsson, S. One-step insertion of low-profile gastrostomy in pediatric patients vs pull percutaneous

endoscopic gastrostomy. *JPEN J Parenter Enteral Nutr.* 2016; 40(3):423–430.

94. Metheny NA, Spies M, Eisenberg P. Frequency of naso-enteral tube displacement and associated risk factors. *Res Nurs Health.* 1986;9(3):241–247.

95. Metheny NA, Titler MG. Assessing placement of feeding tubes. *Am J Nurs.* 2001;101(5):36–45.

96. Harrison AM, Clay B, Grant MJ, et al. Nonradiographic assessment of enteral feeding tube position. *Crit Care Med.* 1997;25(12):2055–2059.

97. Welch SK, Hanlon MD, Waits M, Foulks CJ. Comparison of four bedside indicators used to predict duodenal feeding tube placement with radiography. *JPEN J Parenter Enteral Nutr.* 1994;18(6):525–530.

98. Metheny N. Preventing respiratory complications of tube feedings: evidence-based practice. *Am J Crit Care.* 2006;15(4): 360–369.

99. Bechtold ML, Nguyen DL, Palmer LB, Kiraly LN, Martin-dale RG, McClave SA. Nasal bridles for securing nasoenteric tubes: a meta-analysis. *Nutr Clin Pract.* 2014;29(5):667–671.

100. US Food and Drug Administration. Safety considerations to mitigate the risks of misconnections with small-bore connectors intended for enteral applications: guidance for industry and Food and Drug Administration staff. https://www.fda.gov /downloads/medicaldevices/deviceregulationandguidance /guidancedocuments/ucm313385.pdf. Published February 2015. Accessed December 29, 2018.

101. US Food and Drug Administration. Medical device connectors. https://www.fda.gov/MedicalDevices/Products andMedicalProcedures/GeneralHospitalDevicesand Supplies/TubingandLuerMisconnections/default.htm #misconnections. Updated September 2018. Accessed December 29, 2018.

102. US Food and Drug Administration. The FDA encourages use of enteral device connectors that reduce risk of misconnection and patient injury [letter]. https://www.fda.gov /downloads/MedicalDevices/ResourcesforYou/Industry /UCM619782.pdf. Published September 7, 2018. Accessed December 29, 2018.

103. Global Enteral Device Supplier Association website. http:// gedsa.org. Accessed December 29, 2018.

104. Stay Connected website. http://stayconnected.org. Accessed December 23, 2018.

105. Speck K, Rawat N, Weiner NC, Tujuba HG, Farley D, Berenholtz S. A systematic approach for developing a ventilator-associated pneumonia prevention bundle. *Am J Infect Control.* 2016;44(6):652–656.

106. Lyman B, Shah SR. Nutrition access. In: Corkins MR, ed. *The A.S.P.E.N. Pediatric Nutrition Support Core Curriculum.* 2nd ed. Silver Spring, MD: American Society for Parenteral and Enteral Nutrition; 2015:567–582.

107. Krenitsky J. Blind bedside placement of feeding tubes: treatment or threat? *Pract Gastroenterol.* 2011;35:32–42.

108. McWey RE, Curry NS, Schabel SI, Reines HD. Complications of nasoenteric feeding tubes. *Am J Surg.* 1988;155(2):253–257.

109. de Aguilar-Nascimento JE, Kudsk KA. Clinical costs of feeding tube placement. *JPEN J Parenter Enteral Nutr.* 2007;31(4):269–273.

110. Patrick PG, Marulendra S, Kirby DF, DeLegge MH. Endoscopic nasogastric-jejunal feeding tube placement in critically ill patients. *Gastrointest Endosc.* 1997;45(1):72–76.

111. Bosco JJ, Gordon F, Zelig MP, Heiss F, Horst DA, Howell DA. A reliable method for the endoscopic placement of a nasoenteric feeding tube. *Gastrointest Endosc.* 1994;40(6):740–743.

112. Mion L, Minnick AF, Leipzig RM, Catrambone C, Johnson M. Patient-initiated device removal in intensive care units: a national prevalence study. *Crit Care Med.* 2007;35(12):2714–2720.

113. Chang LY, Wang KWK, Chao YF. Influence of physical restraint on unplanned extubation of adult intensive care patients. *Am J Crit Care.* 2008;17(5):408–415.

114. George DL, Falk PS, Umberto Meduri G, et al. Nosocomial sinusitis in patients in the medical intensive care unit: a prospective epidemiological study. *Clin Infect Dis.* 1998;27(3):463–470.

115. Metheny NA, Hinyard LJ, Mohammed KA. Incidence of sinusitis associated with endotracheal and nasogastric tubes: NIS database. *Am J Crit Care.* 2018;27(1):24–31. doi:10.4037/ajcc2018978.

116. Lynch CR, Fang JC. Prevention and management of complications of percutaneous endoscopic gastrostomy (PEG) tubes. *Pract Gastroenterol.* 2004;28:66–77.

117. Safadi BY, Marks JM, Ponsky JL. Percutaneous endoscopic gastrostomy. *Gastrointest Endosc Clin N Am*. 1998;8(3):551–568.

118. Wojtowycz MM, Arata JA, Micklos TJ, Miller FJ. CT findings after uncomplicated percutaneous gastrostomy. *AJR Am J Roentgenol*. 1988;151(2):307–309.

119. James A, Kapur K, Hawthorne AB. Long-term outcome of percutaneous endoscopic gastrostomy feeding in patients with dysphagic stroke. *Age Ageing*. 1998;27(6):671–676.

120. Akkersdijk WL, van Bergeijk JD, van Egmond T, et al. Percutaneous endoscopic gastrostomy (PEG): comparison of push and pull methods and evaluation of antibiotic prophylaxis. *Endoscopy*. 1995;27(4):313–316.

121. Abdelhadi RA, Rahe K, Lyman B. Pediatric enteral access device management. *Nutr Clin Pract*. 2016; 31:748–761.

122. McClave SA. Managing complications of percutaneous and nasoenteric feeding tubes. *Techniques Gastrointest Endosc*. 2001;3(1):62–68.

123. Cyrany J, Rejchrt S, Kopacova M, Bures J. Buried bumper syndrome: a complication of percutaneous endoscopic gastrostomy. *World J Gastroenterol*. 2016;22(2):618.

124. Segal D, Michaud L, Guimber D, Ganga-Zandzou PS, Turck D, Gottrand F. Late-onset complications of percutaneous endoscopic gastrostomy in children. *J Pediatr Gastroenterol Nutr*. 2001;33(4):495–500.

125. Venu RP, Brown RD, Pastika BJ, Erikson LW. The buried bumper syndrome: a simple management approach in two patients. *Gastrointest Endosc*. 2002;56(4):582–584.

126. Walton GM. Complications of percutaneous gastrostomy in patients with head and neck cancer—an analysis of 42 consecutive patients. *Ann R Coll Surg Engl*. 1999;81(4):272–276.

127. Ma MM, Semlacher EA, Fedorak RN, et al. The buried gastrostomy bumper syndrome: prevention and endoscopic approaches to removal. *Gastrointest Endosc*. 1995;41(5):505–508.

128. Boyd JW, DeLegge MH, Shamburek RD, Kirby DF. The buried bumper syndrome: a new technique for safe, endoscopic PEG removal. *Gastrointest Endosc*. 1995;41(5):508–511.

129. Cruz I, Mamel JJ, Brady PG, Cass-Garcia M. Incidence of abdominal wall metastasis complicating PEG tube placement in untreated head and neck cancer. *Gastrointest Endosc*. 2005;62(5):708–711.

130. McSweeney ME, Kerr J, Jiang H, Lightdale JR. Risk factors for complications in infants and children with percutaneous endoscopic gastrostomy tubes. *J Pediatr.* 2015;166:1514–1519.

131. Suksamanapun N, Mauritz FA, Franken J, van der Zee DC, Herwaarden-Lindeboom MY. Laparoscopic versus percutaneous endoscopic gastrostomy placement in children: results of a systematic review and meta-analysis. *J Minim Access Surg.* 2017;13(2):81–88. doi:10.4103/0972-9941.181776.

132. Aumar M, Lalanne A, Guimber D, et al. Influence of percutaneous endoscopic gastrostomy on gastroesophageal reflux disease in children. *J Pediatr.* 2018;197:116–120.

133. Onwubiko C, Weil BR, Bairdain S, et al. Primary laparoscopic gastrojejunostomy tubes as a feeding modality in the pediatric population. *J Pediatr Surg.* 2017;52:1421–1425.

134. Maple J, Baron T, Petersen B. The frequency, severity, and spectrum of adverse events associated with direct percutaneous endoscopic jejunostomy (DPEJ). *Gastrointest Endosc.* 2005;61(5):AB80.

135. Kim CY, Engstrom BI, Horvath JJ, et al. Comparison of primary jejunostomy tubes versus gastrojejunostomy tubes for percutaneous enteral nutrition. *J Vasc Int Radiol.* 2013; 24(12):1845–1852.

136. Dandeles LM, Lodolce AE. Efficacy of agents to prevent and treat enteral feeding tube clogs. *Ann Pharmacother.* 2011;45(5):676–680.

137. Lord L. Maintaining hydration and tube patency in enteral tube feedings. *Safe Pract Patient Care.* 2012;592:1, 5–11.

138. Arriola TA, Hatashima A, Klang MG. Evaluation of extended-release pancreatic enzyme to dissolve a clog. *Nutr Clin Pract.* 2010;25(5):563–564.

139. Fisher CB, Blalock B. Clogged feeding tubes: a clinician's thorn. *Pract Gastroenterol.* 2014;38:16–22.

140. Marcuard SP, Stegall KS. Unclogging feeding tubes with pancreatic enzyme. *JPEN J Parenter Enteral Nutr.* 1990;14(2): 198–200.

141. Marcuard SP, Stegall KL, Trogdon S. Clearing obstructed feeding tubes. *JPEN J Parenter Enteral Nutr.* 1989;13(1):81–83.

142. Lazar J. Treatment of feeding tube occlusions [abstract]. *Nutr Clin Pract.* 2011;26(1):94–102.

143. Boullata JI. Drug administration through an enteral feeding tube. *Am J Nurs.* 2009;109(10):34–43.

CHAPTER 4

Enteral Formulas for Adult Patients

Introduction

This chapter reviews the composition of enteral formulas, applications of enteral nutrition (EN) formulas in clinical practice, the rationale for the use of specialized formulas in adult patient care, and the development of an enteral product formulary. The focus of this chapter is EN for adult patients, although the general information on formula composition, food allergies and intolerances, and developing an enteral product formulary is also applicable in the pediatric setting. Pediatric and infant formulas are discussed in greater depth in Chapter 5.

Today, more than 100 enteral formulas are available in the United States. These products vary greatly with respect to concentration, macronutrient and micronutrient composition, fiber content, and elements proposed to support

TABLE 4-1. Terms Commonly Used in the Classification of Enteral Formulas

Term	Definition
Standard or polymeric formula	Formula containing intact macronutrients.
Blenderized tube feeding (BTF)	Type of tube feeding used for patients who cannot tolerate semisynthetic formulas or who wish to consume whole foods. BTFs are formulated with a mixture of blenderized food sources, with or without the addition of commercial enteral formula. They are recommended for patients with a healed feeding site and for those who adhere to recipe instructions, food safety practices, and tube maintenance.
Elemental and semi-elemental formula	Formula containing partially or completely hydrolyzed nutrients to maximize nutrient absorption.
Disease-specific formula	A formula used for patients with an organ dysfunction or a specific metabolic condition.
Modular	Product used for supplementation, to create a formula, or to add to nutrient content of a formula.

immune function. Table 4-1 reviews terms commonly used to classify EN formulas.

Federal Regulations

Under federal law, enteral formulas are not considered drugs or conventional foods. Instead, they are categorized as medical foods. A *medical food* is defined in the 1988 Orphan Drug Act as follows:[1]

> A food which is formulated to be consumed or administered enterally under the supervision of a physician and which is intended for the specific dietary management of a disease or condition for which distinctive nutritional requirements, based on recognized scientific principles, are established by medical evaluation.

Manufacturers can include "structure and function" claims about enteral formulas on product labels without the approval of the US Food and Drug Administration. Enteral formulas are also not required to meet Nutrition Facts labeling requirements mandated for conventional foods.[2] As discussed in Chapter 5, federal regulation of infant formulas is more stringent.

Formula Selection Algorithm

Limited direct data are available regarding the efficacy and outcomes associated with the use of specific enteral formulas. This lack of efficacy data makes it challenging for nutrition support clinicians to select the best enteral formula for an individual patient. Figure 4-1 is an algorithm that clinicians may use to select formulas for adult patients.[3] It may be used when EN is first initiated or as the EN prescription is reevaluated throughout the patient's medical care.

Formula Composition

Most enteral formulas are complete nutrition, containing macro- and micronutrients in proportions to meet the nutrient requirements of most patients. See Table 4-2 for common macronutrient sources in EN formulas.

FIGURE 4-1

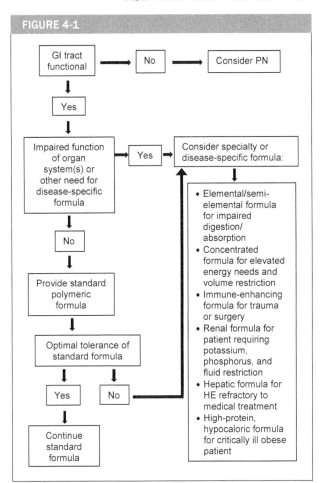

Suggested algorithm for enteral formula selection. This algorithm is not intended to assist with complex clinical decisions. Use clinical judgment to determine which formula to use in cases of multiple organ systems dysfunction and/or if a disease-specific formula is warranted. GI, gastrointestinal; HE, hepatic encephalopathy; PN, parenteral nutrition. Adapted with permission from reference 3: Escuro AA, Hummell AC. Enteral formulas in nutrition support practice: is there a better choice for your patient? *Nutr Clin Pract.* 2016;31(6):709–722.

TABLE 4-2. Macronutrient Sources in Enteral Formulas

Macronutrient	Polymeric Formula	Hydrolyzed Formula
Carbohydrate	• Corn syrup solids • Hydrolyzed cornstarch • Maltodextrin • Sucrose • Fructose • Sugar alcohols	• Cornstarch • Hydrolyzed cornstarch • Maltodextrin • Fructose
Protein	• Casein • Sodium, calcium, magnesium, and potassium caseinates • Soy protein isolate • Whey protein concentrate • Lactalbumin • Milk protein concentrate	• Hydrolyzed casein • Hydrolyzed whey protein • Crystalline L-amino acids • Hydrolyzed lactalbumin • Soy protein isolate
Fat	• Borage oil • Canola oil • Corn oil • Fish oil • High-oleic sunflower oil • Medium-chain triglycerides • Menhaden oil • Mono- and diglycerides • Palm kernel oil • Safflower oil • Soybean oil • Soy lecithin	• Fatty acid esters • Fish oil • Medium-chain triglycerides • Safflower oil • Sardine oil • Soybean oil • Soy lecithin • Structured lipids

Carbohydrate

Carbohydrate is the primary macronutrient and principal energy source in most enteral formulas. Carbohydrate typically supplies 28% to 90% of the energy in enteral formulas, and it contributes to the osmolality, digestibility, and sweetness of the formula.[4] Most formulas contain oligosaccharides or polysaccharides. Polymeric formulas use primarily corn syrup solids as their source of carbohydrate, whereas hydrolyzed formulas use maltodextrin or hydrolyzed cornstarch.[4,5] Oral products contain simpler or less-complex carbohydrates such as sucrose to increase the palatability of the product. Because of the prevalence of lactose intolerance, most adult formulas do not contain lactose.[5]

Fiber

Fiber is added to some enteral formulas. When selecting an enteral formulation for a patient, it is important to note whether the product is supplemented with soluble or insoluble fiber. Most formulations contain a combination of both soluble and insoluble fiber. Soluble fiber is fermented by the gut microbiota in the distal intestine to produce short-chain fatty acids (SCFAs). SCFAs are a source of energy for colonocytes, help increase intestinal mucosal growth, and may help control diarrhea by increasing sodium and water absorption.[5] Insoluble fiber is not effectively fermented by the gut microbiota, but it may help to decrease transit time by increasing fecal weight.[5]

Some enteral formulas contain prebiotic fibers, fructooligosaccharides (FOS), and inulin. These products may provide benefits to some patients by promoting growth of beneficial bacteria in the distal bowel to produce SCFAs.[6]

The patient's tolerance of fiber-supplemented enteral formulas should be monitored closely, particularly in critically ill patients. Cases of bowel obstruction from the use of these formulas have been reported.[7,8] For patients who are critically ill and at risk for bowel ischemia (eg, in cases of hemodynamic instability or vasopressor therapy), administering a fiber-free formula may be a safer option.[9,10]

A number of clinical studies have examined the effects of fiber-containing formulas on gut function; their findings have been inconsistent. A meta-analysis confirmed that the incidence of enteral feeding–related diarrhea is reduced by the inclusion of fiber into enteral diets.[11] However, when intensive care unit (ICU) and non-ICU patients were analyzed separately, no differences in the incidence of diarrhea were shown in ICU patients. Mixed-fiber formulas were found to be better tolerated than single-fiber types of formulas. The same review found that fiber may also speed up transit time, increase fecal bulk, reduce constipation, and improve gut barrier function through the stimulation of colonic bacteria in both healthy volunteers and hospitalized patients.[11] See Table 4-3 for practice recommendations on managing diarrhea with fiber.[10,12]

Fat

The fat component of enteral formulas is a concentrated source of energy and a source of essential fatty acids (ie, linoleic acid and linolenic acid). Long-chain triglycerides (LCTs) and medium-chain triglycerides (MCTs) may be found in enteral formulas. Corn and soybean oil are the most common sources of LCTs; safflower, canola, and fish oils are also used in enteral formulas.[4,5]

Palm kernel and coconut oil may be included in enteral formulas as a source of MCTs. MCTs are absorbed in the portal circulation and do not require chylomicron formation. MCTs are cleared from the bloodstream rapidly, and,

---

TABLE 4-3. Practice Recommendations: Managing Diarrhea with Fiber[a]

AND Evidence Analysis Library recommendations:
- Diarrhea may be reduced in the adult critically ill patient when guar gum is included in the EN regimen (Grade II, fair).
- The impact of other types of fiber on reducing diarrhea is unclear due to variations in the fiber combinations and amounts used in studies (Grade II, fair).

SCCM/ASPEN recommendations:
- We suggest that EN not be automatically interrupted for diarrhea but rather that feeds be continued while evaluating the etiology of diarrhea in an ICU patient to determine appropriate treatment (expert consensus).
- Consider use of a commercial mixed-fiber-containing formulation if there is persistent diarrhea (expert consensus).
- Avoid both soluble and insoluble fiber in critically ill patients at high risk for bowel ischemia or severe dysmotility (expert consensus).
- Consider 10–20 g of a fermentable soluble fiber supplement given in divided doses over 24 hours as adjunctive therapy if there is evidence of diarrhea (expert consensus).

Abbreviations: AND, Academy of Nutrition and Dietetics; ASPEN, American Society for Parenteral and Enteral Nutrition; EN, enteral nutrition; ICU, intensive care unit; SCCM, Society of Critical Care Medicine.

[a]Refer to the original sources for guidance on evidence grading.

Source: Adapted from references 10 and 12.

once in the cell, they can cross the mitochondrial membrane for oxidation without the need for carnitine.[5] However, MCT oil provides no essential fatty acids; therefore, most enteral formulas contain a mixture of LCT and MCT.

Some enteral formulas contain structured lipids as their fat source. Because structured lipids feature a mixture of long-chain fatty acids (LCFAs) and medium-chain fatty acids (MCFAs) on the same glycerol molecule, they offer the advantages of MCFAs and include enough LCFAs to meet essential fatty acid needs.

Some enteral formulas have been designed with an altered ratio of ω-6 to ω-3 fatty acids to include more ω-3 fatty acids. The rationale is that ω-3 fatty acids are metabolized to prostaglandins of the 3 series and leukotrienes of the 5 series, which have anti-inflammatory properties, whereas ω-6 fatty acids are metabolized to prostaglandins of the 2 series and leukotrienes of the 4 series, which tend to be proinflammatory and immunosuppressive.[4]

Protein

Protein is a source of nitrogen and energy in enteral formulas. Enteral formulas may contain intact protein, hydrolyzed protein, or free amino acids.[5]

Intact protein refers to whole protein or protein isolates. Casein and soy protein isolates are the most commonly used types of intact protein. Lactalbumin, whey, and egg albumin are also sources of intact protein. Formulas with intact protein require normal levels of pancreatic enzymes for digestion and absorption.

Formulas with hydrolyzed protein, small peptides, dipeptides and tripeptides, and free amino acids are referred to as *semi-elemental* or *elemental* formulas.[4] These types of formulas are intended for patients with malabsorption, pancreatic dysfunction, or prolonged bowel rest following major abdominal surgery or other evidence of gastrointestinal (GI) dysfunction.

Vitamins and Minerals

Most adult enteral formulas provide adequate amounts of vitamins and minerals to meet the Dietary Reference Intakes (DRIs) when provided in volumes of 1000 to

1500 mL/d. However, some disease-specific enteral formulas may have amounts of specific vitamins and minerals that are higher or lower than the DRI.[5] When considering the adequacy of micronutrients in the individualized EN prescription, it is important to assess the amount of vitamins and minerals being provided by all sources of nutrition relative to the needs of the specific patient.[3] It is the clinician's responsibility to carefully evaluate the products available in the formulary to select the most appropriate EN formula to avoid adverse clinical outcomes associated with inadequate or excessive micronutrient intakes.

Water

Adult enteral formulas contain roughly 70% to 85% water by volume.[13,14] In general, the more energy dense the formula is, the less water it contains.

Enteral formulas are not intended to meet the patient's fluid needs. When calculating the patient's total fluid intake, only the volume of water in the formula is considered. For example, if a formula is 75% water by volume, 1000 mL of formula would count as 750 mL of fluid. Most patients receiving EN require an additional source of water to meet their hydration needs. Supplemental free water is often provided through the feeding tube as flushes for hydration and to maintain feeding tube patency. Intravenous (IV) fluids must be accounted for and adjusted as required while a patient is receiving EN. Chapter 6 presents sample calculations for determining the contributions of enteral formula and flushes to daily fluid goals.

Osmolality

Osmolality is the concentration of free particles, molecules, or ions in a given solution, and it is expressed as milliosmoles per kilogram of water (mOsm/kg).[15] The osmolality of adult enteral formulas typically ranges from 280 to 875 mOsm/kg.[4]

Hypertonic enteral formulas (osmolality >320 mOsm/kg) have frequently been blamed for problems related to formula intolerance (eg, diarrhea). However, the osmolality of an enteral formula has little to do with formula tolerance. GI tolerance or diarrhea is often related to the severity of illness, comorbid conditions, or the concomitant use of hypertonic medications administered through the enteral access device.[16] Some items included in clear and full liquid diets routinely used by hospitalized patients, as well as many medications, are more hyperosmolar than enteral formulas. Refer to Chapter 9 for further information on enteral feeding complications and tolerance.

Food Allergies and Intolerances

To minimize the risk for adverse reactions to ingredients in enteral formulas, it is important that the patient undergo a comprehensive nutrition assessment, including evaluation of any reports of food allergies or intolerances in the medical records or diet history (see Chapter 1). True food *allergies* involve an adverse immune system response to a food protein.[17] In the United States, about 4% of adults and 5% of children have food allergies.[18] Food *intolerances*, such as lactose intolerance, are adverse reactions to foods that do not involve the immune system.[17]

Most enteral formulas do not contain gluten or lactose. However, they may contain common allergens such as egg, corn, casein, whey, or soy. The Food Allergen Labeling and Consumer Protection Act (FALCPA) of 2004, which applies to medical foods (including enteral formulas), requires that the label of a food that contains an ingredient that is or contains protein from a "major food allergen" declare the presence of the allergen in the manner described by the law.[2] FALCPA identifies 8 foods or food groups as the major allergens: milk, eggs, fish, crustacean shellfish, tree nuts, peanuts, wheat, and soybeans.

Manufacturers periodically change ingredients in formulas. When selecting EN for patients with food allergy or food intolerance, the clinician should always refer to the most recent product label.

Formulas for Specific Diseases or Conditions

Specialized formulas cover a wide range of formulas designed for a variety of clinical scenarios. Some are intended for patients with specific disease states such as acute kidney injury (AKI), diabetes, hepatic disease, or pulmonary disease. Others are marketed for use in hypermetabolic disease and inflammatory states such as those occurring in critical illness.

> The brand names mentioned in this chapter do not constitute a comprehensive list of all relevant products on the market in the United States or other countries. Mention of a product does not imply an endorsement.
>
> Manufacturers periodically introduce, withdraw, and alter products. Before using any product, nutrition support clinicians should review the label and product website for current information on ingredients, nutrient composition, and instructions for use. If those resources are insufficient, contact the manufacturer or the formulary manager for additional information. Selected manufacturer websites are listed at the end of the chapter.

Gastrointestinal Disorders and Malabsorption

Elemental and semi-elemental formulas have partially or completely hydrolyzed macronutrient content and are designed for patients with known GI disorders or for those who exhibit signs and symptoms of intolerance to standard polymeric formulas.[4-6] Before assuming that a patient cannot tolerate a formula, nutrition support clinicians should thoroughly investigate the etiology of a patient's diarrhea or malabsorption (ie, assess types and formulations of medications, mode of EN delivery, and possible infectious causes).[10] See Chapter 9 for additional information on diarrhea and other complications of EN.

Elemental and semi-elemental formulas may be useful in patients with malabsorption, pancreatic dysfunction, or prolonged bowel rest following major abdominal surgery (see Table 4-4 for examples of these products). In these products, carbohydrate is included as hydrolyzed cornstarch, maltodextrin, or fructose; protein is provided as hydrolyzed casein, hydrolyzed whey, soy protein isolate, or crystalline amino acids; and lipids are from fatty acid esters or MCTs.

The use of peptide-based formulas has not been extensively evaluated, and available findings are inconsistent. Two studies found that the incidence of diarrhea was reduced by using a peptide-based formula,[19,20] but other studies found that the frequency of diarrhea increased or stayed the same following the change to a peptide-based formula.[21,22] A few of these elemental and semi-elemental formulations also contain components such as ω-3 fatty acids, glutamine, and prebiotics such as FOS and inulin.[4] A small, prospective randomized pilot study found significantly fewer days with adverse events and undesired GI complications using a specialized peptide-based formula containing ω-3 fatty acids compared to a standard polymeric formula.[23] Further research is warranted on the

TABLE 4-4. Selected Enteral Formulas Marketed for Use in Gastrointestinal Disorders and Malabsorption

Product	Manufacturer
Peptamen	Nestlé
Peptamen 1.5	Nestlé
Peptamen 1.5 with Prebio1	Nestlé
Peptamen AF	Nestlé
Peptamen Intense VHP	Nestlé
Peptamen with Prebio1	Nestlé
Peptide 1.5	Kate Farms
Pediatric Peptide 1.5	Kate Farms
Tolerex	Nestlé
Vital 1.0 Cal	Abbott
Vital 1.5 Cal	Abbott
Vital AF 1.2 Cal	Abbott
Vital High Protein	Abbott
Vital Peptide 1.5 Cal	Abbott
Vivonex Plus	Nestlé
Vivonex RTF	Nestlé
Vivonex T.E.N.	Nestlé

The brand names mentioned in this table may not constitute a comprehensive list of all relevant products on the market in the United States or other countries. Mention of a product does not imply an endorsement.

efficacy of specialized formulas for GI disorders containing added components such as prebiotics and ω-3 fatty acids. See Table 4-5 for practice recommendations on formula selection for critically ill patients with GI disorders and malabsorption.[10]

Wound Healing

Wound healing is a complex process that involves a cascade of events to repair and heal damaged tissue. Enteral formulas marketed for oral intake or tube feeding in patients with wounds or pressure injuries contain a combination of nutrients that are thought to aid the healing process (see

TABLE 4-5. Practice Recommendations: Enteral Formula Selection for Critically Ill Patients with Gastrointestinal Disorders and Malabsorption[a]

SCCM/ASPEN recommendations:
- Avoid the routine use semi-elemental or elemental formulas in critically ill patients because no clear benefit to patient outcome has been shown in the literature (expert consensus).
- Consider use of small-peptide formulas in the patient with persistent diarrhea, with suspected malabsorption or lack of response to fiber (expert consensus).

Abbreviations: ASPEN, American Society for Parenteral and Enteral Nutrition; SCCM, Society of Critical Care Medicine.

[a]Refer to the original article for guidance on evidence grading.

Source: Adapted from reference 10.

TABLE 4-6. Selected Enteral Formulas Marketed for Use in Wound Healing

Product	Manufacturer
Impact®	Nestlé
Impact® Peptide 1.5	Nestlé
Replete®	Nestlé
Replete with Fiber®	Nestlé
Perative®	Abbott
Pivot 1.5® Cal	Abbott
Promote®	Abbott
Promote® with Fiber	Abbott

The brand names mentioned in this table may not constitute a comprehensive list of all relevant products on the market in the United States or other countries. Mention of a product does not imply an endorsement.

Table 4-6). Energy; protein; vitamins A, C, and E; zinc; copper; iron; and arginine have all been linked to the wound-healing process.[24] Several studies demonstrate that malnutrition adversely affects wound healing and adequate nutrition is required for healing to occur.[25,26]

A meta-analysis by Cereda and colleagues found that individuals with pressure injuries expended more energy compared with controls and were usually characterized as having negative nitrogen balance.[27] For adults with a pressure injury who are identified as being at risk for malnutrition, the National Pressure Ulcer Advisory Panel (NPUAP) recommends an energy goal of 30–35 kcal per kg body weight per day.[24] The NPUAP practice guidelines also recommend that energy intake be adjusted based on a patient's weight change or level of obesity, and that individuals who have had significant unintended weight loss may need additional energy intake.[24]

Protein is vital for growth and maintenance of cells, promotion of positive nitrogen balance, and provision of structure. All stages of wound healing require adequate protein for wound closure, and increased protein levels have been linked to improved healing rates.[26,28] For adults with existing pressure injury, as well as those at risk for pressure injury and malnutrition, NPUAP recommends providing 1.25 to 1.5 g protein per kg body weight per day.[24] Reassessment of a patient's protein requirement is recommended as the patient's condition changes.[24]

A 2014 systematic review concluded that research on nutrition supplements enriched with various nutrients to promote wound healing should be interpreted with caution because the studies were small, included heterogeneous populations with high dropout rates, and examined various types of oral nutrition supplements.[29] The authors noted that this conclusion should not be interpreted to mean that nutrition interventions have no effect on pressure injury healing; to the contrary, they emphasized that individuals at risk for malnutrition and those identified as malnourished should receive nutrition interventions based on a nutrition assessment.

Another systematic review, published in 2017, evaluated 3 studies on the use of formulas enriched with arginine, zinc, and antioxidants as oral supplements and tube feedings. The authors of this review found that, compared with control interventions, the use of these formulas was associated with significantly higher reduction in pressure injury area; also, a higher proportion of patients using the formulas had a 40% or greater reduction of pressure injury size at 8 weeks when compared with controls.[30]

Diabetes/Glucose Intolerance

Enteral formulas designed for glucose intolerant patients typically contain less carbohydrate (33% to 40% of total energy) and more fat (44% to 49% of total energy) than a standard polymeric formula; diabetes-specific formulas also include 14 to 15 g fiber per liter.[31,32] These formulas are based on the premise that the reduced carbohydrate content, greater amount of fat (particularly monounsaturated fats), and inclusion of fiber will result in better glycemic control. However, the American Diabetes Association (ADA) no longer recommends specific percentages of macronutrients for the hospitalized patient.[33]

Table 4-7 lists selected formulas marketed for use in patients with diabetes or glucose intolerance. These formulas

TABLE 4-7. Selected Enteral Formulas Marketed for Use in Patients with Diabetes or Glucose Intolerance

Product	Manufacturer
Diabetisource®	Nestlé
Glucerna®	Abbott
Glytrol®	Nestlé

The brand names mentioned in this table may not constitute a comprehensive list of all relevant products on the market in the United States or other countries. Mention of a product does not imply an endorsement.

may contain pureed foods, arginine, ω-3 fatty acids, or fructose; they may also be high in monounsaturated fats with reduced amounts of saturated fat. Diabetes-specific products tend to be more costly than standard formulas.

Recommendations about the use of specialized formulas for patients with diabetes or glucose intolerance are varied (see Table 4-8). The Society of Critical Care Medicine/ American Society of Parenteral and Enteral Nutrition

---

TABLE 4-8. Practice Recommendations: Enteral Formula Selection for Patients with Diabetes[a]

SCCM/ASPEN recommendations (critically ill patients):
- Use a standard polymeric formula when initiating EN in ICU (expert consensus).
- Avoid routine use of all specialty formulas (expert consensus).

ACG recommendations (hospitalized patients):
- A standard polymeric or high-protein standard formula should be routinely used in the hospitalized patient requiring EN (conditional recommendation, very low level of evidence).
- Routine use of disease-specific formulas (diabetes) is discouraged (conditional recommendation, very low level of evidence).

ADA recommendations (hospitalized patients with diabetes):
- Diabetes-specific formulas appear to be superior to standard formulas in controlling postprandial glucose, A1C, and insulin response.

CPG recommendations (critically ill patients):
- Data are insufficient to recommend high fat/low CHO enteral nutrition for critically ill patients.

Abbreviations: A1C, hemoglobin A1C; ACG, American College of Gastroenterology; ADA, American Diabetes Association; ASPEN, American Society for Parenteral and Enteral Nutrition; CHO, carbohydrate; CPG, Canadian Clinical Practice Guidelines; EN, enteral nutrition; ICU, intensive care unit; SCCM, Society of Critical Care Medicine.

[a]Refer to the original sources for guidance on evidence grading.

Source: Adapted from references 10 and 33–35.

(SCCM/ASPEN),[10] American College of Gastroenterology (ACG),[34] and the Canadian Clinical Practice Guidelines (CPG) for Nutrition Support in the Mechanically Ventilated, Critically Ill Adult[35] from the Clinical Evaluation Research Unit in Kingston, Ontario, oppose their use, whereas ADA[33] is supportive.

The differences in recommendations are at least partly explained by the distinctive missions of the organizations that published them; also, the recommendations do not all focus on the same target populations. Guidelines from SCCM/ASPEN and CPG are for critically ill patients.[10,35] Hospitalized patients are the target for the ACG guidelines,[34] which were derived from those developed for critically ill patients. ADA guidelines are for hospitalized patients with diabetes.[33]

Based on expert consensus, SCCM/ASPEN guidelines recommend avoiding the routine use of most specialty formulas, including diabetes-specific products, in critically ill patients, citing the lack of benefit in patient outcomes.[10] The ACG guideline for hospitalized patients is identical to that from SCCM/ASPEN, stating that routine use of disease-specific (ie, diabetes-specific) enteral formulas should be avoided.[34]

Having identified only 3 studies for evaluation, the CPG guideline states that data are insufficient to recommend high-fat, low-carbohydrate enteral formulas.[35] Notably, the objective of the CPG was not to evaluate the effectiveness of diabetes-specific formulas but to determine the impact of high-fat, low-carbohydrate *pulmonary* enteral formulas in reducing ventilator days in critically ill patients. However, a study involving a diabetes-specific formula was part of the analysis for this guideline, and that study showed better glycemic control with the diabetes-specific product. On the other hand, the diabetes-specific formula did not alter clinical outcomes (mortality, infections, intensive care length of stay, and number of ventilator days). Consequently, CPG notes that glycemic control may be better in critically ill patients who receive a diabetes-specific formula.[35]

For hospitalized patients with diabetes requiring EN, ADA recommends the use of diabetes-specific enteral formulas, rather than standard enteral formulas, for better control of postprandial glucose, hemoglobin A1C (HbA1C), and insulin response. In support of this recommendation, ADA references the results of several meta-analyses evaluating the effects of diabetes formulas compared with standard products in individuals with diabetes.[33]

For example, ADA considered an early (2005) meta-analysis, in which diabetes formulas were identified as those containing >60% fat, monounsaturated fatty acids, fructose, and fiber; this review demonstrated improved glycemic control with these specialty formulas.[36] However, it is difficult to apply the findings of this meta-analysis to present-day EN therapy because the current diabetes-specific formulas have a lower fat content (44%–49%).

ADA also cited a 2014 systematic review by Ojo and Brooke of 5 studies comparing diabetes-specific vs standard formulas in patients with diabetes.[37] The authors found that use of diabetes-specific formulas resulted in improved postprandial glucose, HbA1c, and insulin response. However, it is difficult to cite these findings to support the use of diabetes-specific enteral formulas for patients with diabetes because the studies evaluated in this meta-analysis had only a few tube-fed patients (n = 46) and these patients had varying degrees of severity of illness while using all feeding administration methods (bolus, intermittent, and continuous feeding).[37]

The ADA recommendation for diabetes-specific enteral formulas does not note any clinical benefit for the patient with diabetes other than improved glycemic control.[33] However, in studies cited by ADA, hyperglycemia persisted, albeit at lower levels, when diabetes-specific formulas were used.[33,38–40] In patients with diabetes who received standard formulas, blood glucose levels were 172.8–223.2 mg/dL vs 156.6–176.4 mg/dL in patients receiving the diabetes-specific products.[38–40] Although these findings were statistically significant, the decline in blood glucose levels associated with diabetes-specific formulas may not be sufficient enough to substantially alter clinical treatment of hyperglycemia in the hospitalized patient. Insulin therapy remains the best way to control hyperglycemia in the hospitalized patient.[33,41]

Research continues to examine the effectiveness of diabetes-specific enteral formulas. Although recent studies have associated diabetes-specific enteral formulas with improvement in glycemic control, the conclusions in each case are not generalizable due to the limitations of the study designs.[42–44] Well-designed research is needed to evaluate the role of EN and diabetes-specific formulas on the management, clinical outcomes, and quality of life of malnourished patients with diabetes or with stress-induced hyperglycemia.

Because there is insufficient evidence to support the routine use of diabetes-specific formulas, it is appropriate to start with a standard enteral formula while closely monitoring the patient's blood glucose levels and using insulin as needed for glycemic control. If glycemic control is difficult to achieve with a standard formula, then a diabetes-specific formula may be tried; however, hyperglycemia may arise from multiple etiologies, and as noted above, insulin is the preferred treatment.

Hepatic Failure

Enteral formulas marketed for use in patients with liver disease (Table 4-9) have increased amounts of branched-chain amino acids (BCAAs). They also have reduced amounts of aromatic amino acids (AAs), total protein, sodium, and fluid.

TABLE 4-9. Selected Enteral Formula Marketed for Use in Patients with Hepatic Failure	
Product	**Manufacturer**
NutriHep®	Nestlé

The brand name mentioned in this table may not be the only relevant product on the market in the United States or other countries. Mention of a product does not imply an endorsement.

In persons with cirrhosis, concentrations of AAAs (phenylalanine, tyrosine, and tryptophan) are increased due to impaired metabolism, and concentrations of BCAAs (valine, leucine, and isoleucine) are decreased because BCAAs are used for glutamine synthesis, which is needed as a source of energy.[45] AAAs compete with BCAAs at the blood-brain barrier, and that leads to a greater number of false neurotransmitters that stimulate additional ammonia production. Development of hepatic enteral formulas is based on the concept that restoration of the plasma BCAA-to-AAA ratio would reduce hepatic encephalopathy (HE) and restore muscle mass.[46]

Guidelines for the use of hepatic formulas vary, depending on the target patient population of the guidelines and the desired outcomes to be achieved by the guidelines (see Table 4-10).[10,34,47] Lactulose and antibiotics can be effective treatments for persons with HE. For this reason, SCCM/ASPEN and ACG do not recommend using BCAA-containing enteral formulas for HE patients.[10,34] The American Association for the Study of Liver Diseases does not support protein restriction in patients with cirrhosis because a chronic inflammatory state is associated with that condition.[47]

Persons with hepatic dysfunction will likely tolerate a standard, polymeric enteral formula. A fluid-restricted formula may be needed if the patient has ascites or edema. If

TABLE 4-10. Practice Recommendations: Enteral Formula Selection for Patients with Hepatic Failure[a]

SCCM/ASPEN recommendations (critically ill patients):
- Use standard polymeric formula in ICU patients with acute and chronic liver disease (expert consensus).
- There is no evidence of further benefit of BCAA formulas on coma grade in the ICU patient with HE who is already getting luminal antibiotics and lactulose (expert consensus).

AASLD recommendations (patients with HE in chronic liver failure):
- Daily protein intake should be 1.2–1.5 g/kg/d (Grade I, A, strong recommendation).
- Oral BCAA supplementation may allow recommended nitrogen intake to be achieved and maintained in patients with HE who are intolerant of dietary protein (Grade II-2, B, weak recommendation).
- Oral BCAA supplementation can be used as an alternative or additional agent to treat patients nonresponsive to conventional therapy (Grade I, B, weak recommendation).

ACG recommendations (hospitalized patients):
- A standard polymeric or high-protein standard formula should be routinely used in the hospitalized patient requiring EN (conditional recommendation, very low level of evidence).
- Routine use of organ-specific formulas (hepatic) is discouraged (conditional recommendation, very low level of evidence).

Abbreviations: AASLD, American Association for the Study of Liver Diseases; ASPEN, American Society for Parenteral and Enteral Nutrition; BCAA, branch-chained amino acid; EN, enteral nutrition; HE, hepatic encephalopathy; ICU, intensive care unit; SCCM, Society of Critical Care Medicine.

[a]Refer to the original sources for guidance on evidence grading.

Source: Adapted from references 10, 34, and 47.

HE is refractory to medical treatment (eg, lactulose, rifaximin), a trial of a hepatic formula may be warranted, but prolonged use of hepatic formulas could worsen malnutrition because these products are low in protein. Nutrition support clinicians must weigh benefits, costs, and efficacy to determine whether a hepatic formula would be a good option.[3]

Immune-Enhancing Nutrition

Enteral formulas marketed as immune-enhancing or immune-modulating nutrition contain supplemental amounts of L-arginine, nucleotides, ω-3 fatty acids, and/or antioxidants in addition to nutrient substrates essential for general nutrition and metabolism (see Table 4-11 for selected products). The goal of immune-enhancing formulas is not only to provide sufficient nutrition but also to modulate immunity during stress in specific patient populations. These formulas vary considerably in composition. Immune-enhancing formulas are the most studied of the specialty enteral formulas; however, the studies lack uniformity in patient populations, formulas studied, and

| TABLE 4-11. Selected Enteral Formulas Marketed as Immune-Enhancing Products ||
Product	Manufacturer
Impact®	Nestlé
Impact® Peptide 1.5	Nestlé
Perative®	Abbott
Pivot® 1.5 Cal	Abbott

The brand names mentioned in this table may not constitute a comprehensive list of all relevant products on the market in the United States or other countries. Mention of a product does not imply an endorsement.

outcomes measured, thus making it difficult to develop recommendations for use.

Specific immune-modulating nutrients have unique roles during stress and trauma (see Table 4-12).[48] Arginine and glutamine are nonessential amino acids under normal circumstances, but they become essential during stress because the demand for them increases and exceeds endogenous supplies.[48] Compared with ω-6 fatty acids, ω-3 fatty acids produce fewer inflammatory prostaglandins and leukotrienes. When consumed, ω-3 fatty acids replace ω-6 fatty acids in cellular membranes, which reduces inflammation during stress.[48]

TABLE 4-12. Functions of Immunonutrients

Immunonutrient	Functions
Arginine	• T-cell lymphocyte proliferation and function • Proline synthesis for wound healing • Substrate for nitric oxide production for blood circulation and vascular tone
Glutamine	• Primary fuel for small bowel, lymphocytes, and macrophages • Gluconeogenesis • Heat shock protein induction to modulate inflammation and oxidation at cellular level
Nucleic acids	• Bases of RNA, DNA, ATP, and other dinucleotides • Cellular proliferation and immunity
ω-3 fatty acids (EPA, DHA)	• Reduction in inflammation

Abbreviations: ATP, adenosine triphosphate; DHA, docosahexaenoic acid; DNA, deoxyribonucleic acid; EPA, eicosapentaenoic acid; RNA, ribonucleic acid.

Source: Adapted from reference 48.

Table 4-13 reviews guidelines regarding the use of immune-enhancing nutrition.[10,34,35] The rationales for the guidelines are based on evidence of reduced infection, shortened length of stay, and potential harm associated with immune-enhancing nutrition.

SCCM/ASPEN suggest using immune-enhancing nutrition containing at least arginine and fish oil in patients with severe trauma, those with traumatic brain injury, and postoperative surgical ICU patients who had major surgery.[10] Routine use of immune-enhancing nutrition in the medical ICU or patients with severe sepsis is not suggested by SCCM/ASPEN because studies do not show clinical benefits.[10]

The guidelines from ACG are similar to those of SCCM/ASPEN. Immune-enhancing formulations containing arginine and fish oil should be used for patients who have had major surgery and are in a surgical ICU setting but not routinely used for patients in the medical ICU.[34]

Formulations containing arginine could worsen hemodynamic instability in a septic patient because arginine is a precursor of nitric oxide. This is the rationale for the guideline from CPG against the routine use of EN with arginine in critically ill patients.[35] However, CPG does not extend this recommendation to the elective surgery patient population.

As noted in Table 4-13, guidelines also exist for EN with glutamine and antioxidants. Because these immunonutrients are in products in various amounts and in different combinations, it is difficult to develop recommendations for their use. CPG does not recommend supplemental enteral glutamine because a large study noted a trend toward a higher mortality rate in critically ill medical patients and a lack of benefit in reducing infections.[35] There is ongoing research to evaluate the effects of immune-enhancing nutrition in the pre- and postoperative periods for various surgical procedures and also during certain disease states.

TABLE 4-13. Practice Recommendations: Use of Immune-Enhancing Enteral Formulas in Critically Ill Patients[a]

SCCM/ASPEN recommendations:

- Immune-modulating enteral formulations (arginine with other agents, including EPA, DHA, glutamine, and nucleic acid) should not be used routinely in MICU patients (very low quality of evidence).
- Data are insufficient to recommend placing a patient with severe acute pancreatitis on immune-enhancing formulation (very low quality of evidence).
- We suggest that immune-modulating formulations containing arginine and fish oil be considered in patients with severe trauma (very low quality of evidence).
- We suggest the use of either arginine-containing immune-modulating formulations or EPA/DHA supplement with standard enteral formula in patients with traumatic brain injury (expert consensus).
- We suggest the routine use of an immune-modulating formula (containing both arginine and fish oils) in the SICU for the postoperative patient who requires EN therapy (moderate to low quality of evidence).
- We suggest providing combinations of antioxidant vitamins and trace minerals in doses reported to be safe for critically ill patients who require specialized nutrition support (low quality of evidence).
- We suggest supplemental enteral glutamine not be added to EN routinely in critically ill patients (moderate quality of evidence).
- We suggest immune-modulating formulas not be routinely used in patients with severe sepsis (moderate quality of evidence).
- No recommendation can be made regarding selenium, zinc, and antioxidant supplementation during sepsis due to conflicting studies (moderate quality of evidence).

(continued)

TABLE 4-13. *(Continued)*

ACG recommendations:
- Immune-enhancing formulas containing arginine and fish oil should be used for patients who have had major surgery and are in SICU (conditional recommendation, very low level of evidence).
- Immune-enhancing formulas containing arginine and fish oil should not be routinely used for patients in MICU (conditional recommendation, very low level of evidence).

CPG recommendations:
- EN supplemented with arginine and other select nutrients is not recommended for critically ill patients.
- EN supplemented with glutamine is not recommended for critically ill patients.

Abbreviations: ACG, American College of Gastroenterology; ASPEN, American Society for Parenteral and Enteral Nutrition; CPG, Canadian Practice Guidelines; DHA, docosahexaenoic acid; EN, enteral nutrition; EPA, eicosapentaenoic acid; MICU, medical intensive care unit; SCCM, Society of Critical Care Medicine; SICU, surgical intensive care unit.

ªRefer to the original sources for guidance on evidence grading.

Source: Adapted from references 10, 34, and 35.

Immune-modulating formulas are probably most beneficial for the following patient populations: patients in the pre- and postoperative periods who are having major elective surgery, critically ill postoperative patients, and those with severe trauma or traumatic brain injury.

Pulmonary Failure and Acute Respiratory Distress Syndrome

Table 4-14 lists selected enteral formulas marketed for use in patients with pulmonary failure or acute respiratory distress syndrome (ARDS). The enteral formulas in this category are intended to help critically ill patients wean off mechanical ventilation.

TABLE 4-14. Selected Enteral Formulas Marketed for Use in Patients with Pulmonary Dysfunction	
Product	**Manufacturer**
Nutren® Pulmonary	Nestlé
Oxepa®a	Abbott
Pulmocare®	Abbott

The brand names mentioned in this table may not constitute a comprehensive list of all relevant products on the market in the United States or other countries. Mention of a product does not imply an endorsement.

aMarketed specifically for patients with acute respiratory distress syndrome.

Pulmonary failure–specific products are high in fat and low in carbohydrate content (55%–56% fat, 26%–28% carbohydrate), which is supposed to reduce carbon dioxide production and respiratory quotient. However, as bedside indirect calorimetry became available, it was theorized that excessive energy intake, not carbohydrate intake, may have been contributing to excess carbon dioxide production. (Notably, excess carbon dioxide production can occur in patients due to fever, thyrotoxicosis, increased catabolism that occurs with sepsis or use of steroids, exercise, or metabolic acidosis without any correlation to nutrition intake.[49]) Also, the high ω-6 fatty acid contents of several pulmonary formulas could worsen inflammation; the ratio of ω-6 fatty acids to ω-3 fatty acids is 4:1.[31,32] Based on these findings, as well as the high cost of specialty EN products, pulmonary failure–specific EN formulas are not recommended (see Table 4-15).[10,34,35]

With increasing understanding of ARDS and acute lung injury, an enteral formula was designed to reduce inflammation, using a high-fat, low-carbohydrate formula as its base with the additions of ω-3 fatty acids (eicosapentaenoic and docosahexaenoic acids); borage oil, which contains γ-linolenic acid (GLA); and antioxidants. When ω-3 fatty acids are provided enterally, they will replace the ω-6

TABLE 4-15. Practice Guidelines: Formula Selection for Patients With Pulmonary Dysfunction[a]

SCCM/ASPEN recommendations:

- Use a standard polymeric formula when initiating EN in the ICU setting (expert consensus).
- Avoid routine use of organ-specialty (pulmonary) formulas in critically ill patients in a MICU and disease-specific formulas in the SICU (expert consensus).
- Specialty high-fat/low-carbohydrate formulas designed to manipulate respiratory quotient and reduce CO_2 should not be used in ICU patients with acute respiratory failure (very low quality of evidence).
- Fluid-restricted, energy-dense EN formula should be considered for patients with acute respiratory failure (especially if in a state of volume overload) (expert consensus).
- We are unable to make a recommendation for routine use of an enteral formula characterized by an anti-inflammatory lipid profile (ω-3 fish oils, borage oil) and antioxidants in patients with ARDS and severe ALI due to conflicting data (low to very low quality of evidence).

ACG recommendations:

- A standard polymeric or high-protein standard formula should be routinely used in the hospitalized patient requiring EN (conditional recommendation, very low level of evidence).
- Routine use of organ-specific formulas (pulmonary) is discouraged (conditional recommendation, very low level of evidence).
- We are unable to make a recommendation for nonarginine anti-inflammatory EN formulas in ARDS/ALI due to conflicting results.

CPG recommendations:

- Unable to make a recommendation for high-fat/low-carbohydrate EN for critically ill patients due to insufficient data.
- Use of EN with fish oils, borage oils, and antioxidants should be considered in patients with ALI and ARDS.

ACG, American College of Gastroenterology; ALI, acute lung injury; ARDS, acute respiratory distress syndrome; ASPEN, American Society for Parenteral and Enteral Nutrition; CO_2, carbon dioxide; CPG, Canadian Clinical Practice Guidelines; EN, enteral nutrition; ICU, intensive care unit; MICU, medical intensive care unit; SCCM, Society of Critical Care Medicine; SICU, surgical intensive care unit.

[a]Refer to the original sources for guidance on evidence grading.

Source: Adapted from references 10, 34, and 35.

fatty acid arachidonic acid in cellular membranes, resulting in production of anti-inflammatory or less-inflammatory eicosanoids.[50] GLA also inhibits production of proin-flammatory metabolites deriving from arachidonic acid. Recommendations for using ω-3 fatty acids and GLA-supplemented pulmonary formulas vary, in part because of variations in the methodologies used to analyze product research (see Table 4-15).[10,34,35]

Fluid-restricted formulas may be beneficial for patients with respiratory failure who are experiencing volume over-load, pulmonary edema, and renal failure with decreasing urinary output. These complications can worsen out-comes.[10] A standard or possibly fluid-restricted enteral for-mula is likely the most cost-effective product for patients with respiratory failure who require mechanical ventila-tion. Additional information on fluid-restricted formulas is presented later in this chapter.

Renal Failure

Enteral formulas developed for use in patients with renal dysfunction are energy dense and have restricted amounts of electrolytes (sodium, potassium, phosphorus, magne-sium). The types and amounts of protein in such formulas vary, depending on the intended use of the product. Some formulas are protein restricted for nondialyzed patients. Other formulas have greater amounts of complete proteins to meet the needs of patients receiving intermittent hemo-dialysis. See Table 4-16 for examples of these products.

The contents of the renal formulas mostly adhere to the electrolyte and fluid recommendations for chronic kidney disease (CKD) developed by the Kidney Disease: Improv-ing Global Outcomes (KDIGO) CKD Workgroup for the nondialysis patient.[51] For the patient with CKD who is

TABLE 4-16. Selected Enteral Formulas Marketed for Use in Patients with Renal Dysfunction

Product	Manufacturer
Nepro®	Abbott
Novasource Renal®	Nestlé
Renalcal®	Nestlé
Suplena®	Abbott

The brand names mentioned in this table may not constitute a comprehensive list of all relevant products on the market in the United States or other countries. Mention of a product does not imply an endorsement.

not receiving dialysis, protein intake should be limited to 0.8 g/kg/d, and sodium, phosphate, and potassium should be restricted, if needed.[51] For persons with CKD who are receiving hemodialysis or peritoneal dialysis, protein intake increases to at least 1.2–1.3 g/kg/d.[52]

AKI is a different disorder than CKD, and there is no formula marketed specifically for it. The National Kidney Foundation Disease Outcomes Quality Initiative and SCCM/ASPEN recommend not restricting protein intake during AKI as an attempt to postpone dialysis.[10,53] According to the KDIGO Work Group for Acute Kidney Injury, suggested protein intakes for patients with AKI are 0.8–1 g/kg/d for noncatabolic, nondialyzed patients; 1–1.5 g/kg/d for patients on renal replacement therapy; and ≤1.7 g/kg/d for patients receiving continuous renal replacement therapy (CRRT) and those who are hypercatabolic.[53] In contrast, SCCM/ASPEN guidelines on AKI use standard ICU recommendations for protein intake: 1.2–2 g/kg/d (using actual body weight) or, if receiving CRRT, ≤2.5 g/kg/d.[10]

Table 4-17 presents practice recommendations for the use of renal disease–specific formulas.[10,34,51–53] Above all,

TABLE 4-17. Practice Recommendations: Selection of Enteral Formulas for Patients with Renal Dysfunction[a]

SCCM/ASPEN recommendations:
- We suggest that ICU patients with AKI should be placed on a standard enteral formula and that standard ICU recommendations for protein (1.2–2 g/kg actual body weight) and energy (25–30 kcal/kg/d) provision should be followed. If significant electrolyte abnormalities develop, a specialty formula designed for renal failure (with appropriate electrolyte profile) may be considered (expert consensus).
- Patients receiving frequent hemodialysis or CRRT should increase protein intake, up to a maximum of 2.5 g/kg/d (very low quality of evidence).
- Protein should not be restricted in patients with renal insufficiency as a means to avoid or delay initiating dialysis therapy (very low quality of evidence).

ACG recommendations:
- A standard polymeric formula or a high-protein standard formula should be used routinely in the hospitalized patient requiring EN (conditional recommendation, very low level of evidence).

KDIGO recommendations:
- We suggest avoiding protein restriction with the aim of preventing or delaying initiation of renal replacement therapy (2D: very low level of evidence).
- CKD (no dialysis): We suggest limiting protein intake to 0.8 g/kg/d and restricting phosphorus, potassium, and sodium (2B for persons without diabetes: moderate quality of evidence; 2C for persons with diabetes: low quality of evidence).
- AKI: Suggested protein intakes are 0.8–1 g/kg/d for noncatabolic, nondialyzed patients, 1–1.5 g/kg/d for dialyzed patients, and up to 1.7 g/kg/d for patients on CRRT and the hypercatabolic patient (2D: very low quality of evidence).

(continued)

TABLE 4-17. *(Continued)*

Ikizler recommendation:
- For patients with CKD who are on hemodialysis or peritoneal dialysis, the suggested minimum protein intake is 1.2–1.3 g/kg/d.

Abbreviations: ACG, American College of Gastroenterology; AKI, acute kidney injury; ASPEN, American Society for Parenteral and Enteral Nutrition; CKD, chronic kidney disease; CRRT, continuous renal replacement therapy; EN, enteral nutrition; ICU, intensive care unit; KDIGO, Kidney Disease: Improving Global Outcomes; SCCM, Society of Critical Care Medicine.

[a]Refer to the original sources for guidance on evidence grading.

Source: Adapted from references 10, 34, and 51–53.

the patient's fluid balance, electrolyte status, use of dialysis, and type of dialysis should be assessed to select the appropriate EN formula. After determining the patient's nutrition prescription, the nutrition support clinician should compare the nutrient contents of the renal disease–specific formulas to those of standard formulas to select the product that will be the best fit for the patient.

Conditions Requiring Fluid Restrictions

Certain patients may need a fluid-restricted enteral formula (see Table 4-18 for examples of these products). Fluid-restricted EN formulas are energy dense (1.5–2 kcal/mL). As noted earlier in this chapter, fluid-restricted EN formulas may be considered for patients with pulmonary failure. They may also be appropriate for persons with other organ dysfunctions such as congestive heart failure or renal failure and for patients with ascites or selected other medical conditions (eg, syndrome of inappropriate antidiuretic hormone secretion, hypervolemic hyponatremia). A fluid-restricted formula may also be used to provide sufficient nutrition without a large volume during specific types of EN administration, such as cyclic or bolus feedings, or

TABLE 4-18. Selected Fluid-Restricted Enteral Formulas	
Product	**Manufacturer**
Isosource® 1.5 Cal	Nestlé
Nutren® 1.5	Nestlé
Nutren® 2.0	Nestlé
Osmolite® 1.5 Cal	Abbott
TwoCal® HN	Abbott

The brand names mentioned in this table may not constitute a comprehensive list of all relevant products on the market in the United States or other countries. Mention of a product does not imply an endorsement.

when transitioning from enteral to oral feedings. However, adequate free water must be provided to prevent dehydration while using concentrated EN for these situations.

The SCCM/ASPEN guidelines include several recommendations for use of fluid-restricted EN for critically ill patients.[10] These guidelines recommend a standard polymeric EN formula rather than disease-specific formulas, unless the use of an immune-modulating formula would be optimal based on the patient's disease state. SCCM/ASPEN's definition of a standard polymeric EN formula is one that is 1.0–1.5 kcal/mL. According to SCCM/ASPEN, 2 kcal/mL formulas are rarely needed unless volume needs to be restricted (ie, in renal failure).[10] Refer to Table 4-19 for practice recommendations.[10]

Obesity and Bariatric Surgery

Specialty enteral formulas have been developed to promote weight loss and provide sufficient protein to promote healing and preserve muscle mass in patients after bariatric surgery (see Table 4-20). These formulations often contain hydrolyzed proteins, fish oil, fiber, and antioxidants. They

TABLE 4-19. Practice Recommendations: Using Fluid-Restricted Enteral Formulas in Critically Ill Patients[a]

SCCM/ASPEN recommendations:

- Use a standard polymeric formula (ie, 1–1.5 kcal/mL) when initiating EN in critically ill patients (expert consensus).
- Use fluid-restricted, energy-dense EN formulations for patients with acute respiratory failure (especially if in a state of volume overload) (expert consensus).

Abbreviations: ASPEN, American Society for Parenteral and Enteral Nutrition; EN, enteral nutrition; SCCM, Society of Critical Care Medicine.

[a]Refer to the original source for guidance on evidence grading.

Source: Adapted from reference 10.

TABLE 4-20. Selected Enteral Formulas Marketed for Use in Patients Requiring Hypocaloric, High-Protein Feedings

Product	Manufacturer
Peptamen Intense® VHP	Nestlé
Vital® High Protein	Abbott

The brand names mentioned in this table may not constitute a comprehensive list of all relevant products on the market in the United States or other countries. Mention of a product does not imply an endorsement.

are therefore also used in the ICU for obese patients who require high-protein, hypocaloric EN and to prevent overfeeding in critically ill patients who are receiving significant amounts of energy from propofol (an IV sedation agent that provides 1.1 kcal/mL infused).

Table 4-21 reviews recommendations related to the use of hypocaloric, high-protein EN.[10,34,35,54] In guidelines on care for patients recovering from bariatric surgery, the American Association of Clinical Endocrinologists (AACE), the Obesity Society (TOS), and the American

TABLE 4-21. Practice Recommendations: Enteral Formula Selection for Patients with Obesity[a]

SCCM/ASPEN recommendations (critically ill obese patients):

- Use high-protein hypocaloric feeding for obese ICU patients (expert consensus).
- If available, use an enteral formula with low caloric density and a reduced NPC:N in the adult obese ICU patient (expert consensus).
- Energy intake: We suggest that, for all classes of obesity, energy intake from EN should not exceed 65%–70% of target energy requirement as determined by IC. If IC is unavailable, we suggest using the weight-based equation 11–14 kcal/kg *actual body weight* per day for patients with BMI in the range of 30–50 and 22–25 kcal/kg *ideal body weight* per day for patients with BMI >50 (expert consensus).
- Protein intake: We suggest that protein should be provided in a range from 2.0 g/kg ideal body weight per day for patients with BMI of 30–40 up to 2.5 g/kg ideal body weight per day for patients with BMI ≥40 (expert consensus).

ACG recommendations (critically ill obese patients):

- Permissive (hypocaloric) underfeeding is an acceptable alternative to full feeding in critically ill obese (BMI >30) patients (conditional recommendation, very low level of evidence).
- Protein intake: 2.0–2.5 g/kg ideal body weight.
- Energy intake: 60%–65% estimated or measured energy expenditure.

CPG recommendations (critically ill obese patients):

- Intentional underfeeding of calories (not protein) should be considered in obese patients at low nutrition risk. However, this recommendation does not apply to patients at high nutrition risk.

(continued)

TABLE 4-21. *(Continued)*

AACE/TOS/ASMBS recommendations (patients receiving early postoperative care following bariatric surgery):

- Protein intake should be individualized, assessed, and guided by an RD (Grade D).
- Minimal protein intake of 60 g/d and up to 1.5 g/kg ideal body weight should be adequate; intake of up to 2.1 g/kg ideal body weight should be assessed on an individualized basis (Grade D).

Abbreviations: AACE, American Association of Clinical Endocrinologists; ACG, American College of Gastroenterology; ASMBE, American Society for Metabolic and Bariatric Surgery; ASPEN, American Society for Parenteral and Enteral Nutrition; BMI, body mass index; CPG, Canadian Clinical Practice Guidelines; EN, enteral nutrition; IC, indirect calorimetry; ICU, intensive care unit; NPC:N, nonprotein calorie–to-nitrogen ratio; RD, registered dietitian; SCCM, Society of Critical Care Medicine; TOS, the Obesity Society.

[a]Refer to the original sources for guidance on evidence grading.

Source: Adapted from references 10, 34, 35, and 54.

Society for Metabolic and Bariatric Surgery (ASMBS) recommend at least 60 g protein intake per day during the early postoperative stage and up to 1.5 g protein per kg ideal body weight. This recommendation is based on studies showing that higher protein intakes (80–90 g/d) are associated with reduced loss of lean body mass.[54] In this guideline, AACE/TOS/ASMBS acknowledge that patients may need EN but make no recommendation for the ideal enteral formula or energy intake level.[54] SCCM/ASPEN, CPG, and ACG recommend high-protein, hypocaloric feedings for critically ill patients with obesity (body mass index >30) because high-protein, hypocaloric nutrition may aid in increasing insulin sensitivity, promote weight loss, reduce ICU and hospital mortality, and improve respiratory function.[10,34,35]

Blenderized Tube Feedings

Blenderized tube feedings (BTFs) are commercially available products and homemade preparations that blend whole food ingredients to a consistency that can be administered through a feeding tube. BTFs can be used for partial, supplemental, or complete EN support.

A variety of commercially prepared BTFs are available (see Table 4-22). Some of these products are made for bolus feeding only. Others may need to be strained or thinned with water for gravity feedings or are intended to supplement commercial formula or food to meet nutrient needs.

TABLE 4-22. Selected Commercial Food-Based Enteral Formulas/Meals

Product	Manufacturer
Compleat®	Nestlé
Compleat® Organic Blends Chicken Garden Blend	Nestlé
Compleat® Organic Blends Plant-Based Blend	Nestlé
Liquid Hope®	Functional Formularies
Real Food Blends™ Beef, Potatoes & Spinach	Real Food Blends
Real Food Blends™ Chicken, Carrots & Brown Rice	Real Food Blends
Real Food Blends™ Quinoa, Kale & Hemp	Real Food Blends
Real Food Blends™ Salmon, Oats & Squash	Real Food Blends

The brand names mentioned in this table may not constitute a comprehensive list of all relevant products on the market in the United States or other countries. Mention of a product does not imply an endorsement.

Homemade BTFs are made from whole foods and usually prepared using a meal plan or recipe. Depending on the patient's nutrient needs, medical condition, and family support, the amount of blended food in homemade tube feeding can range between 1% and 100%.[55] A patient might choose to use a commercial food-based enteral formula or add a small amount of blended food to his or her current feeding plan, while another patient may desire to have 100% of nutrition provided by blended food.

To promote the safe initiation of a BTF regimen and choose the appropriate BTF recipe or product, the nutrition support clinician must assess the patient, with emphasis on the following factors:[3,55–57]

- Medical history
- Tolerance or intolerance of current or past enteral feeding regimen
- Food intolerances and food allergies
- Lifestyle
- Ethnic and religious preferences
- Ability to obtain and store ingredients and tools for preparing a homemade BTF

After a patient begins a BTF regimen, a trained registered dietitian should perform periodic nutrition reassessments and offer continuing patient education on safe preparation, administration, and storage of the formula.[56] Chapter 11 provides additional information on the use of BTFs in the home setting.

Modular Products

Many modular products are available to fortify EN, including protein powders and liquids, liquid fat, MCT oil, soluble fiber, and specific amino acids (eg, glutamine, arginine) (see Table 4-23). Liquid modular products are often hyperosmolar.

Instructions for mixing and administering modulars must be carefully followed because many of these products can occlude feeding tubes. Modular products can be diluted or dissolved in an appropriate volume of water and administered via the feeding tube. Additional water flushes before and after the modular is administered help maintain patency of the enteral access device. See Chapter 3 for additional information on preventing tube occlusion.

In the home setting, administering modular products for the person receiving EN will be an additional task for the caregiver; the ease of providing modulars at home will depend on the caregiver's capabilities and the time dedicated for feeding administration. See Chapter 11 for further information on EN in the home setting.

TABLE 4-23. Selected Examples of Modular Products

Nutrient(s)	Product	Manufacturer
Protein	Beneprotein®	Nestlé
	ProMod® Liquid Protein	Abbott
	ProSource® No Carb	Medtrition
	ProSource® Plus Liquid Protein	Medtrition
	ProSource® Protein Powder	Medtrition
	ProSource® TF	Medtrition
	Pro-Stat® Max	Nutricia
	Pro-Stat® Sugar Free	Nutricia
	Pro-Stat® Sugar Free AWC	Nutricia
Fiber	Fiber-Stat®	Nutricia
	NutriSource® Fiber	Nestlé
Protein and fiber	Pro-Stat® Renal Care	Nutricia
Fat	MCT Oil®	Nestlé
	Microlipid™	Nestlé

The brand names mentioned in this table may not constitute a comprehensive list of all relevant products on the market in the United States or other countries. Mention of a product does not imply an endorsement.

Protein modulars, which provide 6 to 15 g of protein per serving, rank as the most widely used of the modular components. This is because many enteral products may not provide adequate protein for certain patient populations (eg, critically ill patients, patients receiving CRRT).[10] Patient-specific factors must be taken into account when choosing between protein modulars.

There are multiple types of protein modulars, including those with complete protein (whey, casein), collagen-based products, and specific amino acids (arginine, glutamine).[58] Only complete protein modulars contain all 9 essential amino acids. Protein modulars that contain only collagen lack tryptophan. Therefore, it may be necessary to supplement tryptophan via other protein modulars in patients receiving collagen-based protein modulars. If indicated, single-entity arginine and glutamine modulars are available.

The other types of modulars are used less frequently. Fermentable soluble fiber may promote bowel health and reduce diarrhea and may be added if the EN formula is fiber-free and supplementation is indicated based on patient status.[10,34] MCT oil can be used to boost energy intake in persons with chylous leaks because it bypasses the lymphatic system for absorption. If enterally fed, these patients receive very-low-fat EN. However, MCT does not contain essential fatty acids. A liquid fat modular can also be used to provide energy, but a high fat intake could promote delayed gastric emptying. Above all, the nutrition support clinician should thoroughly assess the patient to determine which modulars, if any, are appropriate for the EN regimen.

Developing an Enteral Product Formulary

Many healthcare organizations choose to develop an enteral formulary to save money, improve patient care, and help with inventory control. A multidisciplinary formula selection committee will represent the perspectives of dietitians, pharmacists, physicians, administrators, and individuals working in the supply chain. The committee can evaluate formulas in each category. Evidence-based research should guide the committee in the selection of products; such research is especially helpful when considering specialty and disease-specific formulas. The following factors should be considered when evaluating an enteral product formulary:

- Patient acuity
- EN formula categories
- Current product utilization
- Contractual requirements
- Substitution list in case of product shortages
- Frequency of enteral product formulary review (eg, every year or every 2 years)

Competitive bidding practices and policies that scrutinize nonformulary requests and encourage automatic substitution for nonformulary products promote formulary adherence and cost containment.[59] It may be most economical to select all products from the same manufacturer if that company can provide an appropriate product for each category.

Product Resources

US Contact Information for Enteral Formula and Modular Manufacturers	
Manufacturer	**Website**
Abbott Nutrition	http://abbottnutrition.com
Functional Formularies	http://functionalformularies.com
Kate Farms	http://katefarms.com
Medtrition	https://www.medtrition.com
Nestlé Nutrition	http://nestlehealthscience.us
Nutricia	https://www.nutricia.com
Real Food Blends	http://realfoodblends.com

References

1. US Food and Drug Administration. Medical foods guidance documents & regulatory information. https://www.fda.gov/Food/GuidanceRegulation/GuidanceDocuments RegulatoryInformation/MedicalFoods/default.htm. Updated December 2017. Accessed November 26, 2018.

2. US Food and Drug Administration. Food guidance regulation. https://www.fda.gov/downloads/Food/Guidance Regulation/GuidanceDocumentsRegulatoryInformation /UCM500094.pdf. Accessed September 24, 2018.

3. Escuro AA, Hummell AC. Enteral formulas in nutrition support practice: is there a better choice for your patient? *Nutr Clin Pract.* 2016;31(6):709–722.

4. Roberts S, Kirsch R. Enteral nutrition formulations. In: Mueller CM, ed. *The ASPEN Adult Nutrition Support Core Curriculum.* 3rd ed. Silver Spring, MD: American Society for Parenteral and Enteral Nutrition; 2017:227–249.

5. Malone AM. Enteral formulations. In: Cresci GA, ed. *Nutrition Support for the Critically Ill Patient.* 2nd ed. Boca Raton, FL: CRC Press; 2015:259–277.

6. Brown B, Roehl K, Betz M. Enteral formula selection: current evidence and implications for practice. *Nutr Clin Pract.* 2015;30(1):72–85.

7. Scaife CL, Saffle JR, Morris SE. Intestinal obstruction secondary to enteral feedings in burn trauma patients. *J Trauma.* 1999;47:859–863.

8. McIvor AC, Meguid MM, Curtas S, Kaplan DS. Intestinal obstruction from cecal bezoar: a complication of fiber-containing tube feedings. *Nutrition.* 1990;6:115–117.

9. McClave SA, Chang WK. Feeding the hypotensive patient: does enteral feeding precipitate or protect against ischemic bowel? *Nutr Clin Pract.* 2003;18:279–284.

10. McClave SA, Taylor BE, Martindale RG, et al. Guidelines for the provision and assessment of nutrition support therapy in the adult critically ill patient: Society of Critical Care Medicine (SCCM) and American Society for Parenteral and Enteral Nutrition (ASPEN). *JPEN J Parenter Enteral Nutr.* 2016;40(2):159–211.

11. Elia M, Engfer MB, Green CJ, Slik DB. Systematic review and meta-analysis: the clinical and physiological effects of

fibre-containing formulae. *Aliment Pharmacol Ther*. 2008;27(2): 120–145.

12. Academy of Nutrition and Dietetics Evidence Analysis Library. Enteral nutrition and fiber. http://www.andeal.org. Accessed May 21, 2018.

13. Malone AM. Enteral formula selection. In: Charney P, Malone A, eds. *Academy of Nutrition and Dietetics Pocket Guide to Enteral Nutrition*. 2nd ed. Chicago, IL: Academy of Nutrition and Dietetics; 2013:120–152.

14. Lipp J, Lord LM, Scholer LH. Fluid management in enteral nutrition. *Nutr Clin Pract*. 1999;14:232–237.

15. Trujillo E. Enteral nutrition: a comprehensive overview. In: Matarese LE, Gottschlich MM, eds. *Contemporary Nutrition Support Practice: A Clinical Guide*. Philadelphia, PA: WB Saunders;1998:192–201.

16. Parrish CR, Krenitsky J, Perkey KG. Enteral feeding challenges. In: Cresci GA, ed. *Nutrition Support for the Critically Ill Patient*. 2nd ed. Boca Raton, FL: CRC Press; 2015:291–311.

17. American Academy of Allergy, Asthma, and Immunology. Food allergies, symptoms, diagnosis and treatment. https://www.aaaai.org/conditions-and-treatments/allergies/food-allergies. Accessed September 24, 2018.

18. National Institute of Allergy and Infectious Diseases. Food allergy. https://www.niaid.nih.gov/diseases-conditions/food-allergy. Accessed September 24, 2018.

19. Mowatt-Larssen CA, Brown RO, Wojtysiak SL, Kudsk KA. Comparison of tolerance and nutritional outcome between a peptide and a standard enteral formula in critically ill, hypoalbuminemic patients. *JPEN J Parenter Enteral Nutr*. 1992;16(1):20–24.

20. Brinson RR, Kolts BE. Diarrhea associated with severe hypoalbuminemia: a comparison of a peptide-based chemically defined diet and standard enteral alimentation. *Crit Care Med*. 1988;16(2):130–136.

21. Dietscher JE, Foulks CJ, Smith RW. Nutritional response of patients in an intensive care unit to an elemental formula vs a standard enteral formula. *J Am Diet Assoc*. 1998;98:335–336.

22. Heimburger DC, Geels VJ, Bilbrey J, Redden DT, Keeney C. Effects of small-peptide and whole-protein enteral feedings on serum proteins and diarrhea in critically ill patients: a randomized trial. *JPEN J Parenter Enteral Nutr*. 1997;21:162–167.

23. Seres DS, Ippolito PR. Pilot study evaluating the efficacy, tolerance, and safety of a peptide-based enteral formula versus a high protein enteral formula in multiple ICU settings (medical, surgical, cardiothoracic). *Clin Nutr.* 2017;36:706–709.

24 National Pressure Ulcer Advisory Panel, Europe Pressure Ulcer Advisory Panel, Pan Pacific Pressure Injury Alliance. *Prevention and Treatment of Pressure Ulcers: Clinical Practice Guideline.* Perth, Australia: Cambridge Media; 2014.

25. Litchford MD, Dorner B, Posthauer ME. Malnutrition as a precursor of pressure ulcers. *Adv Wound Care.* 2014;3(1):54–63.

26. Posthauer ME, Dorner B, Schols JMGA. The role of nutrition for pressure ulcer management: National Pressure Ulcer Advisory Panel, European Pressure Ulcer Advisory Panel, and Pan Pacific Pressure Injury Alliance white paper. *Adv Skin Wound Care.* 2015;28(4):175–188.

27. Cereda E, Klersy C, Rondanelli M, Caccialanza R. Energy balance in patients with pressure ulcers: a systematic review and meta-analysis of observational studies. *J Am Diet Assoc.* 2011;111(12):1868–1876.

28. Posthauer ME, Marian M. Wound healing. In: Mueller CM, ed. *The ASPEN Adult Nutrition Support Core Curriculum.* 3rd ed. Silver Spring, MD: American Society for Parenteral and Enteral Nutrition; 2017:419–434.

29. Langer G, Fink A. Nutritional interventions for preventing and treating pressure ulcers. *Cochrane Database Syst Rev.* 2014;(6):CD003216.

30. Cereda E, Neyens JCL, Caccialanza R, Rondanelli M, Schols JMGA. Efficacy of a disease-specific nutritional support for pressure healing: a systematic review and meta-analysis. *J Nutr Health Aging.* 2017;21(6):655–661.

31 Abbott Nutrition website. http://Abbottnutrition.com. Accessed October 2, 2018.

32. Nestlé Health Science website. http://www.NestleHealthScience.us. Accessed October 2, 2018.

33. American Diabetes Association. Standards of medical care in diabetes 2018. *Diabetes Care.* 2018;14(Suppl 1):S1–S172.

34. McClave SA, DiBaise JK, Mullin GE, Martindale RG. ACG clinical guideline: nutrition therapy in the adult hospitalized patient. *Am J Gastroenterol.* 2016;111:315–334.

35. Critical Care Nutrition at the Clinical Evaluation Research Unit. Canadian clinical practice guidelines for nutrition

support in the mechanically ventilated, critically ill adult 2015. http://www.criticalcarenutrition.org. Accessed April 30, 2018.

36. Elia M, Ceriello A, Laube H, Sinclair AJ, Engfer M, Stratton RJ. Enteral nutritional support and use of diabetes-specific formulas for patients with diabetes. *Diabetes Care.* 2005;28(9):2267–2279.

37. Ojo O, Brooke J. Evaluation of the role of enteral nutrition in managing patients with diabetes: a systematic review. *Nutrients.* 2014;6(11):5142–5152.

38. Mesejo A, Acosta JA, Ortega C, et al. Comparison of a high protein disease-specific enteral formula with a high-protein enteral formula in hyperglycemic critically ill patients. *Clin Nutr.* 2003;22(3):295–305.

39. Ceriello A, Lansink M, Rouws CHFC, van Laere KMJ, Frost GS. Administration of a new diabetes-specific enteral formula results in an improved 24 h glucose profile in type 2 diabetic patients. *Diabetes Res Clin Pract.* 2009;84(3):259–266.

40. Alish CJ, Garvey WT, Maki KC, et al. A diabetes-specific enteral formula improves glycaemic variability in patients with type 2 diabetes. *Diabetes Technol Ther.* 2010;12(6):419–425.

41. Corsino L, Dhatariay K, Umpierrez G. Management of diabetes and hyperglycemia in hospitalized patients. In: Endotext [internet]. National Library of Medicine website. http://www.ncbi.nlm.nih.gov/books/NBK279093. Accessed October 15, 2018.

42. Hamdy O, Ernst FR, Baumer D, Mustad V, Partridge J, Hegazi R. Differences in resource utilization between patients with diabetes receiving glycemia-targeted specialized nutrition vs standard nutrition formulas in U.S. hospitals. *JPEN J Parenter Enteral Nutr.* 2014;38(2 suppl):86S–91S.

43. Lansink M, Hofman Z, Genovese S, Rouws CH, Ceriello A. Improved glucose profile in patients with type 2 diabetes with a new, high-protein, diabetes-specific tube feed during 4 hours of continuous feeding. *JPEN J Parenter Enteral Nutr.* 2017;41(6)968–975.

44. Mesejo A, Monteio-Gonzalez JC, Vaquerizo-Alonso C, et al. Diabetes-specific enteral formula in hyperglycemic, mechanically ventilated, critically ill patients: a prospective, open-label, blind-randomized, multi-center study. *Crit Care.* 2015;9:390. doi:10.1186/s13054-015-1108-1.

45. Abdelsayed GG. Diets in encephalopathy. *Clin Liver Dis.* 2015;19:497–505.

46. Bémeur C, Desjardins P, Butterworth RF. Role of nutrition in the management of hepatic encephalopathy in end-stage liver failure. *J Nutr Metab.* 2010;2010:489823. doi:10.1155/2010/489823.

47. Vilstrup H, Amodio P, Bajaj J, et al. Hepatic encephalopathy in chronic liver disease: 2014 practice guideline by the American Association for the Study of Liver Diseases and the European Association for the Study of the Liver. *Hepatology.* 2014;60:715–735.

48. Rosenthal MD, Vanzant EL, Martindale RG, Moore FA. Evolving paradigms in the nutritional support of critically ill surgical patients. *Curr Probl Surg.* 2015;52(4):147–182. doi:10.1067/j.cpsurg.2015.02.003.

49. Feller-Kopman DJ, Schwartzstein RD. Mechanisms, causes, and effects of hypercapnia. UpToDate website. https://www.uptodate.com/contents/mechanisms-causes-and-effects-of-hypercapnia. Published Sept 8, 2017. Accessed October 25, 2018.

50. Shirai K, Yoshida S, Matsumaru N, Toyoda I, Ogura S. Effect of enteral diet enriched with eicosapentaenoic acid, gamma-linolenic acid, and antioxidants in patients with sepsis-induced acute respiratory distress syndrome. *J Intensive Care.* 2015;3(1):24.

51. Kidney Disease: Improving Global Outcomes (KDIGO) CKD Work Group. KDIGO 2012 clinical practice guideline for the evaluation and management of chronic kidney disease. *Kidney Int Suppl.* 2013;3(1):1–150.

52. Ikizler TA. A patient with CKD and poor nutritional status. *Clin J Am Soc Nephrol.* 2013;8(12):2174–2182.

53. Kidney Disease: Improving Global Outcomes (KDIGO) Acute Kidney Injury Work Group. KDIGO clinical practice guideline for acute kidney injury. *Kidney Int Suppl.* 2012;2(1):1–138.

54. Mechanick JI, Youdim A, Jones DB, et al. Clinical practice guidelines for the perioperative nutritional, metabolic, and nonsurgical support of the bariatric surgery patient—2013 update: cosponsored by American Association of Clinical Endocrinologists, the Obesity Society, and American Society for Metabolic & Bariatric Surgery. *Surg Obes Relat Dis.* 2013;9(2):159–191.

55. Walia C, Van Hoorn M, Edlbeck A, Feuling MB. The registered dietitian nutritionist's guide to homemade tube feeding. *J Acad Nutr Diet.* 2017;117(1):11–16.

56. Escuro AA. Blenderized tube feeding: suggested guidelines to clinicians. *Pract Gastroenterol.* 2014;38(12):58–66.

57. Carter H, Johnson K, Johnson TW, Spurlock A. Blended tube feeding prevalence, efficacy, and safety: what does the literature say? *J Am Assoc Nurs Pract.* 2018;30(3):150–157.

58. Castellanos VH, Litchford MD, Campbell WW. Modular protein supplements and their application to long-term care. *Nutr Clin Pract.* 2006;21:485–504.

59. Wildish DE. Enteral formulary management: a cost-effective approach. *Can J Diet Pract Res.* 2006;67(4):193–198.

CHAPTER 5

Enteral Formulas for Pediatric Patients

Introduction

Choosing the appropriate formula is particularly important when caring for a growing and developing pediatric patient. To select the best enteral nutrition option for a patient, the nutrition support clinician must first perform a complete nutrition assessment and identify any nutrition-related diagnoses or symptoms and medical conditions that may affect the individual's energy and nutrient needs (see Chapter 1). This chapter focuses on formula selection for pediatric and infant patients. Chapter 4 provides general information on formula composition, food allergies and intolerances, and developing an enteral product formulary.

The brand names mentioned in this chapter do not constitute a comprehensive list of all relevant products on the market in the United States or other countries. Mention of a product does not imply an endorsement.

Manufacturers periodically introduce, withdraw, and alter products. Before using any product, nutrition support clinicians should review the label and product website for current information on ingredients, nutrient composition, and instructions for use. If those resources are insufficient, contact the manufacturer or the formulary manager for additional information. Selected manufacturer websites are listed at the end of the chapter.

Federal Regulations

Medical Foods

Under US law, enteral formulas (adult and pediatric) are classified as medical foods. A *medical food* is defined in the 1988 Orphan Drug Amendments as follows:[1]

A food which is formulated to be consumed or administered enterally under the supervision of a physician and which is intended for the specific dietary management of a disease or condition for which distinctive nutritional requirements, based on recognized scientific principles, are established by medical evaluation.

The US Food and Drug Administration (FDA) regulates the manufacturing of medical foods. However, it does not require the inclusion of Nutrition Facts on the product label of a medical food. Also, manufacturers do not need FDA approval to make structural or functional claims about medical foods. Even without prior FDA approval, these claims cannot be misleading or disease related. An example of an allowed claim is "This product contains short-chain fructooligosaccharides to stimulate the growth of beneficial bacteria in the colon." There is scientific evidence that this claim is true. However, although we understand that beneficial bacteria in the gut play a role in immune health, a manufacturer cannot claim that the product "strengthens your immune system." The American Society for Parenteral and Enteral Nutrition (ASPEN) recommends that nutrition support clinicians interpret the content and health claims of enteral formulas with caution until more specific regulations are in place.[2]

Infant Formulas

An infant formula is defined by the Federal Food, Drug, and Cosmetic Act as "a food which purports to be or is represented for special dietary use solely as a food for infants by reason of its simulation of human milk or its suitability as a complete or partial substitute for human milk."[1] Compared with enteral products, infant formulas are more highly regulated with regard to quality control, labeling, nutrient requirements, formula recall, notification of new products, and exempt products.

An infant formula is considered exempt if it is designed to meet the nutrition needs of a specific population, such as premature infants. This designation does not exempt the formulas from regulation. Instead, they need to meet criteria established for the specific need of the population for which they are intended.

In 2014, the FDA finalized a rule that established standards to ensure all manufactured infant formula is safe and supports healthy growth. Under these regulations, whenever a new formula is released to the market or an already available formula undergoes any major formulation changes, the manufacturer needs to file notification with the FDA and have studies that show infants have normal growth on the petitioned formulas. Additionally, the new standards require testing for the harmful pathogens *Salmonella* and *Cronobacter,* and infant formulas must be tested for the content of every nutrient in every lot of finished infant formula, both before entering the market and at the end of the products' shelf life.[3]

In response to the incidence of *Enterobacter sakazakii* (now called *Cronobacter sakazakii*) infection resulting in meningitis, necrotizing enterocolitis, and bacteremia in neonates fed cow's milk–based powdered infant formulas, the Centers for Disease Control and Prevention (CDC) and FDA recommend that powdered infant formulas not be used in neonatal intensive care settings unless there is no alternative available.[4,5] The American Academy of Pediatrics (AAP) also warns against the use of powdered infant formulas in term infants less than 2 months of age and infants with underlying medical conditions.[6] The infection risks and associated recommendations have resulted in hospitals implementing policies to primarily feed neonates and high-risk infants the commercially sterile liquid forms of formulas (ie, ready-to-feed [RTF] and concentrated products) when available.

Formula Composition

For an overview of enteral formula composition (ie, carbohydrate, fiber, fat, protein, vitamins, minerals, water, and osmolality), refer to Chapter 4. Specific information about the composition of pediatric and infant formulas is presented later in this chapter.

Pediatric Enteral Formulas

Pediatric enteral formulas are designed for children from 1 to 13 years of age who require tube feedings to meet nutrient needs. These formulas are designed to meet the needs of children 1–8 years old in 1000 mL/d and children 9–13 years old in 1500 mL/d. Most types of pediatric formulas are reviewed in this chapter. One exception is products for children with inborn errors of metabolism; the treatment of those patients is beyond the scope of this handbook.

Adult specialty formulas can be considered when an appropriate pediatric formula is not available. However, when considering the use of these products, nutrition support clinicians must pay special attention to the nutrition needs for growth and development in the pediatric patient.

General Purpose (Polymeric) Pediatric Formulas

General purpose or polymeric pediatric formulas are designed to meet the nutrition needs for growth and development of children when used as the sole source of nutrition (see Table 5-1). These products are available in various energy concentrations from 0.63 kcal/mL to 1.5 kcal/mL and typically meet the Dietary Reference Intakes (DRIs) for children ages 1–8 years in 1000 mL/d and ages 9–13 years in 1500 mL/d. Most polymeric products are available with or without fiber, are considered appropriate for lactose intolerance, are gluten free, and are kosher.[7] Manufactured pediatric blenderized enteral products are considered a subcategory of polymeric formulas (see next section of this chapter).

Polymeric formulas primarily contain intact proteins and typically require normal digestion.[8] These products can be orally consumed or administered into the stomach or the small intestine, and they are typically well tolerated in

TABLE 5-1. Examples of General Purpose/Polymeric Enteral Formulas Marketed for Pediatric Patients

Indications for Use	Characteristics	Product Examples (Manufacturers)
• Supplemental or sole source of nutrition for children without food allergies or significant malabsorption issues	• Intact macronutrients • May or may not contain fiber • May be made with whole foods	• Boost Kid Essentials (Nestlé)[a] • Boost Kid Essentials 1.5 (Nestlé)[a] • Compleat Pediatric (Nestlé) • Compleat Pediatric Reduced Calorie (Nestlé) • Compleat Pediatric Organic Blends (Nestlé) • Nutren Junior (Nestlé)[a] • Pediasure Enteral Formula 1.0 Cal (Abbott)[a] • Pediasure 1.5 (Abbott)[a] • Pediasure Grow and Gain Therapeutic Shake (Abbott)[a] • Pediasure SideKicks 0.63 Cal Shake (Abbott) • Pediatric Standard 1.2 (Kate Farms)

The brand names mentioned in this table may not constitute a comprehensive list of all relevant products on the market in the United States or other countries. Mention of a product does not imply an endorsement.

[a]Available with or without fiber.

patients with normal digestive capacity. They usually contain cow's milk as the protein source in the form of milk protein concentrate, whey protein concentrate, and/or sodium and calcium caseinates. The blenderized products may contain other nonmilk sources of protein; therefore, careful attention to the label and current formulation of these enteral products is important (as it is with all formula products).

Common carbohydrate sources for polymeric products are maltodextrin and sugar. Compared with formulas for enteral use only, oral products or products for both oral and tube feeding usually contain more sugar or added sweeteners for taste. It is important to note that sugar and sweeteners can increase the osmolality of the enteral formula. Fiber sources are usually a combination of soluble and insoluble fibers, including oat fiber, soy fiber, fructooligosaccharides, pea fiber, and inulin.

Sources of fat in polymeric products include soybean oil, canola oil, soy lecithin, and medium-chain triglycerides (MCTs). Some products may contain the long-chain polyunsaturated fatty acids (LCPUFAs) docosahexaenoic acid (DHA) and arachidonic acid (ARA), which are found in human milk (HM) and are associated with neurodevelopment in infants. LCPUFAs are discussed in further detail in the Infant Formulas section of this chapter.

Blenderized Tube Feedings

Blenderized tube feedings (BTFs) have recently regained their popularity in the pediatric population. The BTF may be made by blending whole foods with added liquid, or a commercially available BTF product containing whole foods may be used. The foods in a BTF may include a variety of table foods and/or baby foods from animal or plant protein sources, grains, fruits, and vegetables. Fat and carbohydrates may be added to meet a patient's essential fatty acid and energy needs. The liquid source may be a commercially available formula, but water, cow's milk, nondairy "milks," and electrolyte-containing fluids are also used. The final blenderized feeding plan must be analyzed to determine whether it is nutritionally complete. There are guidelines on recipe development as well as when it is appropriate for a patient to receive a BTF.[9–12]

There are reports of BTFs being especially beneficial in children with intestinal failure, as well as those following the ketogenic diet, those with food sensitivities, and those whose tolerance of commercial formulas is poor.[13,14] Multiple reports indicate that BTFs help improve retching, gagging, dumping syndrome, and constipation.[9,15,16] Some families prefer this type of feeding because it uses whole foods and offers customizability for children who follow a vegetarian or gluten-free diet or have other food preferences or restrictions.

Vieira and associates conducted a cross-sectional study in Brazil comparing contamination of 33 samples of commercial BTFs (some RTF formulas and some powdered products reconstituted with water) and 33 samples of home-blenderized formulas in the home care setting. *Escherichia coli* and mesophilic and coliform bacteria were detected in samples from all 3 groups. The bacteria counts in the home-blenderized formula and reconstituted powdered formula samples were higher than in the RTF samples. The authors attributed contamination in the reconstituted formula samples to the water used in mixing.[17] Refer to Chapters 4, 8, and 11 for additional information on BTFs.

Semi-Elemental (Peptide-Based) Pediatric Formulas

Semi-elemental or peptide-based pediatric formulas are designed for children with impaired gastrointestinal (GI) function or those who had trouble tolerating the polymeric formula.[18] Most are marketed for use in children between the ages of 1 and 13 years; there is also a peptide-based product marketed for adolescents ages 14 years and older (see Table 5-2). These products are *not* intended for the treatment or prevention of allergies or allergic reactions. Like the polymeric products, the peptide-based pediatric products typically meet the DRIs for children 1–8 years old in 1000 mL/d and children 9–13 years old in 1500 mL/d. The product marketed for use in adolescents meets the DRIs for 14- to 18-year-old adolescents in 1000 mL/d.

Peptide-based formulas are acceptable for patients with lactose intolerance and are gluten free. Some, but not all, products meet kosher guidelines; compliance will be clearly

TABLE 5-2. Examples of Semi-Elemental/Peptide-Based Formulas Marketed for Pediatric Patients

Indications for Use	Characteristics	Product Examples (Manufacturers)
• Intolerance of polymeric formulas • May be indicated for patients with malabsorption disorders	• Cow's milk protein hydrolyzed to peptides • May contain plant-based protein • Some fat may be from medium-chain triglycerides • May or may not contain fiber	• Pediasure Peptide 1.0 Cal (Abbott) • Pediasure Peptide 1.5 Cal (Abbott) • Pediatric Peptide 1.5 (Kate Farms) • Peptamen Junior (Nestlé)[a] • Peptamen Junior 1.5 (Nestlé)[a] • Peptamen Junior with Prebio (Nestlé) • Peptamen Junior HP (Nestlé) • Vital Peptide 1.5 Cal (Abbott)[b]

The brand names mentioned in this table may not constitute a comprehensive list of all relevant products on the market in the United States or other countries. Mention of a product does not imply an endorsement.

[a]Available with or without fiber.

[b]Marketed for use in adolescents ages ≥14 years.

indicated on the label. Some products used for oral or tube feeding are flavored.

Peptide-based formulas contain partially hydrolyzed protein, resulting in di- or tri-peptides and other short-chain peptides.[7,18] Research comparing outcomes of peptide-based formulas compared to polymeric formulas is limited, and many studies show no difference in outcomes.[8] The protein source is hydrolyzed cow's milk protein (hydrolyzed whey protein, hydrolyzed sodium caseinate) or plant-based protein. Carbohydrate sources are maltodextrin, hydrolyzed cornstarch, and sugar. Sources of fat include soybean oil, canola oil, soy lecithin, structured lipids, and MCTs. Some products contain soluble fibers or prebiotics in the form of fructooligosaccharides, guar gum, and inulin.

Elemental Pediatric Formulas

Pediatric elemental formulas may be appropriate for patients with malabsorption disorders and GI impairment, including short bowel syndrome or intestinal failure; severe food allergies, such as food protein–induced enterocolitis syndrome; and eosinophilic GI disorders (see Table 5-3). Pediatric elemental products are designed for children 1 year of age or older. Note: Most pediatric ("Junior") elemental formulas have an infant formula counterpart. The ingredients in these paired products and their manufacturing processes are similar, with the intention of making the transition from the infant formula to the pediatric product relatively straightforward.

Because elemental products are amino acid based, they are considered hypoallergenic. The most common carbohydrate source is corn syrup solids; less-common carbohydrate sources include potato starch and tapioca starch. Fat sources include high-oleic safflower oil, refined or modified palm kernel and/or coconut oil for MCT content, MCT

TABLE 5-3. Examples of Elemental Enteral Formulas Marketed for Pediatric Patients		
Indications for Use	**Characteristics**	**Product Examples (Manufacturers)**
• Malabsorption disorders and GI impairment • Short bowel syndrome or intestinal failure • Severe food allergies • Eosinophilic GI disorders	• Amino acid based • Some fat is from MCTs	• Alfamino Junior (Nestlé) • Elecare Junior (Abbott) • Neocate Junior (Nutricia) • Neocate Junior with Prebiotics (Nutricia) • Vivonex Pediatric (Nestlé)

Abbreviations: GI, gastrointestinal; MCT, medium-chain triglyceride.

The brand names mentioned in this table may not constitute a comprehensive list of all relevant products on the market in the United States or other countries. Mention of a product does not imply an endorsement.

oil, soy oil, DHA, and ARA. The percentage of MCT varies from product to product; if fat malabsorption is a concern, read the product information to make the best choice for the patient. As of 2019, 1 product containing prebiotics was available in the US market (see Table 5-3). Similar to polymeric and semi-elemental products, elemental products may be flavored or unflavored.

Modified-Fat Pediatric Formulas

Modified-fat formulas are designed for use in patients with long-chain oxidative disorders and chylous leaks (see Table 5-4). The protein sources are intact cow's milk whey and caseinates. Carbohydrate sources include maltodextrin and corn syrup solids. These products usually contain a lower percentage of calories from fat, and approximately 80% of

TABLE 5-4. Examples of Modified-Fat Formulas Marketed for Use in Pediatric Patients		
Indications for Use	**Characteristics**	**Product Examples (Manufacturers)**
• Long-chain oxidative disorders and chylous leaks	• Intact protein • Low fat with a high percentage of medium-chain triglycerides	• Lipistart (Vitaflo) • Monogen (Nestlé)

The brand names mentioned in this table may not constitute a comprehensive list of all relevant products on the market in the United States or other countries. Mention of a product does not imply an endorsement.

the fat is from MCT. MCT is transported via the portal system while long-chain triglycerides (LCTs) are transported through the lymphatic system. Fat sources are modified palm kernel oil and/or coconut oil, which are high in MCTs, and walnut oil, which is a fat rich in LCTs. To prevent essential fatty acid deficiency, it is important to provide at least 10% of total energy intake as fat and 2%–4% of total energy intake as the essential fatty acid linoleic acid.[19] In addition, DHA and ARA may be added. Manufacturers recommend monitoring the essential fatty acid status of patients using these products.

Renal Pediatric Formulas

In the United States, 1 pediatric formula product is marketed to meet the specific nutrition needs of children with acute kidney injury or chronic kidney disease (see Table 5-5). This product is available in powdered form and is a high-calorie product with limited amounts of protein, calcium, chloride, phosphorus, potassium, and vitamin A. The protein source is whey protein concentrate with some free amino acids, and the carbohydrate source is glucose

TABLE 5-5. Example of an Enteral Formula Marketed for Use in Pediatric Patients with Renal Disease		
Indications for Use	**Characteristics**	**Product Example (Manufacturer)**
• Acute kidney injury • Chronic kidney disease	• High calorie with limited amounts of protein, calcium, phosphorus, chloride, potassium, and vitamin A	• Renastart (Vitaflo)

The brand name mentioned in this table may not be the only relevant product on the market in the United States or other countries. Mention of a product does not imply an endorsement.

syrup solids. Fat is from palm kernel, palm, canola, and sunflower oils, and the product contains DHA and ARA.

Infant Formulas

The AAP states that HM is the preferred source of nutrition for all term and preterm infants for the first year of life.[20] According to the CDC, as of 2015, the percentage of US infants ever receiving HM was 83.2%, which exceeds the Healthy People 2020 breastfeeding rate objective of 81.9%.[21,22]

Still, many infants in the United States rely on infant formula for some portion of their nutrition. Infant formula is designed to be similar in composition to HM, the optimal nutrition for a growing infant.[23] Although infant formulas differ in exact composition, those regulated under the Infant Formula Act have all been shown to promote normal physical growth.[24] Compared with HM, infant formula typically contains higher concentrations of macro- and micronutrients to compensate for the potentially lower bio-availability of nutrients from formula.

Infant formulas are available in RTF, concentrated liquid, and powdered forms. The first 2 forms are commercially sterile, whereas powdered forms are not. RTF products do not require mixing and are the easiest to use. Concentrated formulas and powdered formulas require the addition of water. When a product is available in multiple forms, the RTF is usually most expensive, concentrated formula is typically less costly, and powdered formula is the least-expensive option.

Additives in Infant Formulas

According to the Infant Formula Act, manufacturers are required to submit new ingredients to the FDA to be approved as a food additive or GRAS (Generally Recognized as Safe) for use in infant formulas. Current infant formulations contain a mixture of some of the following functional ingredients: DHA and ARA; probiotics, prebiotics, and synbiotics; nucleotides; and milk fat globule membranes (MFGMs). However, manufacturers are unable to make formulas that provide the hormones, immunoglobulins, enzymes, and live cells found in HM.[25]

DHA and ARA

As mentioned earlier in this chapter, DHA and ARA are LCPUFAs found in HM. They can also be converted in the body from the essential fatty acids alpha-linolenic acid and linoleic acid. The amounts of DHA and ARA in HM vary depending on maternal intake. DHA and ARA are important components of cell membrane structure and neural tissue structure and function.[26] They are the most abundant LCPUFAs in the brain and are considered important in cognitive development.[27] Most infant formulas in the United States have added DHA and ARA.

Prebiotics, Probiotics, and Synbiotics

Prebiotics are carbohydrates that are fermentable and not fully digested in the small intestine. The most common prebiotics in HM and infant formulas are fructooligosaccharides and galactoligosaccharides. These ferment and produce short-chain fatty acids, which are energy for the colonocytes. The prebiotic fibers stimulate the growth of the normal bacteria in the colon while preventing the growth of the pathogenic bacteria.[28,29]

Probiotics are live bacteria that adhere to the colon and increase the barrier function of the intestine. Prebiotics combined with probiotics are called *synbiotics*, and they may enhance the immunological function of the gut.[29] Infant formulas with prebiotics and/or probiotics have been shown to decrease duration of diarrhea related to an illness and may be protective against necrotizing enterocolitis.[28,30]

Nucleotides

Nucleotides are considered "conditionally essential" during infancy because of the increased need for them during periods of accelerated growth. These nonprotein nitrogenous compounds are precursors of nucleic acids and a component of coenzymes.[31] Research suggests that nucleotide supplementation in infant formulas supports immune function in the GI tract and may enhance mucosal recovery after intestinal injury.[32]

Milk Fat Globule Membranes

MFGMs are the newest additive to infant formulas. MFGMs are found in both HM and cow's milk. Because MFGMs are naturally present in cow's milk, they are found to some extent in any cow's milk–based infant formula. However, processing denatures MFGMs, which lessens their concentration in infant formula. Therefore, manufacturers may choose to supplement products with additional MFGMs.[33,34]

Components of the MFGMs are biologically active and important in immune function, development of the central nervous system, and digestion.[34,35] Infant formula supplemented with MFGMs appears to narrow the cognitive development gap seen between breastfed and formula-fed infants.[35]

Standard Cow's Milk–Based Formulas for Term Infants

Standard infant formulas (Table 5-6) are designed to resemble the nutrient composition of HM. In HM,

TABLE 5-6. Examples of Standard Term Infant Formulas

Indications for Use	Characteristics	Product Examples (Manufacturers)
• When human milk is unavailable or contraindicated • Human milk supplementation	• Derived from cow's milk • Designed to resemble the nutrient composition of human milk	• Enfamil NeuroPro (Mead Johnson) • Enspire (Mead Johnson) • Gerber Good Start Gentle (Gerber)[a] • Similac Advance (Abbott) • Similac Pro-Advance (Abbott)

The brand names mentioned in this table may not be the only relevant products on the market in the United States or other countries. Mention of a product does not imply an endorsement.

[a]100% partially hydrolyzed protein.

approximately 6% of energy is from protein, 40%–45% is from carbohydrate, and 50% is from fat. Term infant formulas have 19 to 20 kcal/oz. Although the energy content of HM varies, it is within a similar range.

Most standard formulas intended for term infants contain intact protein derived from cow's milk. One standard formula contains 100% partially hydrolyzed protein. (Other partially hydrolyzed formulas are further discussed later in this chapter.) The protein content in term infant formulas ranges from 2 to 2.2 g per 100 kcal and provides 8%–12% of energy. The amount of protein in term infant formula is higher than in HM to compensate for lower bioavailability.

The ratio of whey-to-casein content in HM is variable (from 80:20 early in lactation to approximately 60:40 in mature milk) but always higher than the ratio in cow's milk (18:82). The whey-to-casein ratio of standard cow's milk–based formulas varies from being the same as its original source, cow's milk protein (18:82) to being more similar to HM (80:20).

The fat source in these formulas is a blend of vegetable oils and typically provides 40%–50% of energy. Lactose is the main carbohydrate source, as it is in HM. Other sources of carbohydrate found in standard infant formula include oligosaccharides, maltodextrin, and sucrose.

Lactose-free and reduced-lactose standard infant formulas are available (Table 5-7); they contain corn syrup solids, maltodextrin, cornstarch, and sucrose as the carbohydrate sources. Because these products contain trace amounts of lactose, they are not indicated in infants with galactosemia.

The AAP recommends that infants who are formula fed receive an iron-fortified infant formula. The AAP also recommends vitamin D supplementation to meet the DRI for all infants whose formula intake is less than 32 oz/d.[25]

TABLE 5-7. Examples of Lactose-Free Standard Term Infant Formulas		
Indications for Use	**Characteristics**	**Product Examples (Manufacturers)**
• Lactose intolerance • *Not* indicated for galactosemia	• Contain trace amounts of lactose	• Similac Sensitive (Abbott) • Similac Pro-Sensitive (Abbott)

The brand names mentioned in this table may not be the only relevant products on the market in the United States or other countries. Mention of a product does not imply an endorsement.

Lower-Calorie (19 kcal/oz) Standard Infant Formulas

Most standard formulas available for term infants in the United States provide 20 kcal/oz; however, lower-calorie standard formulas (19 kcal/oz) have recently been made available. The rationale for lower-calorie products is based on published data measuring the calorie content in HM[36] and donor HM[37] as well as concerns about the incidence of childhood obesity.

In 2015 Abrams and Hawthorne conducted a systematic review of 4 European controlled trials in full-term infants to assess growth outcomes when infants were fed formulas lower in protein and energy than traditional cow's milk protein–based infant formulas.[38] Although the formulas in this investigation differed from formulas historically available in the United States, their concentrations of energy and protein were similar to calorie and protein levels in recently introduced lower-calorie products in the United States. The authors concluded that the range of protein and energy delivery from the lower-energy, lower-protein formulas is associated with adequate growth despite small variances in growth and body composition differences. The studies in the systematic review showed that full-term infants receiving formula lower in protein and energy content grew similar to breastfed infants. However, Abrams and Hawthorne suggest cautious use of these products, especially in former preterm infants and infants born small for gestational age, until further long-term studies are conducted.[38]

Notably, the Special Supplemental Nutrition Program for Women, Infants, and Children has not approved the use of 19 kcal/oz formulas. Therefore, some powdered, concentrated liquid, and RTF products may be available for both retail purchase and hospital use in both 19 kcal/oz and 20 kcal/oz concentrations. These products may have similar labels, which could lead to confusion among consumers.

Soy-Based, Lactose-Free Infant Formulas

Soy-based infant formulas (Table 5-8) contain soy protein isolate. One product contains partially hydrolyzed soy protein as the protein source. L-methionine, taurine, and L-carnitine are added to compensate for the naturally low content of these amino acids in soy protein. Soy-based infant formulas are available as 19 and 20 kcal/oz products. The protein content is 2.45–2.66 g per 100 kcal, which is slightly higher than the protein content of cow's milk–based infant formulas to compensate for the lower quality of soy protein. The fat source of soy-based infant formulas is a blend of vegetable oils. These formulas are lactose free and contain corn syrup solids, corn maltodextrin, and sucrose as the carbohydrate sources. Soy-based formulas are lower in osmolality than cow's milk–based formulas.

Soy protein isolate contains phytates, which may inhibit mineral absorption (primarily calcium, phosphorus, iron, and zinc). To compensate, the calcium and phosphorus

TABLE 5-8. Examples of Soy Protein–Based Infant Formulas

Indications for Use	Characteristics	Product Examples (Manufacturers)
• Galactosemia • Transient lactase deficiency • Cow's milk allergy if not associated with soy protein allergy • Caregiver's preference for vegetarian option	• Lactose free	• Enfamil Prosobee (Mead Johnson) • Gerber Good Start Soy (Gerber)[a] • Similac for Diarrhea (Abbott)[b] • Similac Soy Isomil (Abbott)

The brand names mentioned in this table may not constitute a comprehensive list of all relevant products on the market in the United States or other countries. Mention of a product does not imply an endorsement.

[a]Partially hydrolyzed soy protein.

[b]Contains fiber.

concentrations of soy-based formulas are approximately 30% higher compared to standard cow's milk–based formula. Soy-based formulas are fortified with iron and zinc, similar to standard cow's milk–based formulas for term infants. Their vitamin D content is similar to that of standard formula.

There has been much debate on the safety of soy-based infant formulas. A systematic review with meta-analysis was published in the *British Journal of Nutrition* in 2014.[39] The authors found that children fed soy-based infant formulas had similar anthropometric growth outcomes as children fed standard cow's milk–based formula or HM. Despite the high levels of phytates and aluminum in soy-based infant formula, the infants' serum zinc and calcium levels and bone mineral content were also found to be similar. The authors concluded that soy-based infant formulas are safe options for term infants requiring this type of formula.[39]

The AAP has provided guidelines on the indications for use of soy-based infant formulas.[40] Because soy formulas are lactose free, they are recommended for infants with galactosemia (hereditary lactase deficiency) and infants with documented transient lactase deficiency. It is also indicated when an infant who is not allergic to soy protein has an immunoglobulin E–associated allergy to cow's milk protein. Soy-based formulas are an acceptable option for a term infant whose parents seek a vegetarian alternative to cow's milk–based formula.

Due in part to the higher phytate and aluminum content of these formulas, the AAP recommends that soy protein–based formulas not be given to preterm infants with birth weights less than 1800 g.[40] These formulas do not promote optimal weight gain, linear growth, or bone mineralization in this population. Preterm infants receiving these formulas have been reported to have lower serum levels of phosphorus, higher serum levels of alkaline phosphatase, and higher frequency of osteopenia. High amounts of aluminum present in soy protein–based formulas compete with calcium absorption and may contribute to osteopenia in preterm infants.

Fruzza and colleagues have reported that soy protein interferes with the absorption of exogenous thyroid hormone used to treat congenital hypothyroidism.[41] Therefore, it is prudent to avoid soy protein–based formulas in the presence of hypothyroidism. The authors state that increased monitoring and increasing the dose of thyroid replacement therapy is warranted when infants with hypothyroidism are receiving soy protein–based formulas.

There are several additional instances when soy protein–based infant formulas are contraindicated. Soy

protein–based infant formulas are not recommended in
the prevention of colic or atopic disease. Infants with food
protein–induced enterocolitis or enteropathy should not be
fed soy-based formula because proteins from both cow's
milk and soy are the most common causes of these conditions, and 25%–64% of affected infants have allergies to
both types of proteins.[40,42] Soy-based formula containing
sucrose is contraindicated in infants with either sucrose-
isomaltase deficiency or hereditary fructose intolerance.[40]

Antiregurgitation Infant Formulas

Two standard cow's milk protein–based infant formulas
contain added rice starch to reduce reflux symptoms (Table
5-9). These products are slightly thicker in viscosity than
standard infant formulas. Because they thicken in the low
pH of the stomach, they may not be as effective when given
with an antacid. Both products are predominately casein-
based and contain 2.14–2.5 g of protein per 100 kcal. One
is lactose free and contains corn syrup solids, rice starch,
and sucrose as the carbohydrate sources. The other has a

TABLE 5-9. Examples of Infant Formulas Marketed to Reduce Regurgitation

Indications for Use	Characteristics	Product Examples (Manufacturers)
• To reduce reflux symptoms	• Contain added rice starch • Slightly higher viscosity than standard formulas	• Enfamil AR (Mead Johnson) • Similac for Spit Up (Abbott)[a]

The brand names mentioned in this table may not constitute a comprehensive list
of all relevant products on the market in the United States or other countries. Mention of a product does not imply an endorsement.

[a]Lactose free.

carbohydrate source of approximately 60% lactose, with the rest of the carbohydrate from rice starch and maltodextrin. Fat sources are vegetable oils, including safflower, sunflower, soy, coconut, and palm olein oils. Unlike standard infant formula mixed with infant cereal or thickeners, these formulas do not provide more energy from carbohydrate than standard formula would, and they flow freely through a standard nipple. Clinicians should be aware that these formulas have a slightly higher viscosity than standard formulas, so they may not flow through a feeding tube as easily, especially if the formula is concentrated.

The North American and European Societies for Pediatric Gastroenterology, Hepatology, and Nutrition updated their clinical guidelines on the management of gastroesophageal reflux disease in 2018.[43] They state that the use of antiregurgitation formula may reduce visible regurgitation; however, it is unclear if this type of formula improves other reflux symptoms or has adverse effects. The guidelines suggest considering the provision of lower volumes of formula to reduce the incidence of reflux symptoms; also, if severe symptoms persist, a trial of an extensively hydrolyzed or amino acid–based formula may be warranted.

Low-Electrolyte/Low-Mineral Infant Formula for Renal Disease

As of 2019, 1 term infant formula is marketed for use in infants with renal disease (Table 5-10). This formula is lower in phosphorus to assist in the management of hypocalcemia and hyperphosphatemia, especially in infants with impaired renal function. Protein sources include whey protein concentrate and sodium caseinate. The protein content is 2.2 g per 100 kcal. The whey-to-casein ratio is 60:40. This product has a slightly lower potential renal solute load (18.3 mOsm per 100 kcal) than standard term infant formulas

TABLE 5-10. Example of a Low-Mineral Infant Formula

Indications for Use	Characteristics	Product Example (Manufacturer)
• Renal disease	• Contains less calcium, phosphorus, and potassium than standard term infant formulas • Contains lactose	• Similac PM 60/40 (Abbott)

The brand name mentioned in this table may not constitute a comprehensive list of all relevant products on the market in the United States or other countries. Mention of a product does not imply an endorsement.

(18.6–19.6 mOsm per 100 kcal) and is isotonic. The carbohydrate source is lactose. Fat sources include safflower, soy, and coconut oils. This product is lower in calcium, phosphorus, and potassium than standard cow's milk–based formulas. It is also low in iron (0.7 mg per 100 kcal). An iron supplement is indicated for infants receiving this formula. DHA and ARA are not added to this formula. This product is available in powdered form only.

Modified-Fat Infant Formula

As of 2019, 1 infant formula that is low in LCTs and high in MCTs is marketed in the United States to meet the needs of infants with chylothorax (Table 5-11). The whey-to-casein ratio is 60:40, and the formula contains 3.5 g of protein per 100 kcal. The product is only available as a RTF commercially sterile liquid and provides 30 kcal/oz; however, the formula can be diluted with water to provide a lower energy density. This formula is lactose free and has corn syrup solids as its carbohydrate source. Fat constitutes 46% of total energy, with MCTs providing 83% of the fat. Soy oil provides the other source of fat as well as essential fatty acids.

TABLE 5-11. Example of a Modified-Fat Infant Formula		
Indications for Use	**Characteristics**	**Product Example (Manufacturer)**
• Chylothorax • Chylous ascites • Intestinal lymphangiectasia	• Low in LCTs and high in MCTs	• Enfaport (Mead Johnson)

Abbreviations: LCT, long-chain triglyceride; MCT, medium-chain triglyceride.

The brand name mentioned in this table may not constitute a comprehensive list of all relevant products on the market in the United States or other countries. Mention of a product does not imply an endorsement.

Partially Hydrolyzed Infant Formulas

Partially hydrolyzed infant formulas (Table 5-12) contain protein in the form of peptides from partially broken-down whey protein or a combination of partially hydrolyzed whey and either casein protein or whey protein concentrate solids. Partially hydrolyzed formulas have a lower concentration of intact cow's milk protein than standard term infant formulas. Compared with formulas containing extensively hydrolyzed protein, the partially hydrolyzed formulas contain cow's milk peptides and thus may elicit an allergic reaction in patients with cow's milk protein allergy.[25] The protein content in these formulas is between 2.2 and 2.3 g per 100 kcal.

These formulas are lactose free or reduced in lactose content compared with HM. In addition to or in place of lactose, other carbohydrate sources may include corn maltodextrin, corn syrup solids, and sucrose. Fat sources for these products include a blend of vegetable oils such as safflower, sunflower, soy, coconut, palm olein, and DHA and ARA.

These low-lactose products are marketed to improve symptoms such as fussiness, crying, and gas associated with

TABLE 5-12. Examples of Partially Hydrolyzed Infant Formulas

Indications for Use	Characteristics	Product Examples (Manufacturers)
• Intended to improve symptoms of fussiness, gas, and colic • *Not* intended for cow's milk protein allergy	• Lower concentration of intact cow's milk protein than in standard term infant formulas	• Enfamil NeuroPro Gentlease (Mead Johnson)[a] • Enfamil Reguline (Mead Johnson)[a] • Gerber Good Start Soothe (Gerber)[a] • Similac Total Comfort (Abbott)[b]

The brand names mentioned in this table may not constitute a comprehensive list of all relevant products on the market in the United States or other countries. Mention of a product does not imply an endorsement.

[a]Reduced lactose.

[b]Trace lactose.

lactose intolerance. Partially hydrolyzed formulas are not considered hypoallergenic, and they are not effective nor indicated for use in infants with cow's milk protein allergy.[42]

Extensively Hydrolyzed Protein Infant Formulas

Infant formulas that are considered hypoallergenic contain extensively hydrolyzed protein. Extensively hydrolyzed protein formulas (Table 5-13) contain whey and casein protein from cow's milk that has been heat-treated for hydrolysis and/or enzymatically hydrolyzed. The extensively hydrolyzed proteins are broken down into short-chain peptides and amino acids. These products are supplemented with amino acids. The protein content is 2.6–2.8 g per 100 kcal.

TABLE 5-13. Examples of Extensively Hydrolyzed Infant Formulas

Indications for Use	Characteristics	Product Examples (Manufacturers)
• Cow's milk allergy • Soy protein allergy • Fat malabsorption if formula contains medium-chain triglycerides	• Considered hypoallergenic • Lactose free	• Gerber Extensive HA (Gerber)[a] • Nutramigen (Mead Johnson) • Pregestimil (Mead Johnson)[a] • Similac Alimentum (Abbott)[a]

The brand names mentioned in this table may not constitute a comprehensive list of all relevant products on the market in the United States or other countries. Mention of a product does not imply an endorsement.

[a]Contains medium-chain triglycerides.

Extensively hydrolyzed formulas are lactose free. The carbohydrate sources are corn syrup solids, corn maltodextrin, tapioca starch, potato starch, modified cornstarch, and sucrose. According to the AAP, formulas labeled as hypoallergenic should demonstrate in clinical trials to not provoke reactions in 90% of infants with confirmed cow's milk allergy with 95% confidence.[42] The AAP recommends use of extensively hydrolyzed infant formulas in infants with cow's milk and soy protein allergies.[42]

One of the formulas in this category is indicated for infants with cow's milk protein allergy and has long-chain fatty acids (LCFAs) as its fat source. The fat source in the other 3 products in this category is a combination of LCFAs and MCTs. Infants with liver disease, cystic fibrosis, chylothorax, and intestinal failure who have fat malabsorption and lack adequate bile salt may benefit from a hydrolyzed formula containing MCTs because MCTs do not require bile salt to form a micelle for absorption.[25] The amount of fat from MCTs in these formulas is 33%–55%.

Amino Acid–Based Infant Formulas

Amino acid–based infant formulas (Table 5-14) contain 100% free amino acids. These formulas contain 2.8–3.1 g of protein per 100 kcal. Amino acid–based infant formulas are also lactose free and contain corn syrup solids and modified tapioca starch as the carbohydrate sources. The fat source is a combination of LCFAs and MCTs, with MCTs providing 33%–43% of the energy from fat. The AAP recommends that a free amino acid–based product is indicated when a formula-fed infant has severe allergies and an extensively hydrolyzed infant formula has not resolved symptoms.[25]

TABLE 5-14. Examples of Amino Acid–Based Infant Formulas		
Indications for Use	**Characteristics**	**Product Examples (Manufacturers)**
• Severe cow's milk allergy • Severe soy protein allergy • Fat malabsorption	• Contain 100% free amino acids	• Alfamino Infant (Nestlé)[a] • Elecare for Infants (Abbott)[a] • Neocate Infant (Nutricia)[a] • Neocate Syneo Infant (Nutricia)[a] • PurAmino (Mead Johnson)

The brand names mentioned in this table may not constitute a comprehensive list of all relevant products on the market in the United States or other countries. Mention of a product does not imply an endorsement.

[a]Contains medium-chain triglycerides.

Preterm Infant Enteral Formulas

Human Milk Fortifiers

The AAP recommends HM for preterm infants and advises that it should be fortified for infants born weighing less than 1500 g.[44] Commercially available pasteurized liquid HM-based fortifiers as well as liquid and powdered cow's milk protein–based fortifiers are used to increase the nutrient content of HM by providing additional energy, protein, iron, vitamin D, calcium, phosphorus, and sodium (Table 5-15).[45]

TABLE 5-15. Examples of Human Milk Fortifiers		
Indications for Use	**Characteristics**	**Product Examples (Manufacturers)**
• To fortify HM	• Concentrated products	• Enfamil HMFAL (Mead Johnson)[a]
		• Enfamil Human Milk Fortifier Powder (Mead Johnson)[a]
		• Prolacta +4 H^{2}MF (Prolacta Bioscience)[b]
		• Similac Human Milk Fortifier Concentrated Liquid (Abbott)[a]
		• Similac HMF HPCL (Abbott)[a]
		• Similac Human Milk Fortifier Powder (Abbott)[a]

The brand names mentioned in this table may not constitute a comprehensive list of all relevant products on the market in the United States or other countries. Mention of a product does not imply an endorsement.

Abbreviations: HM, human milk; HMFAL, human milk fortifier acidified liquid; HMF HPLC, human milk fortifier hydrolyzed protein concentrated liquid.

[a]Derived from cow's milk.

[b]Derived from HM.

The AAP, FDA, and CDC advise against the use of powdered formulas in neonatal intensive care units (NICUs).[4,6]

Preterm Infant Formulas

Preterm infant formulas (Table 5-16) are higher in protein, calcium, phosphorus, vitamins A and D, sodium, and other nutrients to meet the high nutrition needs of the preterm infant. They are only available as sterile liquid. They are available in 20, 24, and 30 kcal/oz RTF forms in 2-oz bottles.

Preterm infant formulas are high in protein and provide a range of 3–3.6 g of protein per 100 kcal. One brand has a whey-to-casein ratio of 80:20, and the other available product has a ratio of 60:40. Lactose is the source of 15%–50% of the carbohydrate; corn syrup

TABLE 5-16. Examples of Infant Formulas Marketed for Preterm Infants

Indications for Use	Characteristics	Product Examples (Manufacturers)
• Oral and enteral feeding of very-low-birth-weight infants when human milk is not sufficiently available	• Higher in protein and select micronutrients than standard term formulas • Available as 20, 24, and 30 kcal/oz ready-to-feed products	• Enfamil Premature High Protein (Mead Johnson) • Similac Special Care High Protein (Abbott)

The brand names mentioned in this table may not constitute a comprehensive list of all relevant products on the market in the United States or other countries. Mention of a product does not imply an endorsement.

solids and maltodextrin provide the rest. Preterm formulas are reduced in lactose because the intestinal lactase content is lower in preterm infants than in term infants. Both available preterm formulas are high in MCTs, with 40%–50% of energy from fat calories provided by MCTs. The other fat sources are coconut, soy, and sunflower oils. These products are designed to be lower in LCFAs because the intestinal content of lipase and bile salts in preterm infants is lower than in term infants.

Preterm infant formulas are indicated for oral and enteral feeding of very-low-birth-weight infants when maternal HM and donor HM are not sufficiently available.[46] These products are not intended for infants who weigh more than 3600 g because the formulas could provide excessive fat-soluble vitamins and protein to such patients.

Preterm Infant Discharge Formulas

Transitional formulas (Table 5-17) contain higher amounts of protein and minerals to support growth in preterm infants at the time of discharge from the NICU and after discharge from the hospital. They are higher in these nutrients compared with standard term infant formula and lower compared with preterm infant formula. Typically, preterm infants are transitioned from preterm infant formula to these formulas as early as 34 weeks' postmenstrual age or when preparing for discharge to home. The standard energy concentration is 22 kcal/oz, and the formulas are available in RTF and powdered forms. There is no consensus on the benefits on growth and development in infants receiving these formulas compared with standard term infant formulas.[47] Preterm infants without significant medical complications and growing well on the preterm discharge formula can be

TABLE 5-17. Examples of Transitional Infant Formulas Marketed for Preterm Infants

Indications for Use	Characteristics	Product Examples (Manufacturers)
• May promote growth in infants born prematurely who are being discharged	• Protein and select micronutrient levels are higher than in standard term formulas but lower than in preterm formulas	• Enfamil Enfacare (Mead Johnson) • Similac Neosure (Abbott)

The brand names mentioned in this table may not constitute a comprehensive list of all relevant products on the market in the United States or other countries. Mention of a product does not imply an endorsement.

transitioned to term infant formulas at 6–9 months of age; however, there is no consensus on the appropriate time to transition.[48] It is important to monitor growth in former preterm infants to allow for individualized nutrition plans.

Increasing the Nutrient Density of Infant Formulas

Infants with increased energy and protein requirements and/or those needing a fluid restriction based on their medical condition may need a formula with an increased energy density. This can be accomplished by mixing powdered infant formula or a liquid concentrate with less water than is required for standard dilution. Another option is to add a modular product. The clinician needs to consider the age and medical condition of the infant along with the components of the infant formula being concentrated when formulating a recipe with increased energy density.[49]

Modular carbohydrate and fat products have the advantage of increasing the energy concentration without significantly increasing the osmolality or renal solute load.[50] This can be important for infants with renal issues. The disadvantage of using modulars is that it alters the proportions of macronutrients in the formula and provides lower micronutrient concentrations.

Increasing the energy density using only the powdered formula or liquid concentrate maintains the macronutrient distribution and increases the micronutrient density as well. This method also increases the osmolality and renal solute load.

When a formula with more than 27 kcal/oz is to be used, consider using modular products. Monitor hydration status of infants receiving infant formulas concentrated to higher energy densities.

Modular Products

Modular products can be used to increase the energy density of infant, pediatric, and adult enteral formulas. They can be added to the formula prior to the administration of the tube feeding or mixed with water and administered as a bolus separate from the tube feeding. Available modular products include fiber, intact or extensively hydrolyzed protein, carbohydrate, MCT, emulsified LCT, and combinations of macronutrients. Specific macronutrient modular products may be used to modify the macronutrient distribution of products to meet the disease-specific needs of a patient.

Practice Resources

Manufacturer Information

Selected Manufacturers of Infant Formulas	
Manufacturer	**URL**
Abbott Nutrition	www.abbottnutrition.com
Earth's Best	https://earthsbest.com
Gerber	https://medical.gerber.com /products/formulas
The Honest Company	www.honest.com
Mead Johnson	www.meadjohnson.com /pediatrics/us-en
Nestlé Health Science	www.nestlehealthscience.us
Nutricia	www.nutriciahealthcare.com
Perrigo Nutritionals (manufacturer of store brands)	www.perrigonutritionals.com
Prolacta Bioscience	www.prolacta.com

Selected Manufacturers of Pediatric Enteral Formulas	
Manufacturer	**URL**
Abbott Nutrition	www.abbottnutrition.com
Functional Formularies	www.functionalformularies.com /nourish.html
Kate Farms	www.katefarms.com/for-clinicians
Nestlé Health Science	www.nestlehealthscience.us
Nutricia	www.nutriciahealthcare.com
RealFood Blends	www.realfoodblends.com
Vitaflo	www.nestlehealthscience.us /vitaflo-usa

ASPEN Guidelines and Resources

Boullata JI, Carrera AL, Harvey L, et al. A.S.P.E.N. safe practices for enteral nutrition therapy. *JPEN J Parenter Enteral Nutr.* 2017;41(1):15–103. doi:10.1177/0148607116673053.

Fallon EM, Nehra D, Potemkin AK, et al. A.S.P.E.N. clinical guidelines: nutrition support of neonatal patients at risk for necrotizing enterocolitis. *JPEN J Parenter Enteral Nutr.* 2012;36(5):506–523.

Jaksic T, Hull MA, Modi B, Ching A, George D, Compher C; A.S.P.E.N. Board of Directors. A.S.P.E.N. clinical guidelines: nutrition support of neonates supported with extracorporeal membrane oxygenation. *JPEN J Parenter Enteral Nutr.* 2010;34(3):247–253.

Jesuit C, Dillon C, Compher C, A.S.P.E.N. Board of Directors, Lenders CM. A.S.P.E.N. clinical guidelines: nutrition support of hospitalized pediatric patients with obesity. *JPEN J Parenter Enteral Nutr.* 2010:34(1):13–20.

Mehta NM, Skillman HE, Irving SY, et al. Guidelines for the provision and assessment of nutrition support therapy in the pediatric critically ill patient: Society of Critical Care Medicine and American Society for Parenteral and Enteral Nutrition. *JPEN J Parenter Enteral Nutr.* 2017;41(5):706–742.

Nehra D, Carlson SJ, Fallon EM, et al. A.S.P.E.N. clinical guidelines: nutrition support of neonatal patients at risk for metabolic bone disease. *JPEN J Parenter Enteral Nutr.* 2013;37(5):570–598.

Sabery N. A.S.P.E.N. clinical guidelines: nutrition support of children with human immunodeficiency virus infection. *JPEN J Parenter Enteral Nutr.* 2009;33(6):588–606.

Wales PW, Allen N, Worthington P, et al. A.S.P.E.N. clinical guidelines: support of pediatric patients with intestinal failure at risk of parenteral nutrition–associated liver disease. *JPEN J Parenter Enteral Nutr.* 2014;38(5):538–557.

References

1. Federal Food, Drug, and Cosmetic Act, §412, Title 21. Code of Federal Regulations 106,107.

2. Bankhead R, Boullata J, Brantley S, et al. Enteral nutrition practice recommendations. *JPEN J Parenter Enteral Nutr.* 2009;33:122–167.

3. 21 CFR 107: Infant formula. US Food and Drug Administration website. https://www.accessdata.fda.gov/scripts /cdrh/cfdocs/cfCFR/CFRSearch.cfm?CFRPart=107& showFR=1. Updated April 1, 2018. Accessed October 9, 2018.

4. American Academy of Pediatrics. CDC, FDA advise against powdered formula in NICUs. *AAP News.* http:// www.aappublications.org/content/20/5/219.1. Published May 1, 2002. Accessed October 9, 2018.

5. American Academy of Pediatrics Committee on Nutrition. Nutritional needs of the preterm infant. In: Kleinman RE, Greer FR, eds. *Pediatric Nutrition.* 7th ed. Elk Grove Village, IL: American Academy of Pediatrics; 2014:83–122.

6. Jason J. Prevention of invasive *Cronobacter* infections in young infants fed powdered infant formulas. *Pediatrics.* 2012;130:1–9.

7. Vermilyea S, Goh VL. Enteral feedings in children: sorting out tubes, buttons, and formulas. *Nutr Clin Pract.* 2016;31: 59–67.

8. Brown B, Roehl K, Betz M. Enteral nutrition formula selection: current evidence and implications for practice. *Nutr Clin Pract.* 2015;30:72–85.

9. Bobo E. Reemergence of blenderized tube feedings: exploring the evidence. *Nutr Clin Pract.* 2016;31(6):730–735. doi:10.1177/0884533616669703.

10. Epp L. Blenderized feeding options—the sky's the limit. *Pract Gastroenterol.* 2018;42(6):30–39.

11. Escuro AA. Blenderized tube feeding: suggested guidelines to clinicians. *Pract Gastroenterol.* 2014;38(12):58–66.

12. Walia C, VanHoorn M, Edlbeck A, Feuling MB. The registered dietitian nutritionist's guide to homemade tube feeding. *J Acad Nutr Diet.* 2017;117(1):11–16. doi:10.1016/j. jand.2016.02.007.

13. Samela K, Mokha J, Emerick K, Davidovics ZH. Transition to a tube feeding formula with real food ingredients in pediatric patients with intestinal failure. *Nutr Clin Pract.* 2017;32(2):277–281. doi:10.1177/0884533616661011.

14. Gallagher K, Flint A, Mouzaki M, et al. Blenderized Enteral Nutrition Diet Study: feasibility, clinical and microbiome outcomes of providing blenderized feeds through a gastric tube in a medically complex pediatric population. *JPEN J Parenter Enteral Nutr.* 2018; 42(6):1046–1060. doi:10.1002/jpen.1049.

15. Pentiuk S, O'Flaherty T, Santoro K, Willging P, Kaul A. Pureed by gastrostomy tube diet improves gagging and retching in children with fundoplication. *JPEN J Parenter Enteral Nutr.* 2001;35(3):375–379. doi:10.1177/0148607110377797.

16. O'Flaherty T, Santoro K, Pentiuk S. Calculating and preparing a pureed-by-gastrostomy-tube (PBGT) diet for pediatric patients with retching and gagging postfundoplication. *ICAN Infant Child Adolesc Nutr.* 2011;3(6):361–364. doi:10.1177/1941406411423702.

17. Vieira MMC, Santos VFN, Bottoni A, Morais TB. Nutritional and microbiological quality of commercial and homemade blenderized whole food enteral diets for home-based enteral nutritional therapy in adults. *Clin Nutr.* 2018; 37(1):177–181. doi:10.1016/j.clnu.2016.11.020.

18. Escuro AA, Hummel AC. Enteral formulas in nutrition support practice: is there a better choice for your patient? *Nutr Clin Pract.* 2016;31:709–722.

19. Mogensen KM. Essential fatty acid deficiency. *Pract Gastroenterol.* 2017;41(6):37–44.

20. American Academy of Pediatrics Section on Breastfeeding. Breastfeeding and the use of human milk. *Pediatrics.* 2012; 129(3):e827–e841. doi:10.1542/peds.2011-3552.

21. Centers for Disease Control and Prevention. Breastfeeding report card. United States 2014. https://www.cdc.gov/breastfeeding/pdf/2014breastfeedingreportcard.pdf. Published July 2014. Accessed October 9, 2018.

22. Healthy People 2020. https://www.healthypeople.gov. Accessed October 9, 2018.

23. Schulman AJ. A concise history of infant formula (twists and turns included). *Contemp Pediatr.* 2003;20(2):91–103. http://

www.contemporarypediatrics.com/pediatrics/concise
-history-infant-formula-twists-and-turns-included. Accessed
October 9, 2018.

24. Rossen LM, Simon AE, Herrick KA. Types of infant formulas consumed in the United States. *Clin Pediatr*. 2016;55(3):278–285.

25. American Academy of Pediatrics Committee on Nutrition. Formula feeding of term infants. In: Kleinman RE, Greer FR, eds. *Pediatric Nutrition*. 7th ed. Elk Grove Village, IL: American Academy of Pediatrics; 2014:61–82.

26. Qawasmi A, Landeros-Weisenberger A, Leckman JF, et al. Meta-analysis of long-chain polyunsaturated fatty acid supplementation of formula and infant cognition. *Pediatrics*. 2012;129:1141–1149.

27. Hadders-Algra M. Effect of long-chain polyunsaturated fatty acid supplementation on neurodevelopmental outcome in full-term infants. *Nutrients*. 2010;2:790–804.

28. Patel RM, Denning PW. Therapeutic use of prebiotics, probiotics and postbiotics to prevent necrotizing enterocolitis: what is the current evidence? *Clin Perinatol*. 2013;40(1):11–25.

29. Murguia-Peniche T, Mihatsch WA, Zegarra J, et al. Intestinal mucosal defense system, part 2: probiotics and prebiotics. *J Pediatr*. 2013;162(3 suppl):S64–S71.

30. Wall R, Ross RP, Ryan CA, et al. Role of gut microbiota in early infant development. *Clin Med Pediatr*. 2009;3:45–54.

31. Hess JR, Greenberg NA. The role of nucleotides in the immune and gastrointestinal systems: potential clinical applications. *Nutr Clin Pract*. 2012;27:281–294.

32. Singhal A, Kennedy K, Lanigan J, et al. Dietary nucleotides and early growth in formula-fed infants: a randomized controlled trial. *Pediatrics*. 2010;126:e946–e953.

33. Hernell O, Timby N, Domellöf M, Lönnerdal B. Clinical benefits of milk fat globule membranes for infants and children. *J Pediatr*. 2016;173(Suppl):S60–S65. doi:10.1016/j.jpeds.2016.02.077.

34. Billeaud C, Puccio G, Saliba E, et al. Safety and tolerance evaluation of milk fat globule membrane-enriched infant formulas: a randomized controlled multicenter non-inferiority trial in healthy term infants. *Clin Med Insights Pediatr*. 2014;8:51–60. doi:10.4137/CMPed.S16962.

35. Timby N, Domellöf E, Hernell O, Lönnerdal B, Domellöf M. Neurodevelopment, nutrition, and growth until 12 mo of age in infants fed a low-energy, low-protein formula supplemented with bovine milk fat globule membranes: a randomized controlled trial. *Am J Clin Nutr.* 2014;99(4):860–868. doi:10.3945/ajcn.113.064295.

36. de Halleux V, Rigo J. Variability in human milk composition: benefit of individualized fortification in very-low-birthweight infants. *Am J Clin Nutr.* 2013;98(suppl):529S–535S.

37. Wojcki KY, Rechtman DJ, Lee ML, Montoya A. Macronutrient analysis of a nationwide sample of donor breast milk. *J Am Diet Assoc.* 2009;109:137–140.

38. Abrams SA, Hawthorne KM. A systematic review of controlled trials of lower-protein or energy-containing infant formulas for use by healthy full-term infants. *Adv Nutr.* 2015; 6(2):178–188.

39. Vandenplas Y, Castrellon PG, Rivas R, et al. Systematic review with meta-analysis: safety of soya-based infant formulas in children. *Br J Nutr.* 2014;111(8):1340–1360.

40. Bhatia J, Greer F, Committee on Nutrition. Use of soy protein-based formulas in infant feeding. *Pediatrics.* 2008; 121(5):1062–1068.

41. Fruzza AG, Demeterco-Berggren C, Jones KL. Unawareness of the effects of soy intake on the management of congenital hypothyroidism. *Pediatrics.* 2012;13(3): e699–e702. doi:10.1542/peds.2011-3350.

42. American Academy of Pediatrics. Committee on Nutrition. Hypoallergenic infant formulas. *Pediatrics.* 2000;106(2): 346–349.

43. Rosen R, Vandenplas Y, Singendonk M, et al. Pediatric gastroesophageal reflux clinical practice guidelines: joint recommendations of the North American Society for Pediatric Gastroenterology, Hepatology, and Nutrition and the European Society for Pediatric Gastroenterology, Hepatology, and Nutrition. *J Pediatr Gastroenterol Nutr.* 2018;66(3):516–554. doi:10.1097/MPG.0000000000001889.

44. American Academy of Pediatrics Committee on Nutrition. Breastfeeding. In: Kleinman RE, Greer FR, eds. *Pediatric Nutrition.* 7th ed. Elk Grove Village, IL: American Academy of Pediatrics; 2014:41–60.

45. Ziegler EE. Human milk and human milk fortifiers. In: Koletzko B, Poindexter B, Uauy R, ed. *Nutritional Care of Preterm Infants: Scientific Basis and Practical Guidelines.* Basel, Switzerland: Karger; 2014:215–227.

46. Hay WW, Hendrickson KC. Preterm formula use in the preterm very low birth weight infant. *Semin Fetal Neonatal Med.* 2017;22(1):15–22. doi:10.1016/j.siny.2016.08.005.

47. Nzegwu NI, Ehrenkranz RA. Post-discharge nutrition and the VLBW infant: to supplement or not supplement? *Clin Perinatol.* 2014;41(2):463–474. doi:10.1016/j.clp.2014.02.008.

48. Andrew B, Pellerite M, Myers P, Hageman J. NICU follow-up: medical and developmental management age 0 to 3 years. *NeoReviews.* 2014;15(4):123–132.

49. Nevin-Folino NL, Loughead JL, Loughead ML. Enhanced-calorie formulas: considerations and options. *Neonatal Netw.* 2001;20(1):7–15.

50. Pereira-da-Silva L, Diaz MP, Virella D, Moreira AL, Serelha M. Osmolality of preterm formulas supplemented with nonprotein energy supplements. *Eur J Clin Nutr.* 2008; 62(2): 274–278.

CHAPTER 6

Enteral Nutrition Orders

Introduction

The process of communicating the enteral nutrition (EN) order involves a number of steps and includes several essential elements, which are also to be included on the patient-specific label for the dispensed EN (see Chapter 7 for additional information on labeling). The goal is to communicate the order to all healthcare providers for the benefit of the patient. The nutrition support clinician ordering EN needs to have an understanding of adult and pediatric nutrient requirements and the potential for ordering errors that can occur with an EN prescription. This chapter reviews general considerations for EN ordering, adult and pediatric nutrient dosing requirements, methods of administration, selected special considerations, and sample calculations.

General Considerations

Ordering decisions should factor in patient-specific variables, such as current disease state, nutrition status, available enteral access, condition of the gastrointestinal (GI) tract, and estimated age-specific nutrition requirements. An institution should construct an EN formulary that is broad enough to provide for the nutrition needs of its patients without becoming overwhelming to manage. See Chapter 1 for discussion of nutrition assessment, Chapter 3 for details about enteral access, and Chapter 4 for additional information on formularies.

Nutrient Requirements

Nutrient requirements for EN can reasonably be based on the Dietary Reference Intakes (DRIs).[1] These nutrient standards are based on data generated from epidemiological, depletion-repletion, and clinical intervention studies using appropriate indicators of nutrient adequacy, including clinical and functional outcome markers. The DRIs—or, more specifically, the Recommended Dietary Allowances (RDAs) and Adequate Intakes (AIs)—are estimates for healthy individuals to prevent deficiencies and minimize the risk from nutrition-related chronic disease and developmental disorders. Therefore, nutrition support clinicians must recognize certain inherent limitations about the application of RDAs and AIs for patients receiving EN. First, the DRIs are designed to be met from a usual diet. Also, although the RDAs and AIs take individual variability into account, the DRIs are not intended for use in people with acute or chronic disease.

Enteral formulas can provide daily vitamin and mineral intakes to achieve requirements for most individuals (adults and pediatrics). However, some patients may require additional micronutrient supplementation. Clinicians should

---

TABLE 6-1. Practice Recommendations for Determining Nutrient Requirements

1. Determination of nutrient requirements should be individualized, based on assessment of body composition and function, and fall within acceptable ranges, while taking physiological and pathophysiological conditions into account.
2. When determining requirements for pediatric patients, also consider the individual's needs with regard to growth and development.

---

assess patients for signs and symptoms of nutrient deficiencies and use clinical judgment regarding the appropriateness of administering micronutrient supplements. See Table 6-1 for practice recommendations related to nutrient requirements.

Adult Patients

The usual maintenance goals for energy and protein for adult patients receiving EN are presented in Table 6-2.[2,3]

According to the third edition of *The ASPEN Adult Nutrition Support Core Curriculum*,[4] initial fluid needs (mL/d) can be estimated for adults by calculating the average of results from the following 2 formulas:

- **Equation 1** (based on body weight and age):
  - Ages 18–55 years: 35 mL × Body Weight (kg)
  - Ages 56–75 years: 30 mL × Body Weight (kg)
  - Ages > 75 years: 25 mL × Body Weight (kg)
- **Equation 2** (Holliday-Segar formula adjusted for age):
  - Ages ≤ 50 years: 1500 mL for First 20 kg Body Weight + [20 mL × Remaining Body Weight (kg)]
  - Ages > 50 years: 1500 mL for First 20 kg Body Weight + [15 mL × Remaining Body Weight (kg)]

TABLE 6-2. Estimated Energy and Protein Requirements for Adult Patients		
Parameter	Critically Ill Patients	Stable Patients
Energy, kcal/kg/d	25–30	20–30
Protein, g/kg/d	1.5–2	1–1.5

Source: Data are from references 2 and 3.

When using such estimates, clinicians must exercise careful clinical judgment regarding the individual's fluid status. Fluid prescriptions should take into account the patient's weight, age, and clinical condition and address any additional fluid losses that require replacement.[4]

Pediatric Patients and Neonates

The usual goals for energy, protein, and fluid intake for pediatric patients are presented in Tables 6-3, 6-4, and 6-5.[5] For guidelines on usual vitamin, mineral, and electrolyte requirements, refer to the DRIs.[1]

TABLE 6-3. Daily Energy Requirements for Pediatric Patients	
Age Group	Energy Requirements,[a] kcal/kg/d
Preterm neonates	90–120
<6 mo	85–105
6–12 mo	80–100
1–7 y	75–90
7–12 y	60–75
12–18 y	30–50

[a]Assumes normal age-related organ function and normal losses.

Source: Adapted with permission from reference 5: Ayers P, Guenter P, Holcombe B, Plogsted S, eds. *A.S.P.E.N. Parenteral Nutrition Handbook*. 2nd ed. Silver Spring, MD: American Society for Parenteral and Enteral Nutrition; 2014:124.

TABLE 6-4. Daily Protein Requirements for Pediatric Patients

Age or Weight Group	Protein Requirements,[a] g/kg/d
Preterm neonates	3–4
Birth to age 1 y	2–3
Weight >10 kg or ages 1–10 y	1–2
Ages 11–17 y	0.8–1.5

[a]Assumes normal age-related organ function and normal losses.

Source: Adapted with permission from reference 5: Ayers P, Guenter P, Holcombe B, Plogsted S, eds. *A.S.P.E.N. Parenteral Nutrition Handbook*. 2nd ed. Silver Spring, MD: American Society for Parenteral and Enteral Nutrition; 2014:124.

TABLE 6-5. Daily Fluid Requirements for Pediatric Patients

Body Weight	Fluid Requirements,[a] mL/kg
<1–1.5 kg	150
1.5–2.5 kg	120
First 10 kg	100
Second 10 kg	50
Each additional kg	20

[a]Assumes normal age-related organ function and normal losses.

Source: Adapted with permission from reference 5: Ayers P, Guenter P, Holcombe B, Plogsted S, eds. *A.S.P.E.N. Parenteral Nutrition Handbook*. 2nd ed. Silver Spring, MD: American Society for Parenteral and Enteral Nutrition; 2014:125.

Methods of Administration

EN may be administered as bolus, intermittent, continuous, or volume-based feedings.

- *Bolus feedings* deliver a specific volume of formula, typically using either a syringe or gravity drip via a feeding container, over a short period of time (eg, <30 minutes). Bolus feeding may be more physiological than intermittent or continuous feedings because bolus feedings tend to mimic the normal intake of an oral diet. Bolus feedings also may help prevent constipation by inducing the gastrocolic reflex.

- *Intermittent feedings* are delivered via a feeding container or bag for 30–60 minutes, with or without the use of an enteral feeding pump.[6]
- *Continuous feedings* are feedings administered using a feeding pump at a constant hourly rate of EN administration; they may be provided around the clock or as a cyclic feeding (eg, administered for 8 hours nightly).
- With *volume-based feedings*, a total volume of EN to be administered in 24 hours is prescribed and there is an option to adjust the administration rate from time to time within the 24-hour period, as long as the required total volume is administered.

Initiation and Advancement of Enteral Feedings

Adult Patients

There are limited prospective data to form strong recommendations regarding the best starting administration rate for initiation of enteral feeding. Stable patients tolerate a fairly rapid progression of EN, generally reaching the established goal within 24 to 48 hours of initiation.[7] Initiating EN with "half-strength" or diluted enteral formulas is unnecessary, and the lower osmolality and higher pH of diluted formulas may increase the risk of microbial contamination.[8]

Bolus Feedings and Intermittent Feedings

Bolus and intermittent feedings are intended for gastric feeding; bolus feeding directly into the small bowel can lead to abdominal pain, distention, and diarrhea. Gastric feedings may be initiated with full-strength formula 3 to 8 times per day, with increases of 60 to 120 mL every 8 to 12 hours, as tolerated, up to the goal volume (ie, the amount of formula that closely meets the patient's predicted nutrient needs). When additional water is necessary to meet fluid requirements, it is administered as intermittent flushes throughout the day. Monitoring of GI tolerance is essential in formula titration toward the goal.

Pump-Assisted Feedings

A pump is generally required for small bowel feedings and is preferred for gastric feedings in critically ill patients because the slower administration rate of continuous feedings often enhances tolerance while decreasing the risks of complications. Pump-assisted feedings are also used when a volume-based feeding protocol is followed.

Conservative initiation and advancement rates are recommended for patients who are critically ill and those who have not been fed enterally for an extended period of time. In practice, formulas are frequently initiated at 10–40 mL/h and advanced to the goal rate in increments of 10–20 mL/h every 8 to 12 hours, as tolerated. This approach can usually be used with isotonic formulas as well as high-osmolality or elemental products.[9] There is some evidence that EN can begin at goal rates in stable, adult patients.[6,10]

Pediatric Patients

When determining the best way to deliver the EN prescription, the patient's status and current clinical condition should be considered. For example, in critically ill patients with labile hemodynamics or children with significant malabsorption, continuous feeds may be the safest course of action and promote optimal nutrient absorption. In stable children, bolus or intermittent feedings will more closely mimic what the child's normal diet would have been if the patient were able to ingest food orally.[11]

Initiation and advancement of enteral feedings in pediatric patients is guided by clinical judgment and institutional practices in the absence of prospective controlled clinical trials. Generally, children are started on an isotonic formula and the rate is advanced based on feeding tolerance, with the goal of providing 25% of total energy needs on Day 1.[12] When giving gastric feedings, it is possible to concentrate formula once feeding tolerance is demonstrated, which allows fluid-restricted children to receive more calories.

For patients fed via the gastric route, bolus feedings can be considered. Bolus feeds should not be given over a shorter period of time than the child would be expected to consume an oral feeding and should not be spaced out at intervals longer than normal age-based mealtimes.

Children may receive a combination of daytime bolus feeds and nighttime continuous feeds. Continuous feeds may be better tolerated overnight due to decreased risk of gastroesophageal reflux. For children at home, continuous feeds overnight may also be a more practical regimen for caregivers.[13]

However, continuous feeds given via short-term enteral access (eg, nasogastric or nasojejunal tubes) should be used with caution, especially in the home setting where 24-hour continuous monitoring may not be available. The feeding tube could be dislodged and pose an aspiration risk if feedings are inadvertently infused above the esophageal-gastric sphincter.

In general, infant feeding intervals should be every 3–4 hours for a total of 6–8 feeds per day. Older children may tolerate their full daily volume with 4–5 bolus feedings per day or a combination of daytime bolus and nighttime continuous feedings. Maximum volumes for continuous and bolus feedings are determined by the child's response to the regimen, weight gains, and overall GI status.

Bolus Feedings

To initiate bolus feeds, first determine the daily goal volume of formula and then divide the volume into the desired number of bolus feeds. Initiate full-strength bolus feeds at 25% of the goal and increase the daily volume by 25%, as tolerated, up to the goal volume.[8] Infants generally eat every 2–3 hours; therefore, bolus feeds should be given in a similar manner, such as a feeding every 3 hours around the clock (~8 feeds per day). Older children may be able to tolerate their full volume in 4–5 feeds per day given every 3–4 hours during the day and not require feedings overnight.

Bolus feedings may be given by several methods. The syringe bolus method involves pouring formula into a standard 60 mL syringe and allowing it to flow into the tube by gravity. The gravity bag method uses special bags with a roller clamp on the tubing that allows the formula to flow faster or slower into the tube; this method usually delivers the feed more slowly than the syringe bolus method. Infants and small children are often given their bolus feeds on a feeding pump. The pump can be set to deliver bolus or intermittent feeds at a predetermined rate. An example of a bolus feed via pump would be 90 mL every 3 hours, given over 1 hour via pump at 90 mL/h.

Pump-Assisted (Continuous) Feedings

Continuous EN administered via pump is required if the patient is being fed postpylorically and is recommended if the patient is critically ill, is hemodynamically unstable, or has significant malabsorption. Full-strength, continuous EN via pump can be initiated at 1 to 2 mL/kg/h and advanced by 1–2 mL/kg/h every 8 hours, as tolerated, until the goal volume is achieved.[14]

Special Considerations

Critically Ill Children

EN is the preferred mode of nutrient delivery and can be safely provided to critically ill infants and children with a wide variety of diagnoses when the GI tract is functional. However, pediatric intensive care unit (PICU) patients may not tolerate the initiation and advancement recommendations for the non–critically ill child.

Achieving at least two-thirds of the prescribed energy intake within 5 to 7 days of PICU admission has been associated with lower 60-day mortality and improved outcomes.[15] Initiating EN within 24–48 hours of PICU admission is recommended[16] and has been associated with improved clinical outcomes. Institutional guidelines using a stepwise, algorithmic approach should be in place to guide initiation and advancement, assess tolerance, and monitor delivery of the prescribed amounts. A nutrition support team, including a dietitian, is an integral part of the PICU team and can help to ensure timely and appropriate nutrition interventions throughout the course of therapy.[16]

The 2017 guidelines for the provision and assessment of nutrition support therapy in the pediatric critically ill patient from the Society of Critical Care Medicine and American Society for Parenteral and Enteral Nutrition (ASPEN) suggest that the gastric route may be preferred for patients in the PICU, based on available observational studies and a weak GRADE (Grading of Recommendations, Assessment, Development, and Evaluations) recommendation.[16] There is not enough evidence to determine whether continuous or intermittent gastric feeding would be optimal. In patients who are unable to tolerate gastric feeding and those at high risk for aspiration, postpyloric feeds may be preferable.

Energy needs in critically ill pediatric patients vary widely, and patients in the PICU should be reevaluated frequently to ensure the appropriateness of the energy prescription. If indirect calorimetry (IC) is available, it should be used to determine the energy requirements and guide daily order adjustments. If IC is unavailable, the use of the RDAs or Harris-Benedict equations is not recommended. The Schofield or Food Agriculture Organization/World Health Organization/United Nations University equations may be used to predict energy expenditure in critically ill pediatric patients.[17–19] Stress factors may be added to these calculations based on the clinical condition of the individual patient.

When predictive equations are used to estimate energy needs, patients should be routinely monitored for potential signs of overfeeding, such as elevations in glucose, triglyceride, or carbon dioxide levels, and signs of underfeeding, such as prolonged ventilator dependence and increased length of PICU stay. Anthropometric measurements such as weight and mid–upper arm circumference can also be used to monitor adequacy of energy prescription, although availability and accuracy of these values can be an issue in the critically ill patient.[16]

Protein requirements are elevated during critical illness; therefore, using the RDA values to determine protein goals is not recommended for critically ill patients. Optimal protein dosages for critically ill pediatric patients are not known. Observational studies have indicated a positive association between higher protein delivery and clinical outcomes. A minimum protein intake of at least 1.5 g/kg/d is recommended to prevent cumulative negative protein balance, with greater amounts recommended for infants and young children.[20,21] Modular protein supplements may be required in addition to the enteral formula to fully meet the elevated protein requirements of critical illness.

Preterm Infants

Infants with growth failure are at risk for poor developmental outcomes. In addition, poor growth can contribute to hospital complications—such as necrotizing enterocolitis (NEC), infection and sepsis, and bronchopulmonary dysplasia—as well as longer-term problems, such as increased incidence of cerebral palsy and neurodevelopmental deficits.[22] Early EN stimulates gut motility and maturation, and human milk (HM), which has important anti-infectious effects, can be protective against feeding intolerance, NEC, and late-onset sepsis.[23,24]

Infants with NEC have been shown to have significantly more neurodevelopmental impairment than age-matched peers.[25] Whether that outcome is inevitable or can be changed by nutrition intervention is not known. Parenteral nutrition is the initial mode of nutrition support for the premature infant and should be started as soon as possible after birth.[26] The timing of the initiation of EN depends on the gestational age of the infant and the patient's clinical condition. The concern about NEC governs the timing and advancement of enteral feedings. Research has been conducted for over 40 years, but investigations to date have failed to identify the optimal feeding method to prevent NEC.[26] Current recommendations include exclusive use of HM, rather than cow's milk–based products or formula; initiating minimal EN within the first 2 days of life; and advancing EN by 30 mL/kg/d for infants weighing 1000 g or more.[27] For infants weighing less than 1000 g, starting EN at a more conservative rate of 15–20 mL/kg/d and advancing the volume by 15–20 mL/kg/d may be warranted.[28] The safety of early EN initiation and the relatively faster advancement rate have been confirmed in recent studies as well as a 2017 Cochrane review of 10 randomized controlled trials involving 3753 infants. That review found no increase in NEC when EN was advanced at a faster rate (30–40 mL/kg/d) versus a slower rate (15–20 mL/kg/d).[29] This meta-analysis also concluded that slower advancement resulted in several days' delay in establishing full EN and may have been associated with an increased risk of invasive infection.[29]

Feeding infants HM exclusively also seems to be protective against NEC. Infants who exclusively receive HM, including those who are provided supplementation with banked donor HM and HM-based fortifier, have demonstrated reduced incidence of NEC compared with infants who receive preterm infant formula or a cow's milk–based fortifier.[30–32] Use of standardized feeding protocols and earlier fortification of HM have been shown to improve growth for infants receiving HM exclusively.[33] However, infants fed HM and HM-based fortifiers exclusively may have poorer rates of weight gain and growth when compared with those who are fed cow's milk–based fortifiers and formula. Consequently, the optimal regimen remains unclear.[34]

The optimal frequency and route of EN delivery is unclear. In theory, postpyloric feedings are advantageous because of the decreased potential for gastroesophageal reflux and aspiration into the lungs. However, feeding by this route may impair the secretion of intestinal hormones and growth factors.[35] This method also bypasses the stomach, whose acidic environment serves as a barrier against potentially pathogenic organisms. Placing a postpyloric feeding tube is a challenge, and there are reports of complications, including intestinal perforation and pyloric stenosis.[36,37] Based on the limited evidence available, postpyloric feeds do not seem to offer increased benefit over the gastric route.

The advantages and disadvantages of continuous vs intermittent EN in preterm infants are also frequently debated. Historical trials have pointed toward a worsening of respiratory complications with bolus feeds.[38,39] The continuous feeding method may reach goal feeding volumes faster and promote a faster weight gain.[40,41] A 2011 Cochrane review tried to answer the question of which feeding method was best for premature infants weighing less than 1500 g.[42] In a review of 7 trials with over 500 infants, the authors did not find adequate evidence to determine the best feeding method for low-birth-weight premature infants. Subgroup analysis did reveal faster weight gain and a trend toward earlier discharge for infants weighing less than 1000 g who were fed continuous nasogastric feeds.[42]

It is important to note that there are varying degrees of NEC, as well as medical vs surgical types. Patients with moderate to severe medical NEC or surgical NEC require extremely conservative initiation and advancement of enteral feedings. See Table 6-6 for additional guidance on feedings for premature infants.[27–29]

Postoperative Initiation of Enteral Feedings

Traditionally, clinicians were taught that postoperative feedings should wait until there is evidence that (a) bowel function has returned (as evidenced by flatus or a bowel movement) and (b) the effects of the anesthetic have diminished enough that the patient can protect the airway when swallowing. This teaching was not based on any studies but reflected the fear that early postoperative feedings were associated with complications. For example, it was thought that narcotic pain control might result in an ileus and a patient who was fed too soon could vomit and aspirate.

These traditional assumptions have been challenged by a variety of studies supporting earlier postoperative initiation of feedings. For example, the change in approach is clearly demonstrated in an article by Collier and colleagues about the enteral feeding of patients with an open abdomen following trauma.[43] In this retrospective review, patients with

> **TABLE 6-6.** Practice Recommendations for Premature Infant Feedings
>
> 1. For premature infants weighing ≥1000 g who are at risk for NEC, minimal EN should be initiated within the first 2 days of life at 30 mL/kg/d and advanced by 30 mL/kg/d to a goal of 150–180 mL/kg/d.
> 2. For premature infants weighing <1000 g at risk for NEC, minimal EN should be initiated within the first 2 days of life at 15–20 mL/kg/d and increased by 15–20 mL/kg/d to a goal of 150–180 mL/kg/d.
> 3. Strong consideration should be given to the exclusive use of human milk and human milk–based fortifiers for premature infants at risk for NEC.
> 4. Institution-specific standardized feeding protocols for initiation and advancement of feeds should be used for preterm infants whenever clinically appropriate.

Abbreviations: EN, enteral nutrition; NEC, necrotizing enterocolitis.

Source: Information is from references 27–29.

an open abdomen who were fed within 4 days of celiotomy had earlier wound closure, fewer fistulas, and lower hospital charges when compared with patients whose enteral feedings were initiated more than 4 days after celiotomy.

The patients of greatest concern with regard to EN complications are those who undergo a form of GI surgery. However, in a randomized controlled trial of patients undergoing elective segmental intestinal or rectal resection, investigators used a protocol to introduce solids the evening of postoperative Day 1, without waiting for flatus or a stool, and found that these patients were discharged earlier and had no increase in complications compared with patients receiving traditional care.[44] Another prospective study began a regular diet at 8 hours after GI surgery and found good tolerance.[45]

In another investigation, patients undergoing gastrectomy for gastric cancers were randomly assigned to either a solid diet on demand or the conventional regimen in which a solid diet was initiated on Day 10 after surgery. Compared with the control group, the patients in the on-demand group had improved clinical outcomes, were able to tolerate an oral diet sooner, and had shorter hospitalizations.[46]

Malhotra and associates studied patients presenting emergently with enteric perforations complicated by sepsis and peritonitis.[47] Half of the participants were randomly assigned to receive nasogastric feedings within 48 hours of surgery. Compared with the controls, the patients who received early feedings had no increase in complications and experienced less weight loss.[47]

In a multicenter prospective trial, newborns begun on small feedings by nasogastric tube within 24 hours of surgery for GI anomalies, without waiting for flatus or stool passage, were compared with a control group who were fasted until resolution of postoperative ileus. The early feeding group tolerated the feedings without complications and were discharged sooner than the control group.[48]

Lewis and colleagues conducted a meta-analysis of 11 studies that began feedings within 24 hours of surgery compared with a standard waiting period. The analysts concluded that there is no advantage to waiting and found that patients receiving early feedings had a lower infection rate and were discharged 0.84 days sooner.[49]

Very few complications have been reported with early postoperative feedings. The most serious complication has been bowel necrosis; a review of 9 studies in which enteral feedings were responsible for bowel ischemia found necrosis rates ranging between 1% and 12%.[50] The authors of this review indicated that abdominal distention, sepsis, or worsening general condition should prompt evaluation and discontinuation of enteral feedings.[50]

The studies reviewed here and others like them are difficult to compare because of the wide variety of surgeries done before the trials. There is also little literature regarding the optimal composition of the first feedings or the rate at which they should be initiated and advanced. See Table 6-7 for practice recommendations for the initiation of EN after surgery.[44,45]

Initiation of Feedings After Placement of a Long-Term Enteral Access Device

Several studies of EN after percutaneous endoscopic gastrostomy (PEG) placements in adults have been published. Two studies with more than 20 patients in each group found no difference in complications with patients fed 3 hours after placement, compared with those fed the following day.[51,52] In another study, adults were administered 50 mL of diatrizoate sodium into PEGs 3 hours after placement, and no evidence of leakage was found in X-ray of the abdomen.[53] In a more rigorous study, adult patients were randomly assigned to receive formula feedings at 4 hours or 24 hours after PEG placement. This study, which had over 50 patients in each group and measured post-feeding residuals, noted no differences in the incidence of complications or in the amount of gastric residuals.[54]

TABLE 6-7. Practice Recommendation for Initiating Feedings Postoperatively

Enteral feedings should be started postoperatively in surgical patients without waiting for flatus or a bowel movement.
The current literature indicates that these feedings can be initiated within 24 to 48 hours.

Source: Information is from references 44 and 45.

In a review paper, Kirby and colleagues described their first 55 PEG placements and stated that they began a trial administration of water at 2 hours postprocedure without increased complications.[55] According to the abstract of an article published in Spanish, a randomized trial compared a group of patients who began feeding within 30 minutes after PEG placement with a control group who were not fed for 24 hours postprocedure, and no notable differences in the complication rates were found between the 2 groups.[56]

EN can be initiated safely in pediatric patients within 6 hours of gastrostomy tube placement, whether the tube was inserted using a percutaneous endoscopic, laparoscopic, or open placement method. Earlier initiation of EN following gastrostomy placement may result in shorter hospital length of stay and is not associated with increased complications.[57] See Table 6-8 for practice recommendations regarding initiation of EN after placement of a gastrostomy tube.[51–57]

Best Practices in Enteral Nutrition Orders

The use of standardized EN orders offers many advantages. These include the prevention of errors of omission/commission, the standardization of terminology, and—most importantly—the protection of patient safety.

TABLE 6-8. Practice Recommendation for Initiating Feedings After Placement of a Gastrostomy Tube

A gastrostomy tube may be used for feedings within several hours of placement. Current literature supports the initiation of feeding within 2 hours in adults and 6 hours in infants and children.

Source: Information is from references 51–57.

Elements of the Order

According to ASPEN recommendations, patient-specific EN orders should always include the following 4 essential elements: (a) patient information; (b) EN formula name; (c) delivery route and access device; and (d) administration method and rate.[8] Additionally, orders should include the water flush type, volume, and frequency and may include other ancillary or supplemental elements. Crucial information about the EN prescription must be provided on the labeled product as well as in the order. (See Chapter 7 for more information on labeling requirements.)

Patient Information

The order should clearly state the patient's name, date of birth, weight, location, and medical record number. Other relevant information such as allergies and dosing weight should be included.[8]

EN Formula Name

The formula should be clearly identified in the order by a descriptive generic name, and the use of product-specific names should be avoided entirely or secondary to the use of the generic term. Examples of generic names (which should be standardized by the organization) include "standard," "isotonic," "calorie-dense," "semi-elemental," and "peptide-based." The rationale for using generic names is to minimize prescriber confusion. For pediatric patients, the final energy concentration (kcal/oz) should be noted with the formula name.[8]

Formula orders should also include options for the administration of modular products used to enhance the protein, carbohydrate, fat, or fiber content of the enteral regimen. In the adult population, these products are usually not added to enteral formula. Instead, they are administered separately to the patient via the enteral access device. Orders for modulars should indicate the prescribed amounts, the frequency of administration, and other instructions. In the neonatal and pediatric population, fluid tolerance limits are a concern; therefore, the base formula is often augmented with a modular macronutrient. When this type of manipulation to infant or pediatric formula is prescribed, the base formula, the modular product, and the base and final concentration of formula per 100 kcal are all considered.[58,59] If modulars are added to infant or pediatric formula in the home setting, it is important to teach the parents or caregivers the proper method to prepare a formula with additives. See Chapters 4, 5, and 7 for additional information on modular products.

Delivery Site (Route) and Enteral Access Device

The order must clearly identify the delivery site (route) for formula administration.[6] This information, which is based on the enteral tube's distal tip position (gastric or small bowel), helps prevent wrong-site connections and errors in administration. Multiple instances of enteral misconnections have been reported in the literature.[60] Additionally, the order must document the specific enteral access device to be used (eg, nasogastric, orogastric, gastrostomy, nasojejunal, orojejunal, jejunostomy, or gastrojejunostomy).[8]

Administration Method and Rate

The administration method (bolus, gravity, or continuous feeds), volume or rate of administration, and timing of formula delivery within a specified period of time (24 hours, cyclic or volume-based rates) should all be clearly set forth in an EN order.[8]

Additional Orders

An EN order can be entered as a single order representing a specific prescription, or multiple orders can be made as part of a larger protocol that directs advancement of EN from initiation to a goal rate or volume that represents a nutritionally adequate endpoint. The inclusion of transitional orders will direct weaning from EN, and supplemental orders may address various patient-care issues related to EN.

Any additional orders that differ from the standard formula rate, route, and volume prescriptions should be clearly documented.[8] These types of orders can include the following:

- *Advancement orders:* These orders direct the progression of an EN regimen from initiation through to an endpoint or goal formula volume over a specified time period. Increases in formula volume or rate of administration to achieve a goal should be clearly stated. EN advancement orders also need to be coordinated with decreases in parenteral nutrition or intravenous fluids.
- *Transitional orders:* These orders document incremental decreases in formula volume over a period of time to accommodate increases in oral intake.
- *Ancillary or supplemental orders:* Routine or ancillary orders depend on both the population and the setting. These orders are based on institutional policies for care of the enterally fed patient, such as orders for flushing the enteral access device, head-of-bed elevation, weight checks, and the monitoring of laboratory parameters. Supplemental orders could also include orders to confirm enteral access device

position, nutrition support service consultation, or pharmacy consult for enteral drug administration.

Enteral Nutrition Order Forms

Orders may be entered through a computerized prescriber order entry (CPOE) system or using a standardized electronic template. When the standardized order is incorporated into an electronic health record, further protection is added against inappropriate orders involving omissions or transcription errors. Paper forms should be used only if CPOE or electronic forms are unavailable. Completely handwritten orders and telephone orders should be avoided to minimize the possibility of transcription errors. Only those abbreviations, acronyms, symbols, and numerical expressions considered acceptable by the institution should be used in the EN ordering process.[8]

Whether built into a CPOE system or on a hard copy, the EN order form must contain the 4 essential elements of an EN order and include transitional and supplemental orders.[8] The example in Figure 6-1 should be adapted to meet the needs of each individual institution.

Many institutional settings use CPOE systems, which should address each of the elements shown in Figure 6-1 (eg, a separate screen in sequence for each element). Ideally, CPOE should also provide clinical decision support. For example, if a postpyloric enteral access device order is selected, the intermittent administration delivery screen(s) would not be an option. These systems should be designed with detailed order sets that promote safety by using drop-down menus within each element of an EN order, including required fields, with limited opportunity to enter any information as free text. Such menus

FIGURE 6-1

INPATIENT ENTERAL NUTRITION ORDER	
Patient Name:_____	Medical Record Number: _____
Room Number:_____	Date of Birth:_____
Dosing Weight (kg):_____	Allergies: _____
Total energy (kcal/day): _____	Total protein (g/day): _____
Total carbohydrate (g/day): _____	Total fat (g/day): _____
Total fluid (mL/day): _____	

ENTERAL NUTRITION FORMULA

□ Standard □ Carbohydrate-controlled
□ Standard high-protein □ Elemental including peptide-based
□ Standard high-calorie □ Immune-modulating
□ Fiber-containing □ Renal—low electrolytes

DELIVERY SITE (Route and Access)

Route:	□ Gastric	□ Small bowel	
Access:	□ Nasogastric	□ Nasoduodenal	□ Nasojejunal
	□ Orogastric	□ Oroduodenal	□ Orojejunal
	□ Gastrostomy	□ Jejunostomy	□ Transgastric G/J tube

ADMINISTRATION (Method and Rate)

Method:	**Rate**:
Continuous	□ Initial _____ mL/h
	□ Advance by _ mL/h every __ h to goal of ___ mL/h
Intermittent	□ Initial __ mL feeding over __ min ____ times daily
	□ Advance by __ mL each day to goal of __ mL feeding over _____ min ____ times daily
Bolus	□ Initial __ mL bolus over ____ min ___ times daily
	□ Advance by __ mL each day to goal of _ mL bolus over ____ min ___ times daily

OTHER

□ Flush feeding tube with _____ mL of water every _____ hours (minimum of 30 mL per flush)
□ Elevate head of bed 30–45 degrees

Example of inpatient enteral nutrition order. G/J, gastrojejunostomy. Adapted with permission from reference 8: Boullata J, Carrera AL, Harvey L, et al. ASPEN safe practices for enteral nutrition therapy. *JPEN J Parenter Enteral Nutr.* 2017;41(1): 15–103. doi:10.1177/0148607116673053.

may facilitate standardized advancement of initial administrations to goal volumes, uniform enteral access device flushing volumes and methods, and population-specific ancillary orders. See Table 6-9 for a summary of practice recommendations for EN ordering.[8]

TABLE 6-9. Practice Recommendations for Enteral Nutrition Ordering

1. Develop and design standardized EN orders (CPOE or editable electronic templates, or paper as a last resort) for adult and pediatric EN regimens to aid prescribers in meeting each patient's nutrition needs and to improve order clarity.
2. Include all critical elements in the EN orders: (1) patient identifiers, (2) the formula name, (3) the EAD site/device, (4) the administration method and rate, plus (5) water flush type, volume, and frequency. Incorporate the feeding advancement order, transitional orders, and implementation of complementary orders into protocols. All elements of the EN order must be completed when EN is modified or reordered.
3. Avoid the use of unapproved abbreviations or inappropriate numerical expressions.
4. Encourage the use of generic terms to describe EN formulas. All elements of the EN order must be completed when EN is modified or reordered.
5. Provide clear instructions related to modular products, including product dose, administration method, rate, and frequency.
6. Establish and enforce policies and procedures that clearly describe the preparation of powdered EN products, including who will evaluate compatibility, measure the dose, reconstitute the product, what diluent and source will be used, the location of preparation, labeling including beyond use date and time, and storage.

Abbreviations: CPOE, computerized prescriber order entry; EAD, enteral access device; EN, enteral nutrition.

Source: Reprinted with permission from reference 8: Boullata J, Carrera AL, Harvey L, et al. ASPEN safe practices for enteral nutrition therapy. *JPEN J Parenter Enteral Nutr.* 2017;41(1):15–103. doi:10.1177/0148607116673053.

Sample Calculations

Figure 6-2 illustrates one method of calculating the appropriate EN prescription of formula and water for an adult patient. Figure 6-3 shows the calculations for a fluid-restricted patient requiring EN with similar provision of energy and protein. Figure 6-4 provides a sample of the calculations for a pediatric patient.

FIGURE 6-2

Case: A 56-year-old male status post cerebrovascular accident with persistent dysphagia and 2 failed swallow studies has a percutaneous endoscopic gastrostomy (PEG) placed. He is to be initiated on continuous enteral nutrition (EN) via PEG. His dosing weight is 60 kg.

Calculations:

1. Select formula for this patient.

   Example: Standard 1.5 kcal/mL formula, 75 g protein per 1000 mL, 775 mL water per 1000 mL formula (77.5% water)

2. Determine the patient's energy requirement (kcal/d).

   Example: 60-kg patient requiring 30 kcal/kg/d = 1800 kcal/d

3. Divide the energy requirement (kcal/d) by the energy concentration in the formula (kcal/mL) to determine the volume of formula needed (mL/d).

   Example: 1800 kcal/d ÷ 1.5 kcal/mL = 1200 mL/d

4. Determine the continuous infusion rate (mL/h) by dividing the volume of enteral formula (mL/d) by 24 hours.

   Example: 1200 mL/d ÷ 24 hours = 50 mL/h

5. Determine the protein dose (g/d) by multiplying the volume of formula to be administered (mL/d) by the formula's protein concentration (g/1000 mL).

   Example: 1200 mL/d × 75 g/1000 mL = 90 g/d

(continued)

FIGURE 6-2 *(Continued)*

6. Determine the patient's fluid requirement (mL/d).

   Example: 1 mL/kcal = 1800 mL/d

7. Determine the formula's water contribution (mL/d) by multiplying the volume of enteral formula to be administered (mL/d) by the percentage of water in the formula.

   Example: 1200 mL/d × 77.5% = 930 mL/d

8. Determine the total volume of water flushes (mL/d) by subtracting the volume of water from formula (mL/d) from the fluid requirement (mL/d).

   Example: 1800 mL/d − 930 mL/d = 870 mL/d

9. Calculate the volume of each flush (mL).

   Example: 870 mL/d ÷ 5 flushes/d = ~175 mL free water/flush

EN order: Initiate EN at 10 mL/h per PEG and advance as tolerated to target rate of 50 mL/h per institutional protocol. Administer free water flushes and ancillary orders per institutional protocol.

Calculating the enteral nutrition for an adult patient on continuous feeds.

FIGURE 6-3

Case: A 62-year-old female with heart failure with reduced ejection fraction is being started on enteral nutrition (EN) via nasogastric (NG) tube after being in the intensive care unit for heart failure exacerbation and pneumonia. Her dosing weight is 72 kg, and her body mass index is 28. The heart failure team would like to limit her to 1200 mL of fluid per day.

Calculations:

1. Select formula for this patient.

   Example: Calorically dense 2 kcal/mL formula, 100 g protein per 1000 mL, 675 mL water per 1000 mL formula (67.5% water)

(continued)

FIGURE 6-3 *(Continued)*

2. Determine the patient's energy requirement (kcal/d).

   Example: 72 kg × 30 kcal/kg/d = 2160 kcal/d

3. Determine the volume of formula (mL/d) needed by dividing the energy requirement (kcal/d) by the energy concentration in the formula (kcal/mL).

   Example: 2160 kcal/d ÷ 2 kcal/mL = 1080 mL/d of formula

4. Determine the continuous infusion rate (mL/h) by dividing the volume of formula (mL/d) by 24 hours.

   Example: 1080 mL/d ÷ 24 hours = 45 mL/h

5. Determine the protein dose (g/d) by multiplying the formula volume (mL/d) by the formula's protein concentration (g/1000 mL).

   Example: 1080 mL/d × 100 g/1000 mL = 108 g/d

6. Determine the formula's water contribution (mL/d) by multiplying the volume of enteral formula to be administered (mL/d) by the percentage of water in the formula.

   Example: 1080 mL/d × 67.5% = 729 mL/d

7. Determine the total volume of water flushes (mL/d) by subtracting the volume of water from formula (mL/d) from the total fluid requirement (mL/d).

   Example: 1200 mL/d − 729 mL/d = 471 mL/d

8. Calculate the volume of individual flushes (mL).

   Example: 471 mL/d ÷ 5 flush/d = ~90–95 mL free water/flush (Note: Also consider the volume of free water flushes administered with medications; this additional amount could be subtracted from scheduled free water flushes.)

EN order: Initiate EN at 10 mL/h via NG tube and advance as tolerated to target rate of 45 mL/h per institutional protocol. Administer free water flushes and ancillary orders per institutional protocol.

Calculating the enteral nutrition prescription for a fluid-restricted adult.

FIGURE 6-4

Case: A 3-year-old male (weight: 14 kg) is admitted with broken jaw, as a result of a bike injury. He requires enteral nutrition (EN) because he is unable to take anything by mouth at this time. He was previously growing well and consuming an age-appropriate diet. No food allergies are noted.

Calculations:

1. Select formula for this patient.

   Example: Standard 1.0 kcal/mL pediatric (ages 1–10 years) formula, 30 g protein per 1000 mL, 850 mL water per 1000 mL formula (85% water)

2. Determine the patient's energy requirement (kcal/d).

   Example: 14 kg × 85 kcal/kg = 1190 kcal/d

3. Determine volume of formula (mL/d) by dividing the energy requirement (kcal/d) by the energy concentration of the formula (kcal/mL).

   Example: 1190 kcal/d ÷ 1.0 kcal/mL = 1190 mL/d

4. Determine the administration rate by dividing the volume of formula (mL/d) by (a) 24 hours (continuous infusion rate [mL/h]) or (b) number of bolus feeds per day.

   Example: 1190 mL/d ÷ 24 hours = 50 mL/h

   Example: 1190 mL/d ÷ 5 bolus feeds/d = 238 mL (1 can) 5 times per day

5. Determine the protein dose by multiplying the volume of formula (mL/d) by the protein concentration in the formula (g/1000 mL).

   Example: 1190 mL/d × 30 g/1000 mL = 35.7 g/d (2.6 g/kg/d)

6. Determine the patient's fluid requirement (mL/d).

   Example: Patient needs 1200 mL/d.

(continued)

FIGURE 6-4 *(Continued)*

7. Determine the water contribution of the formula by multiplying the percentage of water in the formula by the volume of formula (mL/d).

   Example: 1190 mL/d × 85% = 1012 mL/d

8. Determine the total volume of water flushes (mL/d) by subtracting the volume of free water provided by the formula (mL/d) from the total fluid requirement (mL/d).

   Example: 1190 mL/d − 1012 mL/d = 178 mL/d

9. Calculate the volume of individual flushes (mL).

   Example: 178 mL/d ÷ 3 flush/d = ~60 mL free water/ flush

EN order: Initiate EN at 60 mL Q4 × 5 feeds per day and advance as tolerated per institutional protocol to goal of 240 mL Q4 × 5 feeds per day via nasogastric tube. Administer free water flushes and ancillary orders per institutional protocol.

Calculating an enteral nutrition prescription for a pediatric patient.

Practice Resources

Resource	URL
Food and Nutrition Information Center DRI Calculator for Professionals	https://fnic.nal.usda.gov/fnic /dri-calculator
Nutrition and Food Web Archive (includes several calculators relevant to calculating enteral nutrition prescriptions)	http://www.nafwa.org

References

1. Institute of Medicine. *Dietary Reference Intakes: The Essential Guide to Nutrient Requirements.* Washington, DC: National Academies Press; 2006.

2. McClave SA, Taylor BE, Martindale RG, et al. Guidelines for the provision and assessment of nutrition support therapy in the adult critically ill patient: Society of Critical Care Medicine (SCCM) and American Society for Parenteral and Enteral Nutrition (ASPEN). *JPEN J Parenter Enteral Nutr.* 2016;40:159–211.

3. A.S.P.E.N. Board of Directors and the Clinical Guidelines Task Force. Guidelines for the use of parenteral and enteral nutrition in adult and pediatric patients. *JPEN J Parenter Enteral Nutr.* 2002;26(suppl):1SA–138SA. (Errata: *JPEN J Parenter Enteral Nutr.* 2002;26:144.)

4. Canada TW, Lord LM. Fluids, electrolytes, and acid-base disorders. In: Mueller CM, ed. *The ASPEN Adult Nutrition Support Core Curriculum.* 3rd ed. Silver Spring, MD: American Society for Parenteral and Enteral Nutrition; 2017:113–138.

5. Ayers P, Guenter P, Holcombe B, Plogsted S, eds. *A.S.P.E.N. Parenteral Nutrition Handbook.* 2nd ed. Silver Spring, MD: American Society for Parenteral and Enteral Nutrition; 2014.

6. Rees RG, Keohane PP, Grimble GK, Frost PG, Attrill H, Silk DB. Tolerance of elemental diet administered without starter regimen. *BMJ.* 1985;290:1869–1870.

7. Doley J, Phillips W. Overview of enteral nutrition. In: Mueller CM, ed. *The ASPEN Adult Nutrition Support Core Curriculum.* 3rd ed. Silver Spring, MD: American Society for Parenteral and Enteral Nutrition; 2017:213–226.

8. Boullata J, Carrera AL, Harvey L, et al. ASPEN safe practices for enteral nutrition therapy. *JPEN J Parenter Enteral Nutr.* 2017;41(1):15–103. doi:10.1177/0148607116673053.

9. Lord L, Harrington M. Enteral nutrition implementation and management. In: Merritt R, ed. *The A.S.P.E.N. Nutrition Support Practice Manual.* 2nd ed. Silver Spring, MD: American Society for Parenteral and Enteral Nutrition; 2005:76–89.

10. Mentec H, Dupont H, Bocchetti M, et al. Upper digestive intolerance during enteral nutrition in critically ill patients:

frequency, risk factors, and complications. *Crit Care Med.* 2001; 29:1955–1961.

11. Monczka J. Enteral nutrition support: determining the best way to feed. In: Corkins M, Balint J, Bobo E, et al, eds. *The A.S.P.E.N. Pediatric Nutrition Support Core Curriculum.* 2nd ed. Silver Spring, MD: American Society for Parenteral and Enteral Nutrition; 2015:583–592.

12. Marchand V. Enteral nutrition tube feedings. In: Baker S, Baker R, Davis A, eds. *Pediatric Nutrition Support.* Boston, MA: Jones and Bartlett; 2007;249–260.

13. Enteral nutrition. In: Kleinman RE, ed. *Pediatric Nutrition Handbook.* 6th ed. Elk Grove Village, IL: American Academy of Pediatrics; 2009:541–556.

14. Bankhead R, Boullata J, Brantley S, et al. Enteral nutrition practice recommendations. *JPEN J Parenter Enteral Nutr.* 2009;33(2):122–167.

15. Mehta NM, Bechard LJ, Cahill N, et al. Nutritional practices and their relationship to clinical outcomes in critically ill children—an international multicenter cohort study. *Crit Care Med.* 2012;40:2204–2211.

16. Mehta NM, Skillman HE, Irving SY, et al. Guidelines for the provision and assessment of nutrition support therapy in the pediatric critically ill patient: Society of Critical Care Medicine and American Society for Parenteral and Enteral Nutrition. *JPEN J Parenter Enteral Nutr.* 2017;41(5):706–742.

17. van der Kuip M, Oosterveld MJ, van Bokhorst-de van Schueren MA, et al. Nutritional support in 111 pediatric intensive care units: a European survey. *Intensive Care Med.* 2004;30:1807–1813.

18. Schofield WN. Predicting basal metabolic rate, new standards and review of previous work. *Hum Nutr Clin Nutr.* 1985; 39(suppl 1):5–41.

19. World Health Organization. *Energy and Protein Requirements: Report of a Joint FAO/WHO/UNU Expert Consultation.* Technical report series 724. Geneva, Switzerland: World Health Organization; 1985.

20. Jotterand Chaparro C, Laure Depeyre J, Longchamp D, et al. How much protein and energy are needed to equilibrate nitrogen and energy balances in ventilated critically ill children? *Clin Nutr.* 2016;35:460–467.

21. Bechard LJ, Parrott JS, Mehta NM. Systematic review of the influence of energy and protein intake on protein balance in critically ill children. *J Pediatr.* 2012;161:333–339.

22. Prince A, Groh-Wargo S. Nutrition management for the promotion of growth in very low birth weight premature infants. *Nutr Clin Pract.* 2013;28(6):659–668.

23. Ziegler EE. Meeting the nutritional needs of the low-birth-weight infant. *Ann Nutr Metab.* 2011;58(suppl 1):8–18.

24. Tsang RC, Uauy R, Koletzko B, et al. *Nutrition of the Preterm Infant: Scientific Basis and Practical Guidelines.* 2nd ed. Cincinnati, OH: Digital Educational; 2005.

25. Rees CM, Pierro A, Eaton S. Neurodevelopmental outcomes of neonates with medically and surgically treated necrotizing enterocolitis. *Arch Dis Child.* 2007;92:F193–F198.

26. Greer FR. Nutrition support of the premature infant. In: Baker SR, Baker RD, Davis AM, eds. *Pediatric Nutrition Support.* Sudbury, MA: Jones and Bartlett; 2007:383–392.

27. Fallon E, Nehra D, Potempkin A, et al. A.S.P.E.N. clinical guidelines: nutrition support of neonatal patients at risk for necrotizing enterocolitis. *JPEN J Parenter Enteral Nutr.* 2012;36(5):506–523.

28. Dutta S, Singh B, Chessell L, et al. Guidelines for feeding very low birth weight infants. *Nutrients.* 2015;7:423–442.

29. Oddie SJ, Young L, McGuire W. Slow advancement of enteral feed volumes to prevent necrotising enterocolitis in very low birth weight infants. *Cochrane Database Syst Rev.* 2017;(8):CD001241. doi:10.1002/14651858.CD001241.pub7.

30. Sullivan S, Schanler RJ, Kim JH, et al. An exclusively human milk-based diet is associated with a lower rate of necrotizing enterocolitis than a diet of human milk and bovine milk-based products. *J Pediatr.* 2010;156:562–567.

31. Cristofalo EA, Schanler RJ, Blanco CL, et al. Randomized trial of exclusive human milk versus preterm formula diets in extremely premature infants. *J Pediatr.* 2013;163:1592–1595.

32. Herrman K, Carroll K. An exclusively human milk diet reduces necrotizing enterocolitis. *Breastfeed Med.* 2014;9:184–190.

33. Huston RK, Markell AM, McCulley EA, et al. Improving growth for infants ≤1250 grams receiving an exclusive human milk diet. *Nutr Clin Pract.* 2018;33(5):671–678. doi:10.1002/ncp.10054.

34. Quigley M, Embleton ND, McGuire W. Formula versus donor breast milk for feeding preterm or low birth weight infants. *Cochrane Database Syst Rev.* 2018;(6):CD002971. doi:10.1002/14651858.CD002971.pub4.

35. Milner RD, Minoli I, Moro G, et al. Growth and metabolic and hormonal profiles during transpyloric and nasogastric feeding in preterm infants. *Acta Paediatr Scand.* 1981;70:9–13.

36. McAlister WH, Seigel MJ, Shackelford GD, et al. Intestinal perforation by tube feedings in small infants: clinical and experimental studies. *Am J Roentgenol.* 1985;145:687–691.

37. Raine PA, Goel KM, Young DG, et al. Pyloric stenosis and transpyloric feeding. *Lancet.* 1982;2:821–822.

38. Blondheim O, Abbasi S, Fox WW, et al. Effect of enteral gavage feeding rate on pulmonary functions of very low birth weight infants. *J Pediatr.* 1993;122:751–755.

39. Nelle M, Hoecker C, Linderkamp O. Effects of bolus tube feeding on cerebral blood flow velocity in neonates. *Arch Dis Child Fetal Neonatal Ed.* 1997;76:F54–F56.

40. Dsilna A, Christensson K, Alfredsson L, et al. Continuous feeding promotes gastrointestinal tolerance and growth in very low birth weight infants. *J Pediatr.* 2005;147:43–49.

41. Silvestre MA, Morbach CA, Brans YW, et al. A prospective randomized trial comparing continuous versus intermittent feeding methods in very low birth weight infants. *J Pediatr.* 1999;134:293–297.

42. Premji SS, Chessel I. Continuous nasogastric milk feeding versus intermittent bolus milk feeding for premature infants less than 1500 grams. *Cochrane Database Syst Rev.* 2011;(11):CD001819. doi:10.1002/14651858.CD001819.pub2.

43. Collier B, Guillamondegui O, Cotton B, et al. Feeding the open abdomen. *JPEN J Parenter Enteral Nutr.* 2007;31:410–415.

44. Delaney CP, Zutshi M, Senagore AJ, Remzi FH, Hammel J, Fazio VW. Prospective, randomized, controlled trial between a pathway of controlled rehabilitation with early ambulation and diet and traditional postoperative care after laparotomy and intestinal resection. *Dis Colon Rectum.* 2003;46:851–859.

45. Lucha PA, Butler R, Plichta J, Francis M. The economic impact of early enteral feeding in gastrointestinal surgery: a prospective survey of 51 consecutive patients. *Am Surg.* 2005;71(3):187–190.

46. Hirao M, Tsujinaka T, Takeno A, Fujitani K, Kurata M. Patient-controlled dietary schedule improves clinical outcome after gastrectomy for gastric cancer. *World J Surg.* 2005; 29:853–857.

47. Malhotra A, Mathur AK, Gupta S. Early enteral nutrition after surgical treatment of gut perforations: a prospective randomized study. *J Postgrad Med.* 2004;50:102–106.

48. Ekingen G, Ceran C, Guvenc BH, Tuzlaci A, Kahraman H. Early enteral feeding in newborn surgical patients. *Nutrition.* 2005;21:142–146.

49. Lewis SJ, Egger M, Sylvester PA, Thomas S. Early enteral feeding versus "nil by mouth" after gastrointestinal surgery: systematic review and meta-analysis of controlled trials. *BMJ.* 2001;323:1–5.

50. Melis M, Fichera A, Ferguson MK. Bowel necrosis associated with early jejunal feeding: a complication of postoperative enteral nutrition. *Arch Surg.* 2006;141:701–704.

51. Brown DN, Miedema BW, King PD, Marshall JB. Safety of early feeding after percutaneous endoscopic gastrostomy. *J Clin Gastroenterol.* 1995;21:330–331.

52. Choudhry U, Barde CJ, Markert R, Gopalswamy N. Percutaneous endoscopic gastrostomy: a randomized prospective comparison of early and delayed feeding. *Gastrointest Endosc.* 1996;44:164–167.

53. Nolan TF, Callon R, Choudry U, Reisinger P, Shaar CJ. Same day use of percutaneous endoscopic gastrostomy tubes: radiographic evidence of safety. *Am J Gastroenterol.* 1994;89:1743.

54. McCarter TL, Condon SC, Aguilar RC, et al. Randomized prospective trial of early versus delayed feeding after percutaneous endoscopic gastrostomy placement. *Am J Gastroenterol.* 1998;93:419–421.

55. Kirby DF, Craig RM, Tsang TK, Plotnick BH. Percutaneous endoscopic gastrostomies: a prospective evaluation and review of the literature. *JPEN J Parenter Enteral Nutr.* 1986;10:155–159.

56. Carmona-Sanchez R, Navarro-Cano G. Percutaneous endoscopic gastrostomy: is it safe to start eating immediately? *Rev Gastroenterol Mex.* 2002;67:6–10.

57. Jensen AR, Renaud E, Drucker NA. Why wait: early enteral feeding after pediatric gastrostomy tube placement. *J Pediatr Surg.* 2017;53:656–660.

58. Klein CJ. Nutrient requirements for preterm infant formulas. *J Nutr.* 2002;132(6 suppl):1395S–1577S.

59. Raiten DJ. LRSO report: assessment of nutrient requirements for formulas. *J Nutr.* 1998;128(11 suppl):2059S–2293S.

60. Guenter P, Hicks RW, Simmons D, et al. Enteral feeding misconnections: a consortium position statement. *Jt Comm J Qual Patient Saf.* 2008;34:285–292.

CHAPTER 7

Preparation, Labeling, and Dispensing of Enteral Nutrition

Introduction

The safe and accurate provision of enteral nutrition (EN), including human milk (HM) for infants as well as infant, pediatric, and adult formulas, within the healthcare setting is critical for ensuring patient safety and promoting positive outcomes.[1,2] Some patients require individualized enteral feeding regimens. In the pediatric setting, fortification of HM or the use of powdered or concentrated liquid formulas may be required to modify the nutrient density of EN (see Chapter 5).[3–5] In both the adult and pediatric settings, modulars may be mixed with water and administered as a bolus separate from the tube feeding. In the pediatric setting, modular products may also be added to formula prior to the administration of the tube feeding (see Chapters 4 and 5 for additional information on modulars).[5] The more extensively enteral feedings are manipulated, the greater the risks are for preparation errors and contamination—and both types of risk may be life threatening.[2,4,6] Consequently, it is imperative that healthcare facilities critically evaluate their processes and implement well-defined procedures that employ best practices for the preparation, labeling, and dispensing of HM and formulas for infant, pediatric, and adult patients.

Microbiology and Contamination of Enteral Nutrition

Microbial contamination of EN may occur at any step in the preparation, dispensing, and administration process: during expression and collection of HM, in the manufacturer's production of formulas, during preparation and storage within the healthcare facility, or when EN is administered to the patient.[1]

Enteral feedings as a source of hospital-associated infections have been reported in the literature.[7–15] HM and enteral formulas provide ideal growth media for microbes (nutrients, moisture, oxygen, and the proper pH).[1] Both normal flora and pathogenic microorganisms are common in the hospital environment.[16,17] Of particular concern are those that are resistant to heat, antibiotics, and disinfectants as well as those that continue to grow at refrigerator temperatures.[8,9,13,17–20] While pathogenic microorganisms are of greatest concern, even the introduction of those not considered pathogenic, such as gram-positive rods (including *Bacillus*), is concerning, especially for immunocompromised patients, because infections and sepsis have been linked to such species in the neonate.[7,21–24] In addition to contamination of feedings during preparation and administration, retrograde contamination has also been described in the literature, potentially affecting up to 85% of EN feedings

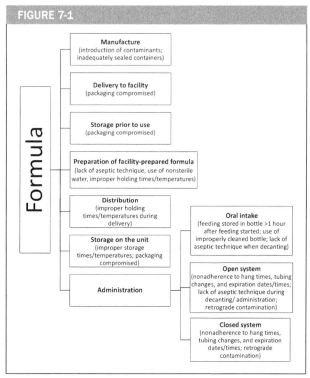

FIGURE 7-1

Potential points of contamination for formula handling in the healthcare setting.
Information is from reference 1.

in the neonatal intensive care setting.[25] Potential points of contamination for EN in the healthcare setting are identified in Figure 7-1 (formula) and Figure 7-2 (HM).

Reducing Risks for Contamination and Preparation Errors

Optimal processes are needed to reduce the risk of enhancing growth of microbes that may be present in nonsterile feedings as well as risk of introducing new microorganisms to sterile and nonsterile feedings.[2] Recommendations

FIGURE 7-2

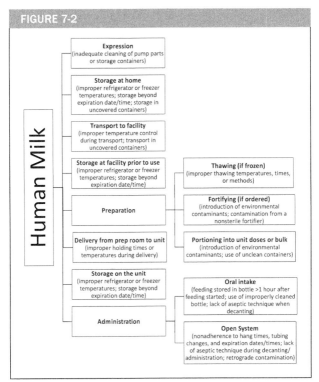

Potential points of contamination for human milk handling in the healthcare setting. All potential points of contamination also apply to donor human milk except for the point of expression and storage at home. Information is from reference 1.

for safe practices in the preparation and dispensing of EN have been widely published, with emphasis on the importance of preparation location, aseptic technique, trained staff, and prevention of misadministration of HM and/or formulas.[1,2,26–28] Individual state regulations and Joint Commission standards require healthcare institutions to prepare food and nutrition products (which includes HM and formulas) under proper conditions, taking sanitation, storage, and security into account.[1,29]

See Table 7-1 for practice recommendations for safe preparation of enteral formulas.[2] Additional recommendations specific to the safe preparation of HM, infant and pediatric formulas, and blenderized tube feedings (BTFs), as well as the labeling of EN, are addressed later in this

---

TABLE 7-1. Practice Recommendations for Safe Preparation of Enteral Nutrition Formulas

1. Use competent personnel trained to follow strict aseptic technique for formula preparation.
2. Establish and follow protocols for preparation, handling, and storage of commercial and handmade EN.
3. Use a closed EN system when possible.
4. If using an open system, use formula decanted from container with a screw cap instead of a flip top, if possible.
5. Use effective hand hygiene and a clean work space when handling enteral formulas. When gloves are used, they must be clean gloves, not having been involved in other unrelated tasks.
6. Use equipment dedicated for EN use only. Keep all equipment as clean and dry as possible. Store clean equipment away from potential sources of contamination.
7. Follow practice recommendations, manufacturer guidelines, and/or facility policies for administration hang times.[a]
8. Use strict aseptic technique for powdered formula preparation.
9. Refrigerate unused formula and use within 24 hours of preparation or opening.
10. Expose reconstituted formulas to room temperature for no longer than 4 hours. Discard unused formula after this time.
11. Use a sterile water source for formula reconstitution.
12. Avoid mixing additives directly into formula when possible.
13. Periodically survey and regularly monitor adherence to safety protocols.

Abbreviation: EN, enteral nutrition.

[a]See Chapter 8 for additional information on hang times.

Source: Information is from reference 2.

chapter. For resources on hand hygiene, refer to the Suggested Reading and Practice Resources section at the end of the chapter.

Formula Selection and Storage

While illness related to contaminated formulas is not common, it is suspected that incidents may be under-reported.[30,31] Furthermore, ingestion of contaminated formulas could result in serious injury or death.[30,31] The US Food and Drug Administration (FDA) is responsible for monitoring microbiological quality of commercial formulas.[32–34] (See Chapters 4 and 5 for additional information on FDA regulation of formula.)

Commercially sealed liquid formulas are sterile as long as the packaging remains intact. Commercial powdered formulas are not sterile at the time of manufacture; therefore, extra care is required to prevent both the proliferation of existing microbes and the introduction of new organisms. Contamination of powdered infant formulas with *Cronobacter* (a gram-negative member of the *Enterobacteriaceae* family that is found in the environment and a variety of foods) and *Salmonella* has been reported in the literature. Powdered formulas should only be used within the healthcare setting if no commercially sterile alternative is available.[1,30,35–37] Liquid formulas are heat sterilized, making them preferable for immunocompromised and hospitalized patients.

Sterile ready-to-feed (RTF) formulas pose the lowest risk with regard to contamination because they require no preparation prior to use; therefore, they should be used in healthcare facilities when nutritionally appropriate.[1] However, care must still be taken to avoid contamination during feeding administration. Research has shown that bedside handling of sterile RTF formulas may still result in microbial growth.[7] As discussed in the next sections of this chapter, use of closed EN systems, when available, and safe practices for hang times further reduce risk of contamination.[1,2,14]

Unopened formulas should be stored in a dry area at room temperature (13°C/55°F to 24°C/75°F) to minimize risks to the products' nutrient and physical integrity. These products should be rotated using "first in, first out" (FIFO) storage techniques.[1,38–40] Storage of opened containers of formula and prepared feedings is discussed later in the chapter.

Closed vs Open Enteral Nutrition Systems

A closed EN system uses a bag or rigid container of liquid formula that is prepackaged by the manufacturer and ready to administer (hang). With an open EN system, formula is decanted into an enteral container before administration. Use of closed EN systems involves less manipulation of enteral formulas and feeding administration sets, which reduces the risk of contamination.[41–45] Using a closed system has also been shown to reduce nursing time.[42] However, closed systems tend to be more expensive and are not appropriate for all situations. When open EN systems are used, hand hygiene, proper handling and storage procedures, and observation of recommended hang times reduce risk of contamination.

According to findings from a survey of American Society for Parenteral and Enteral Nutrition members published in 2017, the use of open systems in acute care was 25% for adults, 62% for pediatrics, and 76% for neonates.[46] These data may reflect the lack of availability of pediatric or infant formulas in closed systems (many infant and pediatric formulas are powders that require reconstitution). In long-term acute care hospitals, closed systems are used

87% of the time; notably, most patients in this setting are adults. In home care, 11% of the survey respondents used closed systems. This finding may reflect the use of bolus feedings in this setting.[46]

Hang Times

Exceeding the recommended hang time for EN is a safety risk whether a closed or open system is used. Manufacturer hang time recommendations for closed EN containers vary but may be up to 48 hours; hang times for EN administered in an open system are considerably shorter (see Chapter 8). Refer to facility-specific policies when determining all hang times.[2]

Effective Use of Technology

Utilization of technology, including use of bar code scanning systems, may reduce risk of preparation errors by automating enteral recipe calculations, automating calculation of expiration dates and times, ensuring proper HM identification, and confirming correct formula and additive product identities.[1,3,6,7,28,47] Furthermore, technology may promote improved staff efficiency while allowing for automated tracking of a variety of metrics, including productivity, compliance, errors and near misses, and product lot numbers in the event of a recall.[1,3,6,7,28,47]

Water Safety

Commercially prepared sterile water as a source of purified water is preferred for formula preparation, hydration, and feeding tube flushes within the acute care setting and with immunocompromised patients due to the potential for contamination of tap water.[2,48] Chilling sterile water prior to formula preparation is recommended to assist the final product in reaching appropriate storage temperatures (≤4°C [≤40°F]) as quickly as possible.[1,49]

If commercial sterile water is not available, tap water may be sterilized by bringing the water to a full rolling boil for 1–2 minutes and allowing to cool. However, sterilizing does not make the water purified; this requires filtration.[2,39,40,50] Knowledge of the lead content of the water supply (available from the Environmental Protection Agency website) is important if tap water is used because lead is known to be harmful to health, particularly in infants, children, and pregnant women.[51]

Additives

Addition of any component to EN increases the risk of introducing microbes into the final product, as well as other risks such as clogged tubing. In the pediatric setting, macronutrient modular products may be added to feedings at the time of preparation. Additives that are considered medications (such as vitamin/mineral preparations and electrolytes) should be administered by appropriately licensed staff; addition of such items is generally considered outside the scope of practice of the feeding preparation room.[1] (See Chapter 10 for additional information on medication administration.) Colorants have been linked to serious adverse outcomes and risk of contamination; therefore, colorants should not be added to feedings for any reason (including detection of aspiration).[52]

Preparation Space, Equipment, and Staffing

The benefits of a dedicated centralized space with dedicated trained staff for the preparation of HM and pediatric formulas have been well documented in the literature.[1,6,7,26,28,47,53,54] Published recommendations for the pediatric setting suggest a preparation space solely designated for preparing enteral feedings that supports aseptic technique and is physically separate from patient care areas.[1,6,7,28,55] The space should allow for an efficient and logical workflow from clean to dirty for optimal function and safety.[1,55,56] Such a model reduces the risk of contamination, preparation errors, and HM errors (use of the wrong patient's HM).[6,7,26,28,47,53,54] Furthermore, many states now require a designated feeding preparation space for new neonatal intensive care unit construction.[55,57–67]

Equipment and Supplies

Refrigerators and Freezers

Refrigerators are necessary both for ingredient storage and for holding of the final prepared product.[1] Facilities preparing HM will also require freezer storage.[1] The overall capacity and number of refrigerators and freezers required will be based on the type of EN managed (HM, pasteurized donor HM, and/or formula), taking into account the space necessary for ingredient storage and volume of feedings prepared daily.[1]

Guidelines for storage times and temperatures for HM provided to healthy infants at home are available from the Centers for Disease Control and Prevention and the Academy of Breastfeeding Medicine.[68,69] Within the healthcare setting, however, the recommended temperature ranges and duration of storage are more conservative to prevent illness in immunocompromised patients.[1,2,27,68] Facility refrigerators must have the ability to maintain temperatures between 2°C and 4°C (35°F and 39°F), while HM storage freezers must sustain temperatures of ≤4°C (≤39°F).[1,2,8,68–70]

Often, laboratory- or pharmacy-grade units are preferred for their ability to better maintain desired temperatures despite frequent opening.[1]

Refrigeration unit temperatures should be confirmed using a thermometer that meets the National Institute of Standards and Technology requirements.[1] A temperature monitoring system with an alarm to alert staff of temperatures outside the desired ranges promotes patient safety and can prevent HM waste in the event of equipment malfunction.[1] It may also be prudent to have HM refrigerators and freezers plugged into outlets that provide emergency power to prevent loss in the event of a power outage.[5,27,70] Once HM has thawed, it must be used within 24 hours or discarded; however, HM that is partially thawed and still contains ice crystals may be refrozen.[1,27]

Refrigerators used to store EN should be regularly cleaned and well organized using FIFO storage methods.[1] Use of plastic bins or resealable plastic bags may help with organization and FIFO and lessens the risk for errors by keeping each individual patient's EN separated from others.[1] This may be particularly important for HM feedings, which, if fed to the incorrect patient, constitute a bodily fluid exposure.[1] Access to EN refrigerators and HM freezers should be limited to authorized staff to reduce risk of error, tampering, and waste.[1,27]

Sinks and Dishwashers

Recommendations for the pediatric setting include use of a separate, hands-free sink for hand hygiene.[1] See Suggested Reading and Practice Resources at the end of the chapter for additional information on hand hygiene.

If nondisposable items are used for EN preparation, proper equipment for sanitation is required. A commercial dishwashing machine, separate from the facility's foodservice dishwasher, is recommended.[1] Wash temperatures of 66°C (150°F) and rinse temperatures of 82°C (180°F) are needed to meet National Sanitation Foundation standards as well as most local codes.[71,72] Alternatively, reusable items may be hand-washed in a single-compartment sink and autoclaved or sanitized using a 3-compartment sink (wash, rinse, and chemically sanitize).[73]

Carts

Delivery carts may be needed to transport prepared feedings from the preparation area to the patient unit(s). Temperature maintenance of 2°C–4°C (35°F–39°F) for facility-prepared EN is critical to prevent microbial growth and possible foodborne illness.[73] The time and distance required for EN delivery will determine the type of cart needed. Feedings may be transported in ice baths; alternatively, insulated carts and temperature-controlled carts are available for appropriate temperature maintenance.[1]

Laminar Flow Hood

While a laminar flow hood may provide an additional barrier to potential contaminants, a hood is *not* required for EN preparation.[1] Commonly used in the preparation of *sterile* pharmaceutical products, use of a laminar flow hood is not required for the preparation of oral (ie, nonsterile) medications, and its use with nonsterile products (including HM and powdered formulas) does not result in a sterile final product.[74,75] If a laminar flow hood is used, staff must be adequately trained and demonstrate competency on well-defined operating procedures.[1]

Measuring and Mixing Devices

All items used in the preparation and storage of pediatric EN should be made of bisphenol A (BPA)–free and di(2-ethylhexyl) phthalate (DEHP)–free food-grade plastic or stainless steel; glass items (such as graduated cylinders or beakers) are not recommended because of the risk of glass particles.[72] Reusable items should be sanitized between uses with different formulas to prevent cross contamination of allergens and between individual patient HM preparations to prevent biological cross contamination. Single-use, disposable items may be preferred for ease and sanitation.

Liquid ingredients should be measured using graduated cylinders, beakers, liquid measuring cups, or syringes.[1] Powdered ingredients should be measured using a gram scale accurate to 0.1 g.[1]

Scoops and household measurements should not be used for EN preparation in healthcare facilities because of the high variability of the measuring devices themselves as well as variability in packing the powder.[1,76] Research has shown that inconsistencies in packing and technique contribute to differences of 10%–25% when scoops or household measurements are used.[77] Calibration of scales should be conducted per manufacturer guidelines and per facility biomedical engineering standards to verify the accuracy of weights.[1]

Whisks with solid handles and immersion blenders with removable blades are both acceptable types of mixing devices because they may be properly cleaned and sanitized.[1,72] Upright blenders are not recommended for the preparation of EN because it is not possible to adequately sanitize parts and gaskets.[1]

Storage Containers

When HM and prepared EN are stored, food-grade and BPA- and DEHP-free storage containers with leak-proof, solid surface lids must be used.[27,78] Single-use containers and syringes must be clean, but they do *not* need to be sterile as there is no evidence that use of nonsterile items results in higher microbial counts in collected HM or prepared EN.[1,27] Reusable containers must be appropriately cleaned and sanitized between uses.[1]

Thawing and Warming Equipment

Microwave ovens must *not* be used for thawing HM or warming EN because there is a potential for nutrient losses and a risk of hot spots within the feeding, which could cause burns.[38,49,79–81] Safe methods of thawing frozen HM and warming prepared EN include use of water baths, bead baths, and commercial milk warmers.[27,81,82] Tap water is a potential source of microbial contamination; therefore, steps must be employed to prevent water from coming into contact with the feeding itself if water baths or water-based commercial warmers are utilized.[82,83]

Staff Hygiene and Apparel

Use of disposable gowns over clean scrubs or other professional attire is recommended when preparing EN.[1] Gowns should be changed between type of formula preparation (such as between milk-based formulas and hypoallergenic formulas) to prevent cross contamination of allergens from residue that may be present on the gown.

Personal protective items such as a bonnet or hairnet and beard cover (if needed) should be used when preparing HM and formulas.[1] As allowed by the facility, a face mask may be used for minor illnesses (if changed frequently); however, staff preparing EN should be in good health and follow the facility's employee health standards.[84]

To minimize risk for infection transmission, EN preparation staff should have short, unpolished, natural nails.[85–87] Gloves are recommended, but they are not required in the handling of HM and EN if effective hand-washing techniques are employed.[1,27] Furthermore, gloves should not be considered a substitute for appropriate hand hygiene.[16]

Preparation, Dispensing, and Administration of Human Milk and Pediatric Enteral Nutrition

Human Milk

Policies for the use of HM within the healthcare setting must address more than breastfeeding.[3] HM for hospitalized infants is typically expressed, stored, thawed, fortified, and fed (either by mouth or via tube).[3] Therefore, systems must be in place to preserve HM nutrients and immune factors during storage and processing and document appropriate expiration dates/times, while reducing risk of contamination, fortification errors, and misadministration.[3,27,88] Expressed HM is not sterile and contains beneficial microorganisms (probiotic organisms and commensal, nonpathogenic organisms that support establishment of optimal gut flora).[1] However, if HM is not collected under sanitary conditions, stored at proper temperatures, and safely transported to the hospital, it may become contaminated by harmful viruses and/or bacteria.[27,89,90] Proper cleaning of breast pumps and personal collection kits is critical to decrease contamination rates at the time of HM expression and subsequent risk of infection, sepsis, and/or feeding intolerance in the preterm or ill infant.[77,88,89,91–95] Donor HM that has been appropriately commercially pasteurized is sterile, but it may still become contaminated during storage, handling, and administration if improper procedures are used.[1]

It is imperative that HM be labeled clearly to prevent administration errors. Preprinted labels and/or bar coding systems may help avoid HM administration errors. See the

Labeling Enteral Nutrition section later in this chapter for additional information on labeling elements for HM.

Preparation Steps in the Healthcare Setting

HM and pediatric enteral formulas should be prepared in a dedicated space that supports aseptic technique by trained staff using well-defined procedures that promote accuracy in fulfillment of the provider order. Table 7-2 provides an overview of steps for HM and pediatric EN preparation within the hospital setting.[1,2] EN in home care is discussed in Chapter 11.

Dispensing and Administration

Closed, food-grade containers should be used to deliver prepared HM and EN; feedings dispensed in single doses reduce risk of contamination by limiting handling at bedside.[1] If bulk volumes (up to a 24-hour supply) are prepared, care must be taken to avoid introduction of contaminants when each feeding is retrieved.[1,16] Temperatures must be maintained during delivery from the preparation area to the patient unit or room.[1] Adherence to proper hang times, tubing changes, and EN expiration times during administration is critical for infection prevention.[2] HM and facility-prepared formulas should not be held at room temperature for more than 4 hours.[2,15,25,96] Sterile RTF formulas should not exceed hang times of 4 hours for neonates (infants younger than 30 days) and immunocompromised infants/children; 8-hour hang times are acceptable for sterile RTF formulas for nonimmunocompromised pediatric patients older than 30 days.[2,15,25,96] Any pediatric EN remaining in the bottle 1 hour after an oral feeding has begun should be discarded due to potential

TABLE 7-2. Steps for Human Milk and Pediatric Enteral Nutrition Preparation

1. Perform hand hygiene:
   - Upon entry into the preparation area;
   - After sanitizing work spaces;
   - Before and after preparing each type of formula and each individual patient's human milk;
   - As needed for ongoing aseptic technique.
2. Don appropriate personal protective gear as outlined by facility policies (such items may include gowns, bonnets or hairnets, beard covers, masks).
3. Confirm the provider's order.
4. Confirm the recipe for fortified human milk or formula.
5. Sanitize preparation surfaces:
   - Prior to initiating feeding preparation;
   - Before and after each type of formula and each individual patient's human milk;
   - As needed for ongoing aseptic technique.
6. Assemble needed supplies and ingredients:
   - Employ first-in-first-out techniques for formulas, fortifiers, modulars, and human milk bottles.
   - Thaw human milk using appropriate techniques, taking care to avoid waste.
   - Perform a double-check procedure to confirm correct human milk before decanting, combining, preparing, or relabeling any human milk. This double-check procedure may be (a) a manual 2-person verification of a minimum of 2 patient identifiers; **or** (b) bar code scanning.
7. Don gloves (following hand hygiene) prior to preparing the human milk or formula feeding.
8. Measure ingredients using appropriate equipment and aseptic technique.
   - Measure human milk, sterile water, and liquid formulas using graduated cylinders, beakers, liquid measuring cups, or syringes.
   - Measure powdered ingredients using a gram scale.
   - Verify that equipment is clean and sanitized to prevent cross contamination of microbes and allergens.

(continued)

TABLE 7-2. *(Continued)*

9. Combine ingredients in a clean disposable container or a reusable clean and sanitized container.

10. Decant prepared enteral nutrition into a closed container for delivery.
    - No more than 24-hour volumes may be prepared.
    - Feedings may be dosed into units for individual feedings or in bulk volumes.
    - New, clean disposable containers may be sterile or nonsterile.
    - Reusable containers must be cleaned and sanitized between uses.

11. Label each container: See the labeling recommendations later in this chapter.

12. Refrigerate prepared human milk or formula immediately in the preparation area, patient unit refrigerator, or patient in-room refrigerator for up to 24 hours after preparation.

Source: Information is from references 1 and 2.

bacterial contamination from the oral flora.[49] See Chapter 8 for additional information on administration and monitoring of EN.

Blenderized Tube Feedings

The term *blenderized tube feeding* may refer to either home-made or commercially prepared blended whole foods. Both types of BTF are gaining popularity with patients receiving EN.[97–99] BTF can be provided exclusively or in conjunction with a standard polymeric formula.

A disadvantage to the use of homemade BTF is the risk of cross contamination and potential for foodborne illness. Once prepared, homemade BTF should be immediately used or refrigerated at appropriate temperatures.[100] Homemade BTF should not be held at room temperature for more than 2 hours due to concerns about bacterial contamination. For this reason, a bolus regimen is recommended instead of continuous infusion.[100] Refrigerated homemade BTF that is not used within 24 hours of preparation should be discarded. Commercially prepared BTFs have longer hang times of 8–12 hours, depending on manufacturer recommendations.[97]

Another disadvantage to homemade BTF is the potential for clogged feeding tubes, which may be related to varying consistencies in the blended formula. The FDA has published recommendations on the preparation of homemade BTF to prevent clogged feeding tubes, including use of high-end blenders or increasing blend time with existing blenders.[101] Additional recommendations on administration of homemade BTF are found in Table 7-3, the practice resources at the end of this chapter, and Chapters 8 and 11.[2] See Chapters 4, 5, and 8 for additional information on commercially prepared BTF products.

TABLE 7-3. Practice Recommendations for Blenderized Tube Feedings

1. Prepare homemade BTF using safe food-handling techniques, and store at refrigerator temperature immediately after preparation. Discard any unused portion after 24 hours.
2. Sanitize mechanical devices (eg, blenders) used to prepare homemade BTF after each use, using an established protocol.
3. Limit the hang time of homemade BTF to ≤2 hours.
4. Limit the hang time of commercial BTF to 8–12 hours or per manufacturer recommendation (similar to other open system EN feeding systems).

Abbreviations: BTF, blenderized tube feeding; EN, enteral nutrition.

Source: Adapted with permission from reference 2: Boullata JI, Carrera AL, Harvey L, et al. ASPEN safe practices for enteral nutrition therapy. *JPEN J Parenter Enteral Nutr.* 2017;41:15–103. doi:10.1177/0148607116673053.

Labeling Enteral Nutrition

Patient-specific, standardized labels for EN decrease potential confusion when a patient is transferred to a different unit within a facility, or when a new staff member takes over a patient's care.[2] For example, "Not for IV Use" helps decrease the risk for an enteral misconnection. Proper labeling also allows for a final check of that enteral formula against the prescriber's order.[2,102] (See Chapter 6 for additional information on EN orders.)

To avoid misinterpretation, EN should be treated as a medication, and a standardized label should be affixed to all EN formula administration containers (bags, bottles, syringes used in syringe pumps). Care should be taken in developing a label that is clear and concise and of a size that fits neatly on the container (see Figures 7-3, 7-4, and

FIGURE 7-3

ENTERAL USE ONLY

Institution and Department Name — Contact Information
Patient name: _____   Patient ID: _____
Room number: _____

Generic (Brand) Formula Name
Formula: _____
_____ grams of protein/_____kcal/container
_____ mL/container

Delivery Site
Route of Delivery: _____
Enteral Access Device: _____

IV   IV

Administration
Method of Administration: Bolus   Intermittent   Continuous
Rate of Administration: _____ mL/hour
Formula Hung by: _____, Nurse   Date: _____   Time: _____
Expiration vs Beyond Use Date: _____   Time: _____

Standard enteral nutrition label template (adult patient). ID, identification; IV, intravenous. Reprinted with permission from reference 2: Boullata JI, Carrera AL, Harvey L, et al. ASPEN safe practices for enteral nutrition therapy. *JPEN J Parenter Enteral Nutr.* 2017;41:15–103. doi:10.1177/0148607116673053.

FIGURE 7-4

ENTERAL USE ONLY

Institution and Department Name — Contact Information

Patient name: _____   Patient ID: _____

Room number: _____

Generic (Brand) Formula Name

Base Formula: _____   _____ kcal/100 mL

_____ mL/container

Fortifier: _____

Final concentration: ____ kcal   _____ mL/container

Prepared by: _____   Date: _____   Time: _____

Delivery Site

IV

Route of Delivery: _____

Enteral Access Device: _____

IV

Administration

Method of Administration: Bolus   Continuous

Rate of Administration: _____ mL/hour

Formula Hung by: _____, Nurse   Date: _____   Time: _____

Expiration Date: _____   Time: _____

Standard enteral nutrition label template (neonatal or pediatric patient). ID, identification; IV, intravenous. Reprinted with permission from reference 2: Boullata JI, Carrera AL, Harvey L, et al. ASPEN safe practices for enteral nutrition therapy. *JPEN J Parenter Enteral Nutr.* 2017;41:15–103. doi:10.1177/0148607116673053.

7-5 for examples).[2] In some institutions it may not be possible to print standardized labels. Some formula manufacturers provide labels to document important elements on the formula container. In all cases, the critical label elements (Table 7-4) should be listed on the enteral product container or label.[2] See Table 7-5 for a summary of practice recommendations for EN labeling.[2]

Quality Assurance

EN handling processes should be routinely evaluated to determine their ongoing quality effectiveness and safety. Examples of methods for quality assurance monitoring include the Hazard Analysis Critical Control Point

FIGURE 7-5

ENTERAL USE ONLY
Institution and Department Name — Contact Information
Patient name: _____   Patient ID: _____
Room number: _____

Human Milk Contents
Fresh or Frozen (circle)
HM Fortifier: _____ kcal/oz and/or _____ to make
_____ (as per prescriber order)
Prepared by: _____   Date:_____   Time: _____

Delivery Site
IV (crossed out)   Route of Delivery: _____   **IV** (crossed out)
Enteral Access Device: _____

Administration
Method of Administration: Bolus   Continuous
Rate of Administration: _____ mL/hour
Formula Hung by: _____, Nurse   Date: _____   Time: _____
Expiration Date: _____   Time: _____

Standard human milk label template (infant patient). HM, human milk; ID, identification; IV, intravenous. Adapted with permission from reference 2: Boullata JI, Carrera AL, Harvey L, et al. ASPEN safe practices for enteral nutrition therapy. *JPEN J Parenter Enteral Nutr.* 2017;41:15–103. doi:10.1177/0148607116673053.

(HACCP) system and the plan-do-check-act (PDCA) process.[7,70,103-105] The HACCP system uses a scientific approach to identify critical control points in the provision of nutrition products and implement safeguards at those points to prevent microbial contamination.[7,70,103,104] Originally used for healthcare food service, many facilities have extended the use of HACCP to EN (including HM).[7,70,103,104] Table 7-6 provides an overview of the HACCP plan process.[70] The steps in the PDCA model proceed in a cyclical manner, allowing for a systematic approach for implementing a new process as well as a method for ongoing monitoring and adjustments.[105]

Policies and procedures should reflect current practice and be easily accessible to provide guidance to staff. Regular assessment of staff competency (both within the

TABLE 7-4. Components of the Formula Label

Labeling of enteral formula:
- Patient's name
- Medical record ID number
- Formula name and strength of formula, if diluted
- Date and time formula prepared[a]
- Date and time formula hung[a]
- Administration route
- Rate of administration expressed as mL/h over 24 hours if continuous administration or "Rate not to exceed _____" or "Volume not to exceed _____"
- Administration duration and rates are to be expressed on the label if the EN is cycled or intermittent
- Initials of who prepared, hung, and checked the EN against the order
- Appropriate hang time (expiration date and time)
- Dosing weight if appropriate
- "Not for IV Use"

Labeling of incoming human milk:
- Infant's name
- Medical record ID number
- Dosing weight
- Date and time that HM was expressed
- Medication or supplements being taken by the mother
- Specify whether HM is fresh or frozen
- Contents in syringe/container (expressed HM)
- If frozen, date and time HM was thawed
- Expiration date (based on whether the HM was fresh or frozen)
- "Not for IV Use"
- Fortified HM also includes:
  - Name of fortifier
  - Final concentration
  - Date and time formula prepared
- Initials of who prepared, hung, and checked the EN against the order

Abbreviations: EN, enteral nutrition; HM, human milk; ID, identification; IV, intravenous.

[a]The date-time of formula prepared and the date-time of formula hung may be different, so note both.

Adapted with permission from reference 2: Boullata JI, Carrera AL, Harvey L, et al. ASPEN safe practices for enteral nutrition therapy. *JPEN J Parenter Enteral Nutr.* 2017;41:15–103. doi:10.1177/0148607116673053.

TABLE 7-5. Practice Recommendations for Labeling of Enteral Nutrition

1. Include all the critical elements of the EN order on the EN label: patient identifiers, formula type, enteral delivery site (route and access), administration method and type, and volume and frequency of water flushes.

2. Standardize the labels for all EN formula containers, bags, or syringes to include who prepared the formula, date/time it was prepared, and date and time it was started.

3. Express clearly and accurately on all EN labels in any healthcare environment what the patient was ordered. Given changes to administration rates/volumes, consider patient-specific labels that state:
   a. "Rate not to exceed _____"
   b. "Volume not to exceed _____"

4. Include on the label of HM stored in the hospital: contents in container, infant's name, infant's medical record number, date and time of milk expressed, maternal medications, fortifiers added, and energy density.

5. State on the HM label whether the milk is fresh or frozen, date and time the milk was thawed, and the appropriate expiration date. Bar codes, special colors, or symbols may be used to further identify the HM.

6. Label commercial enteral containers "Not for IV Use" to help decrease the risk for an enteral misconnection.

7. Carefully check commercial enteral container labeling against the prescriber's order. Be aware of sound-alike or look-alike product names that may be mixed up on the order or during selection of the product.

Abbreviations: EN, enteral nutrition; HM, human milk.

Adapted with permission from reference 2: Boullata JI, Carrera AL, Harvey L, et al. ASPEN safe practices for enteral nutrition therapy. *JPEN J Parenter Enteral Nutr.* 2017;41:15–103. doi:10.1177/0148607116673053.

TABLE 7-6. Steps in a Hazard Analysis Critical Control Point Plan
1. Assessment of potential hazards
2. Identification of critical control points (CCPs)
3. Establishment of policies and procedures for CCPs
4. Monitoring of CCPs
5. Planning for procedure failures and corrective actions
6. Verification that systems and procedures are working
7. Record keeping

Source: Information is from references 1, 7, 70, 103, and 104.

preparation room and at bedside) is crucial to verify compliance and identify gaps in training or the process.

Suggested Reading and Practice Resources

Hand Hygiene

- Centers for Disease Control and Prevention. When and how to wash your hands. https://www.cdc.gov/handwashing/when-how-handwashing.html. Updated March 2016. Accessed November 8, 2018.
- Association for Professionals in Infection Control and Epidemiology. Guide to hand hygiene programs for infection prevention. http://www.apic.org/Professional-Practice/Implementation-guides#HandHygiene. Published 2016. Accessed November 8, 2018.
- World Health Organization. WHO guidelines on hand hygiene in health care: a summary. http://apps.who.int/iris/bitstream/10665/70126/1/WHO_IER_PSP_2009.07_eng.pdf. Published 2009. Accessed November 8, 2018.

Human Milk and Infant/Pediatric Formulas

- Steele C, Collins EA, eds. *Infant and Pediatric Feedings: Guidelines for Preparation of Human Milk and Formula in Health Care Facilities.* 3rd ed. Chicago, IL: Academy of Nutrition and Dietetics; 2018.
- Centers for Disease Control and Prevention. How to keep your breast pump kit clean: the essentials. https://www.cdc.gov/healthywater/hygiene/healthychildcare/infantfeeding/breastpump.html. Updated August 2017. Accessed November 8, 2018.

Blenderized Tube Feedings

- Fessler TA. Home tube feeding with blenderized foods. Oley Foundation website. https://oley.org/page/hometf_blenderfoods?&terms=%22blenderized%22. Updated September 2016. Accessed November 8, 2018.
- Escuro A. Blenderized tube feeding: suggested guidelines to clinicians. *Pract Gastroenterol.* 2014;38(12):58–66. https://www.practicalgastro.com/article/144773/Blenderized-Tube-Feeding-Suggested-Guidelines. Accessed November 8, 2018.
- Epp L. Blenderized feeding options—the sky's the limit. *Pract Gastroenterol.* 2018;42(6):30–39. https://www.practicalgastro.com/article/183989/Blenderized-Feeding-Options-Skys-the-Limit. Accessed December 30, 2018.

References

1. Steele C, Collins EA, eds. *Infant and Pediatric Feedings: Guidelines for Preparation of Human Milk and Formula in Health Care Facilities.* 3rd ed. Chicago, IL: Academy of Nutrition and Dietetics; 2019.

2. Boullata JI, Carrera AL, Harvey L, et al. ASPEN safe practices for enteral nutrition therapy. *JPEN J Parenter Enteral Nutr.* 2017;41:15–103. doi:10.1177/0148607116673053.

3. Steele C, Czerwin A, Bixby C. Breast milk bar code scanning results in time savings and staff efficiency. *J Acad Nutr Diet.* 2015;115(1):23–26.

4. Vermilyea S, Goh VL. Enteral feedings in children: sorting out tubes, buttons, and formulas. *Nutr Clin Pract.* 2016; 31(1):59–67.

5. Drenckpohl M, Bowers L, Cooper H. Use of the Six Sigma methodology to reduce incidence of breast milk administration errors in the NICU. *Neonatal Netw.* 2007;26(3): 161–166.

6. Steele C, Bixby C. Centralized breastmilk handling and bar code scanning improve safety and reduce breastmilk administration errors. *Breastfeed Med.* 2014;9(9):426–429. doi:10.1089/bfm.2014.0077.

7. Steele C, Short R. Centralized infant formula preparation room in the neonatal intensive care unit reduces incidence of microbial contamination. *J Am Diet Assoc.* 2008;108: 1700–1703.

8. Iversen C, Forsythe SJ. Comparison of media for the isolation of *Enterobacter sakazakii. Appl Environ Microbiol.* 2007;73: 48–52.

9. Kandhai MC, Reij MW, Grognou C, van Schothorst M, Gorris LGM, Zwietering MH. Effects of preculturing conditions on lag time and specific growth rate of *Enterobacter sakazakii* in reconstituted powdered infant formula. *Appl Environ Microbiol.* 2006;72:2721–2729.

10. Marino LV, Goddard E, Whitelaw A, Workman L. Prevalence of bacterial contamination of powdered infant feeds in a hospital environment. *S Afr Med J.* 2007;97:534–537.

11. Buyukyavuz BI, Adiloglu AK, Onal S, Cubukcu SE, Cetin H. Finding the sources of septicemia at a neonatal

intensive care unit: newborns and infants can be contaminated while being fed. *Jpn J Infect Dis.* 2006;59:213–215.

12. Giovannini M, Verduci E, Ghisleni D, Salvatici E, Riva E, Agostoni C. *Enterobacter sakazakii:* an emerging problem in paediatric nutrition. *J Int Med Res.* 2008;36:394–399.

13. Iversen C, Lane M, Forsythe SJ. The growth profile, thermotolerance and biofilm formation of *Enterobacter sakazakii* grown in infant formula milk. *Lett Appl Microbiol.* 2004;38:378–382.

14. Mathus-Vliegen L, Binnekade J, de Hann R. Bacterial contamination of ready-to-use 1-L feeding bottles and administration sets in severely compromised intensive care patients. *Crit Care Med.* 2000;28:67–73.

15. Perry J, Stankorb S, Salgueiro M. Microbial contamination of enteral feeding products in thermoneutral and hyperthermal ICU environments. *Nutr Clin Pract.* 2015;30:128–133.

16. Boyce JM, Pittet D. Guideline for hand hygiene in healthcare settings: recommendations of the Healthcare Infection Control Practices Advisory Committee and the HICPAC/SHEA/APIC/IDSA Hand Hygiene Task Force. *Infect Control Hosp Epidemiol.* 2002;23(12 Suppl):S3–S40.

17. Goff HD. Microbial growth. Dairy science and technology education series. University of Guelph Food Science website. https://www.uoguelph.ca/foodscience/book-page/microbial-growth. Accessed November 9, 2018.

18. Centers for Disease Control and Prevention. Diagnosis and management of foodborne illnesses: a primer for physicians. *MMWR Morb Mortal Wkly Rep.* 2001;50(RR-02):1–69.

19. Nair MK, Joy J, Venkitanarayanan KS. Inactivation of *Enterobacter sakazakii* in reconstituted infant formula by monocaprylin. *J Food Prot.* 2004;67(12):2815–2819.

20. Brett MM, McLauchlin J, Harris A, et al. A case of infant botulism with a possible link to infant formula milk powder: evidence for the presence of more than one strain of *Clostridium botulinum* in clinical specimens and food. *J Med Microbiol.* 2005;54:769–776.

21. Hilliard NJ, Schelonka RL, Waites KB. *Bacillus cereus* bacteremia in a preterm neonate. *J Clin Microbiol.* 2003;41:3441–3444.

22. Adler A, Gottesman G, Dolfin T, et al. *Bacillus* species sepsis in the neonatal intensive care unit. *J Infect.* 2005;51(5):390–395.

23. Ko KS, Oh WS, Le MY, et al. *Bacillus infantis* sp. nov. and *Bacillus idriensis* sp. nov., isolated from a patient with neonatal sepsis. *Int J Syst Evol Microbiol.* 2006;56(Pt 11):2541–2544.

24. Boyle RJ, Robins-Browne RM, Tang MLK. Probiotic use in clinical practices: what are the risks? *Am J Clin Nutr.* 2006; 83:1256–1264.

25. Hurrell E, Kucerova E, Loughlin M. Neonatal enteral feeding tubes as loci for colonization by members of the *Enterobacteriaceae. BMC Infect Dis.* 2009;9:146.

26. National Association of Neonatal Nurses. The use of human milk and breastfeeding in the neonatal intensive care unit. Position statement #3065. http://nann.org/about/position -statements. Published 2015. Accessed November 8, 2018.

27. Jones F. *Best Practice for Expressing, Storing and Handling Human Milk in Hospitals, Homes, and Child Care Settings.* 3rd ed. Fort Worth, TX: Human Milk Banking Association of North America; 2011.

28. Moro GE, Arslanoglu S, Bernito E, et al. Human milk in feeding premature infants: from tradition to bioengineering. *J Pediatr Gastroenterol Nutr.* 2015;61(Suppl 1):S1–S19. doi:10.1097/MPG.0000000000000897.

29. The Joint Commission. The Joint Commission Comprehensive Accreditation and Certification Manual 2017 (E-dition). https://e-dition.jcrinc.com. Accessed May 3, 2017.

30. Food and Agriculture Organization of the United Nations/ World Health Organization. *Enterobacter sakazakii* and other microorganisms in powdered infant formula. Food and Agriculture Organization website. http://www.fao.org/docrep /007/y5502e/y5502e00.htm. Published 2004. Accessed November 9, 2018.

31. US Food and Drug Administration. FDA and CDC update: investigation of *Cronobacter* bacteria illness in infants. https://www.cdc.gov/media/releases/2011 /s1230_Cronobacter.html. Published December 30, 2011. Accessed December 30, 2018.

32. US Food and Drug Administration. Code of Federal Regulations. Title 21: Food and Drugs. Part 106: infant formula requirements pertaining to current good manufacturing practice, quality control procedures, quality factors, records and reports, and notifications. Part 107: infant formula. April 1, 2016. https://www.accessdata.fda.gov/scripts

/cdrh/cfdocs/cfcfr/CFRSearch.cfm. Accessed November 13, 2017.

33. US Food and Drug Administration. Code of Federal Regulations. Title 21: Food and Drugs. Part 113: thermally processed low-acid foods packaged in hermetically sealed containers. https://www.accessdata.fda.gov/scripts/cdrh/cfdocs/cfcfr/CFRSearch.cfm?CFRPart=113. Accessed November 14, 2017.

34. US Food and Drug Administration. Current Good Manufacturing Practices, quality control procedures, quality factors, notification requirements, and records and reports, for infant formula; correction. a rule by the Food and Drug Administration on 7/15/2014. *Federal Register*. 2014;79:41127. https://www.federalregister.gov/documents/2014/07/15/201416476/current-good-manufacturing-practices-quality-control-procedures-quality-factors-notification. Accessed November 9, 2018.

35. Food and Agriculture Organization of the United Nations/World Health Organization. Safe preparation, storage and handling of powdered infant formula. World Health Organization website. http://www.who.int/foodsafety/publications/powdered-infant-formula/en. Published 2007. Accessed November 9, 2018.

36. Jason J. Prevention of invasive *Cronobacter* infection in young infants fed powdered infant formulas. *Pediatrics*. 2012;130(5):e1076–e1084.

37. Forsythe S. *Cronobacter* species. *Culture*. 2010;31(1):1–8.

38. US Food and Drug Administration. FDA takes final step on infant formula protections. https://www.fda.gov/ForConsumers/ConsumerUpdates/ucm048694.htm. Published June 4, 2014; updated January 4, 2018. Accessed April 26, 2018.

39. Abbott Nutrition. How to make a bottle. Similac website. https://similac.com/baby-feeding/formula/how-to-make-bottle. Accessed November 9, 2018.

40. Abbott Nutrition. Recommended storage guidelines for Abbott Nutrition pediatric products. https://static.abbottnutrition.com/cms-prod/abbottnutrition-2016.com/img/13-14_Recommended_Storage_Guidelines_for_Abbott_Nutrition_Pediatric_Products_tcm1310-72819.pdf. Accessed November 9, 2018.

41. Beattie TK, Anderton A. Decanting versus sterile prefilled nutrient containers—the microbiological risks in enteral feeding. *Int J Environ Health Res.* 2001;11:81–93.

42. Marlon ND, Rupp ME. Infection control issues of enteral feeding systems. *Curr Opin Clin Nutr Metab Care.* 2000;3(5):363–366.

43. Vanek V. Closed versus open enteral delivery systems: a quality improvement study. *Nutr Clin Pract.* 2000;15(5):234–243.

44. Phillips W. Economic impact of switching from an open to a closed enteral nutrition feeding system in an acute care setting. *Nutr Clin Pract.* 2013;28(4):510–514.

45. Lyman B, Gebhards S, Hensley C, Roberts C, San Pablo W. Safety of decanted enteral formula hung for 12 hours in a pediatric setting. *Nutr Clin Pract.* 2011;26:451–456.

46. Read J, Guenter P. *ASPEN Enteral Nutrition by the Numbers: EN Data Across the Healthcare Continuum.* Silver Spring, MD: American Society for Parenteral and Enteral Nutrition; 2017.

47. Oza-Frank R, Kachoria R, Dail J, Green J, Walls K, McClead RE. A quality improvement project to decrease human milk errors in the NICU. *Pediatrics.* 2017;139(2 suppl):S1–S13.

48. US Environmental Protection Agency. The Safe Drinking Water Act. https://www.epa.gov/sdwa. Accessed November 9, 2018.

49. American Academy of Pediatrics Committee on Nutrition. Formula feeding of term infants. In: Kleinman RE, Greer FR, eds. *Pediatric Nutrition.* 7th ed. Elk Grove Village, IL: American Academy of Pediatrics; 2014:66–68.

50. American Academy of Pediatrics. How to safely prepare formula with water. https://www.healthychildren.org/English/ages-stages/baby/feeding-nutrition/Pages/How-to-Safely-Prepare-Formula-with-Water.aspx. Updated July 3, 2018. Accessed November 9, 2018.

51. US Environmental Protection Agency. Basic information about lead in drinking water. https://www.epa.gov/ground-water-and-drinking-water/basic-information-about-lead-drinking-water. Accessed November 9, 2018.

52. Corkins MR, Griggs KC, Groh-Wargo S, et al. Standards for nutrition support: pediatric hospitalized patients. *Nutr Clin Pract.* 2013;28(2):263–276.

53. Paul E. Minimizing patient safety events through a multidisciplinary approach to human milk management. *ICAN Infant Child Adolesc Nutr.* 2015;7(5):258–261.

54. Gabrielski L, Lessen R. Centralized model of human milk preparation and storage in a state-of-the-art human milk lab. *ICAN Infant Child Adolesc Nutr.* 2011;3:225–232.

55. Facilities Guidelines Institute. Standard A2.1-7.2.3.2(3) and Standard 2.1-7.2.3.3(5). In: *Guidelines for Design and Construction of Hospital and Health Care Facilities.* Washington, DC: American Institute of Architects; 2014:91–92.

56. White RD, Smith JA, Shepley MM. Recommended standards for newborn ICU design. *J Perinatol.* 2013;33(suppl): S2–S16.

57. Massachusetts Department of Public Health. Compliance checklist IP6: neonatal intensive care unit. http://www.mass .gov/eohhs/docs/dph/quality/hcq-plan-review/ip06.pdf. Published May 2015. Accessed November 8, 2018.

58. Oklahoma State Department of Health. OAC 310:667-49-4 General medical surgical hospital construction requirements— nurseries. https://www.ok.gov/health2/documents/Medical %20Surgical%20Hospital_Nurseries.docx. Accessed November 8, 2018.

59. Texas Administrative Code. Title 25 health services, part 1, Department of State Health Services, chapter 133 hospital licensing, subchapter 1 physical plant and construction requirements, rule 133.163 spatial requirements for new construction. http://texreg.sos.state.tx.us/public/readtac $ext.TacPage?sl=T&app=9&p_dir=F&p_rloc=149501& p_tloc=237062&p_ploc=222130&pg=17&p_tac=&ti=25& pt=1&ch=133&rl=163. Accessed November 8, 2018.

60. US Department of Defense. DOD space planning criteria. Chapter 430: neonatal intensive care unit June 1, 2016. Whole Building Design Guide website. https://www.wbdg .org/FFC/DOD/MHSSC/spaceplanning_healthfac_430 _2016.pdf. Accessed November 8, 2018.

61. Georgia Department of Community Health. 2010 guidelines for design and construction of health care facilities. https://weblink.dch.georgia.gov/WebLink8/1/doc/307664 /Electronic.aspx. Accessed November 8, 2018.

62. Oregon Health Authority. FPS newborn nursery units rulesheet. https://public.health.oregon.gov/ProviderPartner Resources/HealthcareProvidersFacilities/FacilitiesPlanning Safety/Documents/FPSHospitalNewbornNurseryUnit RuleTemplate.pdf. Accessed November 8, 2018.

63. Michigan Department of Consumer and Industry Services Bureau of Health Systems Division of Health Facilities and Services. 2007 minimum design standards for health care facilities in Michigan. https://www.michigan.gov/documents/mdch/bhs_2007_Minimum_Design_Standards_Final_PDF_Doc._198958_7.pdf. Accessed November 8, 2018.

64. Office of Statewide Health Planning and Development. Interior environment. In: 2016 California Building Code. 2016:662. California Building Standards website. http://www.bsc.ca.gov/Codes.aspx. Accessed November 8, 2018.

65. Illinois General Assembly. Title 77: public health, chapter I: Department of Public Health, subchapter b: hospitals and ambulatory care facilities, part 250 hospital licensing requirements, section 250.1830 general requirements for all obstetric departments. http://ilga.gov/commission/jcar/admincode/077/077002500O18300R.html. Accessed November 20, 2016.

66. New York City Department of Health. Article 115 Prescription Formula Preparation Facilities. https://www1.nyc.gov/assets/doh/downloads/pdf/about/healthcode/health-code-article115.pdf. Accessed November 8, 2018.

67. Office of the Revisor of Statutes. Minnesota administrative rules. https://www.revisor.mn.gov/rules/?id=4645.1200. Published 2000. Accessed November 9, 2018.

68. Eglash A, Simon L, Academy of Breastfeeding Medicine. ABM clinical protocol #8: human milk storage information for home use for full-term infants, revised 2017. *Breastfeed Med.* 2017;12:390–395.

69. Centers for Disease Control and Prevention. Proper handling and storage of human milk. https://www.cdc.gov/breastfeeding/recommendations/handling_breastmilk.htm. Updated September 2018. Accessed November 9, 2018.

70. Cossey V, Jeurissen A, Thelissen MJ, Vanhole C, Schuermans A. Expressed breast milk on a neonatal unit: a hazard analysis and critical control points approach. *Am J Infect Control.* 2011;39(10):832–838.

71. NSF International, American National Standards Institute. NSF/ANSI 3: Commercial warewashing equipment. In: *NSF International Standard/American National Standard for Food Equipment.* Ann Arbor, MI: NSF International; 2012.

72. NSF International, American National Standards Institute. NSF/ANSI 51: Food equipment materials. In: *NSF International Standard/American National Standard for Food Equipment.* Ann Arbor, MI: NSF International; 2015.

73. US Food and Drug Administration. FDA food code. 2013. https://www.fda.gov/food/guidanceregulation/retail foodprotection/foodcode/default.htm. Accessed May 4, 2017.

74. United States Pharmacopeial Convention. USP 795 pharmaceutical compounding—nonsterile preparations. In: *USP Compounding Compendium 2016.* Rockville, MD: United States Pharmacopeial Convention; 2016:31–38.

75. United States Pharmacopeial Convention. USP 797 Pharmaceutical compounding—sterile preparations. In: *USP Compounding Compendium 2016.* Rockville, MD: United States Pharmacopeial Convention: 2016:39–84.

76. Renfrew MJ, Ansell P, Macleod KL. Formula feed preparation: helping reduce the risk; a systematic review. *Arch Dis Child.* 2003;88:855–858.

77. Bower A, Wiesenfeld HC, Kloesz JL, et al. *Cronobacter sakazakii* infection associated with feeding extrinsically contaminated expressed human milk to a premature infant—Pennsylvania, 2016. *MMWR Morb Mortal Wkly Rep.* 2017;66(28):761–762.

78. Chang JC, Chen CH, Fang LJ, Tsai CR, Chang YC, Wang TM. Influence of prolonged storage process, pasteurization, and heat treatment on biologically-active human milk proteins. *Pediatr Neonatal.* 2013;54:360304366.

79. De la Fuente M, Olano A, Juraz M. Mineral balance in milk heated using microwave energy. *J Agric Food Chem.* 2002;10:2274–2277.

80. Mohrenschlager M, Weigl LB, Haug S, et al. Iatrogenic burns by warming bottles in the neonatal period: report of two cases and review of the literature. *J Burn Care Rehabil.* 2003;24(1):52–55.

81. Bransburg-Zabary S, Virozub A, Mimouni F. Human milk warming temperatures using a simulation of currently available storage and warming methods. *PLoS One.* 2015;10(6):1–13.E0128806. doi:10.1371/journal.pone.0128806.

82. Steele C, Gonzalez B, Gornick W. Thawing human milk for hospitalized infants: use of a laboratory bead bath may

be an effective method for large quantities. *J Acad Nutr Diet.* 2018;118(5):801–804.

83. Cervia JS, Ortolano GA, Canonica FP. Hospital tap water: a reservoir of risk for health care-associated infection. *Infect Dis Clin Pract.* 2008;16(6):349–353.

84. Centers for Disease Control and Prevention. Prevention strategies for seasonal influenza in healthcare settings. https://www.cdc.gov/flu/professionals/infectioncontrol/healthcaresettings.htm. Published February 13, 2018. Accessed April 26, 2018.

85. McNeil SA, Foster CL, Hedderwick SA, Kauffman CA. Effect of hand cleansing with antimicrobial soap or alcohol-based gel on microbial colonization of artificial fingernails worn by health care workers. *Clin Infect Dis.* 2001;32: 367–372.

86. Association of Perioperative Registered Nurses. Hand hygiene. http://www.aorn.org/guidelines/clinical-resources/clinical-faqs/hand-antisepsis-hygiene. Accessed May 19, 2017.

87. Moolenaar RL, Crutcher M, San Joaquin VH, et al. A prolonged outbreak of *Pseudomonas aeruginosa* in a neonatal intensive care unit: did staff fingernails play a role in disease transmission? *Infect Control Hosp Epidemiol.* 2000;21:80–85.

88. Peters MD, McArthur A, Munn Z. Safe management of expressed breast milk: a systematic review. *Women Birth.* 2016;29(6):473–481.

89. Centers for Disease Control and Prevention. How to keep your breast pump kit clean: the essentials. https://www.cdc.gov/healthywater/hygiene/healthychildcare/infantfeeding/breastpump.html. Updated August 2017. Accessed November 8, 2018.

90. Lawrence RM. Transmission of infectious diseases through breast milk and breastfeeding. In: Lawrence RA, Lawrence RM, eds. *Breastfeeding: A Guide for the Medical Profession.* 7th ed. Maryland Heights, MO: Elsevier Mosby; 2011:406–473.

91. Becker GE, Smith HA, Cooney F. Methods of milk expression for lactating women. *Cochrane Database Syst Rev.* 2015;(2): CD006170. doi:10.1002/14651858.CD006170.pub4.

92. Boo NY, Nordiah AJ, Alfizah H, Nor-Rohaini AH, Lim VK. Contamination of breast milk obtained by manual expression and breast pumps in mothers of very low birthweight infants. *J Hosp Infect.* 2001; 49(4):274–281.

93. Smith SL, Serke L. Case report of sepsis in neonates fed expressed mother's milk. *J Obstet Gynecol Neonat Nurs*. 2016; 45:699–705.

94. Karimi M, Eslami Z, Shamsi F, Moradi J, Ahmadi AY, Baghianimoghadam B. The effect of educational intervention on decreasing mothers' expressed breast milk bacterial contamination whose infants are admitted to neonatal intensive care unit. *J Res Health Sci*. 2013;l13(1):43–47.

95. Weems MF, Dereddy NR, Arnold SR. Mother's milk as a source of *Enterobacter cloacae* sepsis in a preterm infant. *Breastfeed Med*. 2015;10(10):503–504.

96. Petersen S, Greisen G, Krogfelt K. Nasogastric feeding tubes from a neonatal department yield high concentrations of potentially pathogenic bacteria—even 1 day after insertion. *Pediatr Res*. 2016;80:395–400.

97. Bobo E. Reemergence of blenderized tube feedings: exploring the evidence. *Nutr Clin Pract*. 2016;31(6):730–735.

98. Martin M, Gardner G. Home enteral nutrition: updates, trends, and challenges. *Nutr Clin Pract*. 2017;32(6):712–721.

99. Epp L, Lammert L, Vallumsetla N, et al. Use of blenderized tube feeding in adult and pediatric home enteral nutrition patients. *Nutr Clin Pract*. 2017;32(2):201–205.

100. Epp L. Blenderized feeding options—the sky's the limit. *Pract Gastroenterol*. 2018;42(6):30–39. https://www.practicalgastro.com/article/183989/Blenderized-Feeding-Options-Skys-the-Limit. Accessed December 30, 2018.

101. US Food and Drug Administration; Guha S, Myers MR, Silverstein J, Antonino MJ, Cooper J. Feeding tubes and transition to ENFit™: creating science around infinite user variables. Stay Connected website. http://stayconnected.org/wp-content/uploads/2017/08/FDA.Blenderized-Update-upload.pdf. Accessed January 2, 2019.

102. Perry AG, Potter PA. *Clinical Nursing Skills & Techniques*. 6th ed. St. Louis, MO: Mosby; 2006:1032.

103. Oliveira M, Batista C, Aidoo K. Application of hazard analysis critical control points system to enteral tube feeding in hospital. *J Hum Nutr Diet*. 2001;14:397–403.

104. Carvalho M, Morais T, Amaral D, Sigulem D. Hazard analysis of critical control point system approach in the evaluation of environmental and procedural sources of contamination

of enteral feedings in three hospitals. *JPEN J Parenter Enteral Nutr.* 2000;24:296–300.

105. American Society for Quality. Plan-do-check-act (PDCA) cycle. http://asq.org/learn-about-quality/project-planning-tools/overview/pdca-cycle.html. Accessed November 9, 2018.

CHAPTER 8

Administration and Monitoring of Enteral Nutrition

Introduction

Clinicians must be cognizant of many factors when developing an individualized enteral nutrition (EN) regimen. For example, EN can be supplemental nutrition for patients who are unable to meet nutrition needs with an oral diet alone, or it can meet 100% of an individual's nutrition needs. It can be administered through a temporary enteral access device (EAD), such as a nasogastric feeding tube, or a long-term EAD, such as a gastrostomy or jejunostomy feeding tube (see Chapter 3). Feeding modalities include the syringe method (also known as bolus feeding), gravity-bag feeding, and pump-assisted feedings. Patients and caregivers vary in terms of their ability and availability to administer EN. An individual's medical history, gastrointestinal (GI) status, and ability to participate in the feeding process will all influence the selection of the optimal EN regimen for that patient.

Insurance coverage is an important consideration, particularly when selecting an EN feeding regimen for the hospitalized patient who will be discharged to receive EN therapy in another setting. Above all, while considering these variables and others, the clinician must remember that, if medically possible, the desired outcome of the EN regimen is to restore the patient's ability to meet nutrition needs via oral diet and end dependency on nutrition support.

Implementation of Enteral Nutrition Feedings

After the patient undergoes a comprehensive nutrition assessment, the nutrition support clinician can develop an individualized EN regimen, establish nutrition goals, and either initiate EN or assist the ordering practitioner with EN initiation. After initiation of the EN regimen, the clinician should closely monitor the safety of EN, the advancement of feedings, and the patient's metabolic and GI tolerance of the prescribed feeding regimen. (See Chapter 6 for information on ordering, initiating, and advancing EN.) While EN is being administered, clinicians must adjust the regimen as needed to prevent complications and achieve nutrition goals. At this time, clinicians may also be required to provide education on feeding administration (eg, hang times, water flushes, and proper feeding administration techniques), patient positioning, or the feeding equipment.

Reducing Microbial Contamination Risks

Microbial contamination of EN formula or administration sets can occur at any step of the feeding delivery process. For example, bacterial contamination of EN has been attributed to touch contamination, formula preparation/addition of modular to commercially manufactured formulas, extended hang times of the enteral formula beyond manufacturer guidelines/facility policy, use of administration sets for more than 24 hours, and endogenous retrograde growth.[1-8] The consequences of EN contamination can be serious. It has been associated with nosocomial infections, feeding intolerance (diarrhea), infectious enterocolitis, vomiting, fever, abdominal distention, aspiration pneumonia, and sepsis.[1,4,5,8,9] See Chapter 7 for discussion of the contamination points in the formula and human milk (HM) preparation processes.

Based on results of testing and reports about microbial contamination, criteria have been established for how long various types of formula preparations can safely hang in ambient environments, the recommended use of administration sets, safe feeding administration procedures, and proper hand hygiene (see Table 8-1 for selected recommendations).[1] At the federal level, the US Food and Drug Administration (FDA) has established standards for unacceptable levels of bacterial contamination in medical foods that FDA inspectors of medical food firms must immediately report (Table 8-2).[10] As discussed in Chapter 5, federal regulations for infant formulas are distinct from those for medical foods such as adult and pediatric enteral formulas.

Environmental Controls and Temperature

The environment in which enteral formula is prepared and ambient temperatures when the formula is administered can affect microbial growth. The American Society for Parenteral and Enteral Nutrition (ASPEN) has recommended that "the environment in which enteral nutrition preparation takes place should be controlled to reduce the risk of contamination."[11] When this recommendation was published in 2009, it was endorsed by the Academy of Nutrition and Dietetics, American Society of Health-System Pharmacists, and Institute for Safe Medication

TABLE 8-1. Practice Recommendations to Promote Safe Handling of Enteral Nutrition

1. Use a closed EN delivery system when possible.

2. Follow the manufacturer's recommendations for duration of infusion through an intact delivery device (container and administration set).

3. Do not reuse the enteral delivery device for open or closed systems (container and administration set in excess of what is recommended by the manufacturer).

4. If open systems are used, follow recommended hang times and avoid topping off remaining formula, which may result in a continuous culture for exponential microbial growth.
   a. Limit infusion time for open EN feeding systems to 4–8 hours maximum (12 hours in the home setting).
   b. Limit infusion time for a reconstituted powder product or modular to 4 hours maximum.
   c. Change the delivery device (container and administration set) according to the manufacturer's recommendations for open systems.

5. Be aware that the addition of modular units to an open feeding system may result in an unacceptable risk of contamination in hyperthermal environments.

6. To limit the risk of microbial growth and biofilm formation, avoid unnecessary additions to the EN administration set. If additional equipment, such as 3-way stopcocks, is used, follow manufacturer recommendations or facility protocol for change and cleaning practices.

7. Establish and follow protocols for preparation, handling, and storage of commercial and handmade EN.
   a. Educate those who prepare and administer EN about hand hygiene (a critical point) and safe handling of EN preparation and administration; extend education to patients and family members/care givers who will continue this practice into the home setting.

(continued)

TABLE 8-1. *(Continued)*

    b. Use effective hand hygiene in all aspects of EN preparation and administration. When gloves are used, they must be clean gloves, not having been involved in other nonrelated tasks. The importance of hand washing in minimizing transference of microbial growth and preventing hospital-acquired infections cannot be overstressed.

    c. Give preference to selecting systems that require minimal handling.

    d. Use a clean work surface for EN preparation.

    e. Use equipment dedicated for EN use only.

    f. Store EN formula according to the manufacturer's instructions. Store prepared or opened ready-to-feed solutions in an appropriate refrigerator, discarding any used solutions within 24 hours of preparation or opening.

8. Periodically survey and regularly monitor adherence to the above-listed protocols. Document findings and take appropriate actions if protocols are not followed.

9. Reduce potential for touch contamination of EN-related equipment as well as risk of exposure to body fluids by reducing interruptions to the system, providing a clean work surface (eg, small clean towel under tube/ administration connection), and, when interruptions are necessary, using only washed hands and gloves.

10. Keep all equipment, including syringes and containers for flush and medication administration, as clean and dry as possible. Store clean equipment away from potential sources of contamination.

11. Consider whether microbial growth related to EN might be implicated as part of the diagnosis when patients have adverse conditions such as diarrhea.

Abbreviation: EN, enteral nutrition.

Source: Reprinted with permission from reference 1: Boullata JI, Carrera AL, Harvey L, et al. ASPEN safe practices for enteral nutrition therapy. *JPEN J Parenter Enteral Nutr*. 2017;41(1):15–103. doi:10.1177/0148607116673053.

TABLE 8-2. FDA Guidance on Inspection of Medical Foods for Contamination

FDA inspectors of firms manufacturing, distributing, or repacking medical foods must immediately report findings of any of the following:

- Any aerobic agar plate growing >10^4 cfu/mL
- Positive for coliform and *Escherichia coli*
- Presence of *Salmonella* spp., *Listeria monocytogenes,* or staphylococcal enterotoxin
- *Bacillus cereus* subsample >1000 organisms/g
- Aerobic plate count subsample >10,000 organisms/g, *or* ≥3 subsamples exceed 1000 organisms/g

---

Source: Adapted from reference 10.

Practices. The ASPEN recommendations for safe practices in EN were updated in 2017.[1]

Hang Times and Administration Set Use

To reduce the risk for contamination, hang time protocols for EN must be enforced. The recommended hang time will vary depending on the type of product administered, the administration system, and the care setting. For example, the FDA has recommended that reconstituted enteral formulas prepared from powdered products (which are not sterile) hang no more than 4 hours; this recommendation was issued in response to deaths of infants who consumed infant formula contaminated with *Cronobacter sakazakii* (formerly called *Enterobacter sakazakii*).[12,13] Other recommendations regarding hang times have been published by ASPEN. See Figure 8-1 for a summary.[1]

The literature suggests that limiting formula hang time lowers the risk for bacterial contamination. Although patient safety is the paramount concern, shortening hang times increases supply costs. Therefore, healthcare

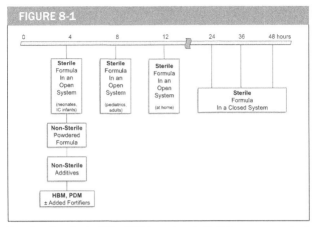

FIGURE 8-1

Hang times for enteral nutrition. HBM, human breast milk; IC, immunocompromised; PDM, pasteurized donor milk. Reprinted with permission from reference 1: Boullata JI, Carrera AL, Harvey L, et al. ASPEN safe practices for enteral nutrition therapy. *JPEN J Parenter Enteral Nutr.* 2017;41(1):15–103. doi:10.1177/0148607116673053.

providers have an incentive to create protocols that promote safety without incurring undue expense. Neely and associates investigated whether the hang time protocol for feeding administration sets in a burn unit could be extended from a very conservative approach of 1 administration set every 4 hours to a longer hang time of 8 hours.[6] The investigation used both commercially prepared formulas and the specialized, hospital-specific standard tube feeding formula (designed for burn patients) made of multiple separate components. The extended hang time was not associated with an increase in microbial load, unacceptable levels of contamination, or a higher rate of nosocomial infections, and changing the protocol to 8-hour hang times reduced supply costs. The investigators suggest that the microbial load did not increase with the 8-hour hang time because the hospital-specific formula was refrigerated after preparation until needed and only 4 hours' worth of formula was administered at a time. In addition, diligent aseptic technique was followed during preparation and during administration of the feedings.

Improper handling of the enteral feeding administration set and feeding port increases the risk for microbial contamination. Touch contamination by the nursing staff is a particular risk because they are typically the personnel most involved in manipulating the enteral feeding system. In a study of handling techniques in a pediatric hospital, Lyman and colleagues estimated contamination rates of enteral formula and/or administration sets to be between 19% and 59% and determined that 17 of the 24 species found to contaminate EN originated from skin or oral flora.[2] This study compared sterile water rinse of administration sets, refrigeration of administration sets that were not rinsed, and ready-to-hang formula with the administration set capped off and left at room temperature. The sterile water rinse and unrinsed refrigerated techniques showed similar bacterial growth of 11.4% and 10.3%, respectively. The ready-to-hang samples had 4.4% bacterial growth. The authors then factored in nursing labor and supply costs for each technique. The sterile water rinse technique significantly increased the overall expense, while ready-to-hang systems were deemed the most effective, in relation to decreasing bacterial contamination, supply, and labor costs.[2]

In a 1992 study, Payne-James and colleagues investigated retrograde contamination with 3 types of administration sets: feeding set without drip chamber, feeding set with drip chamber, and feeding set with antireflux ball valve. The authors found that the drip chamber on the administration set showed less bacterial growth than the no-drip chamber and drip chamber with antireflux ball valve.[14]

A potential source of bacterial contamination of EN is endogenous retrograde growth stemming from secretions of the throat, lungs, and stomach that enter the feeding tube and migrate toward the connection site of the administration set.[8] Mathus-Vliegen and colleagues found that feeding containers and/or administration sets tested positive for the same predominant bacteria found from the cultures of the throat, lung and stomach, including 4 pathogenic species that are mobile and can easily grow upstream.[8]

One high-risk group for microbial infections is neonates. Hurrell and associates reported that opportunistic pathogens (including *Enterobacteriaceae* spp.) were found growing in 76% of neonatal enteral feeding tubes tested after being in place for <6 hours to >48 hours.[15] The feeding regimen (HM, fortified HM, ready-to-feed formula, reconstituted powdered formula, or a mixture) did not seem to affect microbial growth. Mehall and colleagues also studied neonatal feeding tubes and found them to be a reservoir for antibiotic-resistant pathogens that could be transmitted to other infants.[16] In that study of 50 tube-fed neonates, formula-fed infants had significant feeding intolerance when fed with contaminated tubes, and 4 infants developed necrotizing enterocolitis that required surgery. Contamination was more prevalent in those infants receiving H_2 receptor antagonists.[16] Juma and Forsythe investigated the colonization of feeding tubes in neonates with a wide range of bacterial and fungal organisms.[17] The potential for these organisms to translocate and cause systemic infections in immunocompromised infants with increased mucosal permeability and underdeveloped gut microflora was explored. See Chapter 7 for guidance on the use of infant formulas and HM in EN.

Modulars

Modulars, especially those in powdered form, are not sterilized at the end of the manufacturing process and may increase the risk of bacterial contamination.[3] Prepared enteral formulas with the addition of modular products should be refrigerated when not in use, and unused product should be discarded after 24 hours of mixing.[1] See Chapter 7 for additional information on preparing enteral formulas as well as infant formulas and HM.

Blenderized Tube Feedings

Microbial contamination of blenderized tube feedings (BTFs) may cause foodborne illness.[9] BTFs can be contaminated at multiple points in the preparation and administration process. Ingredients in BTFs may be contaminated, or improper food handling techniques may be used during preparation of the BTF, while cleaning equipment, in food storage, or during feeding administration.[7,18]

Research on the incidence of bacterial contamination of BTFs and associated infections is scant. In a study conducted in Iran, where BTFs are widely used in hospitals, Jalali and associates studied samples of BTFs prepared in a hospital kitchen under the supervision of a nutritionist and then delivered to patient wards in closed containers and refrigerated until time of use. In 76 samples collected immediately after preparation, variable counts of coliform and *Staphylococcus aureus* were found in all samples. In 76 samples taken at 18 hours after preparation, 68 samples (90%) were positive for coliform and 72 samples (95%) were positive for *S. aureus*. Tests did not detect *Salmonella* spp. or *Listeria monoocytgenes*.[7]

In a study by Gallagher et al, 20 pediatric patients who were fed via gastrostomy tubes were switched to a blenderized food diet from commercial enteral formulas.[19] These patients exhibited improved GI tolerance (patients with >1 episode of vomiting per week decreased from 76% to 53%, and patients experiencing gagging or retching decreased from 82% to 47% by the end of the study). Investigators also reported increased intestinal bacterial diversity. Patients did require 50% more energy intake while fed with BTFs.

To reduce the risk for microbial contamination, hospital- or home-prepared BTFs should be treated in the same manner as reconstituted powdered formulas with respect to preparation in a controlled environment, handling, storage, and administration. The Academy of Nutrition and Dietetics has published guidelines to minimize contamination of BTFs from preparation to administration and meet food safety standards.[20] It is recommended that BTFs should be prepared and handled according to safe food handling and preparation guidelines; hospital-prepared or home-blended products must be refrigerated until administered and between feedings; and unused portions must be discarded after 24 hours. The maximum hang time for home- or hospital-blended BTFs at room temperature is 2 hours.[1,20] Hang times for commercial BTFs may be different.

Enteral Feeding Pumps

The first commercial enteral feeding pump, which used rotary and linear peristaltic mechanisms to compress and decompress fluid against rollers, was introduced in 1956. Use of enteral pumps took off in the 1970s, coinciding with the development of commercially manufactured enteral formulas. Pump design advanced to use volumetric mechanisms that improved the accuracy of measuring a preset volume of formula into a cassette before delivering the formula at a controlled rate into the infusion tubing. By the late 1990s, enteral feeding pumps were enhanced with safety features, including microprocessor controls, display screens, programming options, alarm alerts, error messages, automatic water flush features, anti-free-flow protection, administration-set security doors, and safeguards against overinfusion.[21] Today, enteral feeding pumps offer even more sophisticated features, such as ambulatory functionality (ie, a battery-operated pump and bag can be carried in a shoulder bag or backpack), delivery of a controlled amount of enteral feedings, automatic priming, dose-volume settings, memory/feeding history information, easy-to-load cassettes, and one-handed pump setup.[21]

Current enteral feeding pumps can be programmed at rates of 0.1 mL/h (a specialized infant feeding pump designed for low-volume/HM feedings) to 600 mL/h. Enteral feeding pumps can be programmed for continuous, intermittent, or bolus feedings. According to manufacturer manuals, the accuracy of flow rates ranges from ±5% to 10%. Flow-rate accuracy depends on hang height, which ranges from about 6 to 18 inches above the pump, depending on the pump model. When the specialized pediatric low-volume/HM feeding pump is used with a feeding rate of <0.1 mL/h, the pump should be level with the patient.

If a feeding pump fails to deliver feedings within the manufacturer's accuracy specification, the pump should be recalibrated. Pump manufacturers recommend that enteral feeding pumps should routinely be recalibrated every 2 years.

Use of enteral feeding pumps is recommended for patients receiving tube feedings into the small bowel.[1] The jejunum secretes fluid in response to hyperosmolar solutions, and rapid infusion of such a formula into the small bowel may result in abdominal distention, hyperperistalsis, and diarrhea.[21] In addition, because the stomach reservoir is bypassed, patients may experience bloating and diarrhea if bolus or gravity feedings are administered through a jejunal tube. A slow, controlled rate of infusion can avoid or reduce these symptoms. The addition of anti-free-flow devices on the administration set protects against the possibility of free-flow incidents, preventing large volumes of feeding from entering the GI tract as a single bolus feeding.[21]

Critically ill patients may also benefit from pump-assisted enteral feedings because continuous infusion of formula may improve tolerance.[1,22] Patients who experience enteral feeding aspiration, gastroesophageal reflux, vomiting, or unresolved diarrhea may benefit from controlled-rate, small-volume feedings administered by an enteral feeding pump.[21,23]

To deliver EN as prescribed, enteral feeding pumps must be used correctly. Walker and colleagues investigated discrepancies between 24-hour enteral feeding pump histories and the hourly EN provision documented by the nursing staff at a facility that had changed which type of enteral feeding pump it used.[24] The researchers determined that the enteral formula was rarely hung according to the manufacturer's specifications and improper hang height accounted for the delivery discrepancies. Improper hang height can result in underfeeding. At the conclusion of this study, nursing staff was trained on the proper hang height for accurate nutrition support delivery, and the facility's EN protocol was updated accordingly.[24] See Table 8-3 for recommendations regarding the use of enteral feeding pumps.[1,25]

Protocols on Preventing Pulmonary Aspiration

Healthcare facilities should have in place protocols to minimize pulmonary aspiration risk in patients receiving EN. For example, clinicians should be trained regarding best practices for positioning the patient during feeding (see Table 8-4).[1,26,27] Protocols related to pulmonary aspiration risk should also address the use of gastric residual volumes (GRVs). ASPEN recommends the following:[1]

GRV measurements may not need to be used as part of routine care to monitor ICU [intensive care unit]

TABLE 8-3. Practice Recommendations for the Use of Enteral Feeding Pumps

- Enteral feeding pumps should deliver the prescribed volume within 10% accuracy for children and adults.
- Enteral feeding pumps should have a flow accuracy within 5% accuracy for neonatal patients.
- Zero the volume delivery amount on the feeding pump at the beginning of a time period, such as usual intake and output assessment period.
- For pediatric patients, pumps should have an alarm for no flow or occlusion (even at low infusion rates) and automatic anti-free-flow protection should the tubing become disconnected from the pump. A lockout feature to prevent settings from being changed is also preferable.[25]
- Ensure that institutional biomedical engineering departments periodically test, according to manufacturer recommendations, whether pumps continue to meet the accuracy rates and whether alarms function.
- Human milk infused at low rates should be administered via syringe pump with the syringe tip elevated.
- Feeding pumps used for patients requiring enteral nutrition at home should have features that promote safety and minimize sleep disturbances.

Source: Information is from references 1 and 25.

---

patients on EN. For those patient care areas where GRVs are still utilized, holding EN for GRVs <500 mL in the absence of other signs of intolerance should be avoided. A gastric residual volume of between 250 and 500 mL should lead to implementation of measures to reduce risk of aspiration.

This recommendation is based on a lack of evidence that GRVs are sufficiently predictive of risk to warrant routine use of the invasive procedure, which "leads to increased EAD clogging, inappropriate cessation of EN, consumption of nursing time, and allocation of healthcare resources

> **TABLE 8-4.** Practice Recommendations on Positioning Patients Receiving Enteral Nutrition
>
> - Elevate the head of the bed at least 30° while patients are receiving EN, unless an elevated position is medically contraindicated. If there is a contraindication, consider the reverse Trendelenburg position.
> - If it is necessary to lower the head of the bed for a procedure or because of a medical contraindication, return the patient to an elevated head-of-the-bed position as soon as possible.
> - Pediatric patients over 12 months of age are to be elevated at least 30° while tube feeding is infusing and for an additional 30 minutes after the feeding, unless elevation is medically contraindicated.[26,27]
> - Infants under 1 year of age should sleep on their backs without the head of the bed being elevated.

Source: Information is from references 1, 26, and 27.

and may adversely affect outcome through reduced volume of EN delivered."[1] Refer to Chapter 9 for further discussion of preventing aspiration risk.

Feeding Tube Patency

Feeding tubes are prone to clogging for a variety of reasons, including an accumulation of formula sediment in the lower portion of the tube, especially during slow administration rates of energy-dense and fiber-containing formulas.[28] To minimize the risk for tube clogging, clinicians should follow protocols for flushing adequate volumes of water through tubes; completely grind medications into a fine powder before dissolving them in purified water; avoid mixing medications together; limit the frequency of GRV checks; and avoid administering acidic fluids through the tube.[1,29,30] See Chapter 10 for information on recommended medication administration techniques.

Nasogastric and jejunostomy tubes are more likely than other tubes to clog because of their long lengths and narrow diameters.[29] Clogging may be caused by the acidic contents of gastric residual aspiration in the feeding tube.[1,29,30] Historically, colas, meat tenderizers, and acidic juices have been used to clear clogs. However, acidic juices may worsen clogs because the proteins in the enteral formula coagulate in an acid environment.[30,31] It is crucial to restore tube patency when a clog is suspected. See Table 8-5[1] and Chapter 3 for additional guidance on the management of tube patency.

TABLE 8-5. Practice Recommendations on Maintaining and Monitoring Feeding Tube Patency

1. Flush feeding tubes with 30 mL of water every 4 hours during continuous feeding or before and after intermittent feedings in adult patients.
2. Limit gastric residual checks as acidic gastric contents may cause protein in enteral formulas to precipitate within the lumen of the tube.
3. Flush the feeding tube with 30 mL of water after gastric residual volume measurements in an adult patient.
4. Flush feeding tubes in neonatal and pediatric patients with the lowest volume of water necessary to clear the tube, unless the patient needs additional fluids to meet fluid needs. In some neonate patients with strict fluid limits, a small amount of air may be used to flush the tube.
5. Purified water is recommended for use in tube flushes in adult and neonatal/pediatric patients before and after medication administration.
6. Adhere to protocols that call for proper flushing of tubes before and after medication administration.
7. Use an enteral feeding pump when patients, such as neonates, require slow rates of enteral feeding, and respond promptly to pump alarms.

Source: Adapted with permission from reference 1: Boullata JI, Carrera AL, Harvey L, et al. ASPEN safe practices for enteral nutrition therapy. *JPEN J Parenter Enteral Nutr.* 2017;41(1):15–103. doi:10.1177/0148607116673053.

Monitoring

Goals and Scope of Monitoring

Careful monitoring of patients receiving EN is imperative to optimize patient safety, assess the effectiveness of nutrition support, and avoid potential deleterious complications. An important part of monitoring is investigating and promptly resolving problems related to EN. To attain positive clinical outcomes related to the provision of EN, the clinician needs a thorough understanding of pathophysiology; energy and macronutrient metabolism; and fluid, electrolyte, and micronutrient disorders.

The preeminent goals of monitoring EN are to (a) evaluate the adequacy of energy, nutrient, and fluid provision; (b) minimize risk factors for feeding intolerance and other complications; and (c) detect and resolve any complications or other problems as soon as possible. In the acute care and subacute care settings, responsibility for monitoring tolerance and identifying complications frequently rests with the nursing staff, who then bring concerns to nutrition support specialists for recommendations. See Chapter 3 for information on mechanical complications and Chapter 9 for a review of GI-related and metabolic complications.

While patients are receiving EN, their nutrition and clinical status must be periodically reassessed. The frequency of reassessment is based on the patient's stability and tolerance of EN. The scope of the nutrition reassessment resembles that of the initial nutrition assessment (see Chapter 1) while being guided by patient-specific goals of the nutrition care plan (eg, to maintain or improve nutrition/clinical status, transition the patient to another care setting, or enhance the patient's quality of life).

The periodic nutrition assessments in the monitoring period should include the following:[1,32,33]

- Medical, surgical, social, and diet histories
- Anthropometric measurements
- Laboratory and diagnostic studies
- Nutrition-focused physical exam
- Handgrip strength and functional status

Surrogate markers such as energy intake, body weight, serum protein levels, nitrogen balance, body composition, and functional status have been used to assess the adequacy of the nutrition support regimen.[34] However, many of these measures are influenced by the patient's clinical status and, therefore, may not accurately reflect the patient's nutrition status. Serum proteins (albumin and prealbumin) and C-reactive protein are indicators of an inflammatory process and may serve as predictors of morbidity and mortality, but they are not accurate measures of nutrition status.[1,35] Nutrition status is an intermediate marker that acts as a stepping-stone to the ultimate goal of achieving positive clinical outcomes (eg, wound healing, weight gain, decreased infectious complications, reduced length of stay).

Table 8-6 summarizes suggested monitoring parameters for patients receiving EN.[1,27,34,36] In addition to monitoring the factors outlined in this table, clinicians monitoring patients receiving EN must verify that the EN regimen includes routine procedures designed to promote safety (Table 8-7).[1] To advance the safety and cost-effectiveness of patient care, the nutrition support clinician must also provide ongoing education related to optimal EN delivery for other members of the healthcare team.[1]

A plan for monitoring EN therapy, including short- and long-term goals, should be documented in the patient's initial nutrition care plan as well as in specific plans of care, such as clinical pathways. Once tolerance of enteral feedings is established, the frequency of monitoring is influenced by the patient's disease, severity of illness, degree of

TABLE 8-6. Monitoring Parameters for Patients Receiving Enteral Nutrition Support

- Nutrition-focused physical exam, including clinical signs of energy, fluid, and nutrient excess or deficiency
- Vital signs
- Actual energy, fluid, and nutrient intake (oral, enteral, and parenteral) vs nutrition goals
- Measurement of output (urine, GI fluids, wound losses, chest tube drainage, etc)
- Weight trends
- Growth trends for infants and children (appropriate weight gain and linear growth, head circumferences for children up to 3 years of age)[36]
- Laboratory data,[a] including:
  ◦ CBC, glucose, BUN, creatinine, electrolytes, calcium, magnesium, phosphorus, LFTs, triglycerides, serum proteins, PT/INR, urine glucose, urine sodium, urine-specific gravity
  ◦ Vitamin D (25,OH) levels in pediatric patients
- Review of medications and any vitamin, mineral, or herbal supplements
- Diagnostic studies
- Changes in GI function indicating tolerance of nutrition therapy (eg, ostomy output, stool frequency and consistency, presence of blood in the stool, presence of abdominal distention/firmness, increasing abdominal girth, nausea, vomiting)
- Signs and symptoms of complications of EN therapy[b]
- For infants and children, apnea and bradycardia with feeds, which may be exacerbated by gastric distention[27]
- Functional status (eg, handgrip strength)
- Skin integrity status

Abbreviations: BUN, blood urea nitrogen; CBC, complete blood count; GI, gastrointestinal; INR, international normalized ratio; LFT, liver function test; PT, prothrombin time.

[a]The burden of the test, including consideration of the blood volume required to do the test, should be balanced by the benefit or usefulness of the results, particularly in those patients who have been on a stable enteral regimen.

[b]Refer to Table 8-7 for additional information on monitoring and preventing EN-related complications.

Source: Information is from references 1, 27, 34, and 36.

TABLE 8-7. Practice Recommendations for Monitoring and Preventing Complications

1. Evaluate all enterally fed patients for risk of aspiration.
2. Use ENFit® feeding sets, tubes, and syringes to avoid misconnections with intravenous lines.
3. Verify that the feeding tube is in the proper position before initiating feedings.
4. Keep the head of the bed elevated at least 30° at all times during the administration of enteral feedings, unless contraindicated.
5. In those facilities where GRV is utilized as a monitoring parameter, a GRV >500 mL should result in holding EN and reassessing patient tolerance by use of an established algorithm including physical assessment, GI assessment, evaluation of glycemic control, minimization of sedation, and consideration of promotility agent use, if not already prescribed.
6. Consider a feeding tube placed well beyond the pylorus when GRVs are consistently measured at >500 mL.

Abbreviations: EN, enteral nutrition; GI, gastrointestinal; GRV, gastric residual volume.

Source: Adapted with permission from reference 1: Boullata JI, Carrera AL, Harvey L, et al. ASPEN safe practices for enteral nutrition therapy. *JPEN J Parenter Enteral Nutr.* 2017;41(1):15–103. doi:10.1177/0148607116673053.

malnutrition, and level of metabolic stress.[37,38] To provide adequate nutrition, it is often necessary to make adjustments based on the patient's clinical status.

The administration of EN may be interrupted for procedures/tests, surgery, medical interventions and therapies, activities of daily living, periods of GI distress, medication administration, and elevated GRVs. Any interruptions that can affect adequate delivery of nutrition support and hydration should be addressed during the monitoring process. Progress toward nutrition goals should be documented within the medical record. If goals of therapy are not being achieved, the nutrition care plan should be revised.[32]

Meeting Targets for Nutrient Delivery

Once enteral feeding orders have been written, it is essential for the nutrition support clinician to verify that the tube feedings are actually being administered as ordered (see Chapter 6 for information on EN orders). Multiple studies show that delivery of EN to hospitalized patients often falls short of established goals.[37–40] Scheduled and unscheduled interruptions, inadequate nutrient prescriptions, or other barriers (eg, mechanical, GI, or infectious complications) are all factors cited that contribute to the inadequate provision of EN.[37] A study in burn patients found that the amount of energy received by patients was significantly less than the prescribed amount on all study days (first 2 weeks of admission).[41] The most common reasons why the EN prescription was not met were EN not being administered at the goal rate (35%); feedings being held for surgery (24%); physician- or nurse-directed interruptions to feedings (16%); and feeding intolerance (11%). The average time per day that EN was not administered was 8.9 hours.[41]

Volume-based feeding is one strategy to meet the EN goal in cases where EN is frequently interrupted. With this technique, a set volume of formula is prescribed for the day and the nurses compensate for the time that the tube feeding is stopped by adjusting the hourly rate of administration as needed to meet the daily goal.[42]

When achievement of the established EN goal is not feasible in critically ill patients, administering a smaller volume of EN during the first week of ICU admission seems to be adequate to achieve positive outcomes.[22,37,38,43,44] Kudsk and colleagues found that adult trauma patients receiving as little as 15 kcal/kg/d via EN demonstrated improved outcomes as compared with patients receiving parenteral nutrition (PN).[43] Others have found that the delivery of approximately 14–18 kcal/kg/d or 60% to 70% of enteral feeding goal has also been favorable.[37,38] However, before this is accepted as the standard of care, larger clinical trials must take place to delineate the optimal timing and critical amount of enteral formulation needed to promote positive outcomes.

Transitional Feedings

Management of a patient's transition from PN to tube feeding or oral intake, or from tube feeding to oral intake, is one of the most challenging aspects of nutrition support. The process of weaning a patient off nutrition support should be individualized, with tactics, goals, and timing that reflect the patient's clinical status.[1]

Parenteral Nutrition to Tube Feedings

When transitioning from PN to tube feeding, a reasonable approach is to begin tapering PN when tube feedings are providing 33% to 50% of the patient's nutrient requirements. As EN progresses, the PN formulation can be decreased such that total intake (ie, EN and PN) meets nutrient requirements. Once tube feedings are well tolerated and provide 60%–75% of nutrient requirements, PN can be discontinued.[33] In pediatric patients whose EN is being advanced at a very conservative rate to the EN goal, it may be necessary to continue PN beyond the point when EN meets 75% of nutrient requirements to provide total intake that adequately promotes optimal growth and development.[45]

Tube Feeding to Oral Intake

Transition from tube feeding to voluntary oral intake also requires careful management. Close monitoring reduces the risk that EN will be discontinued prematurely, which can lead to nutrient inadequacy and weight loss. After EN is discontinued, it may be prudent to delay removing the EAD until it is confirmed that the transition to oral intake is a success; this conservative approach to EAD removal can minimize the risks associated with device reinsertion in the event that the patient must resume EN because appetite and oral intake do not continue to improve as expected. On the other hand, continuing EN when a patient is consuming an adequate amount orally could potentially interfere with the patient's appetite and motivation to eat and may cause overfeeding.

The transition phase from EN to oral intake may begin as soon as a patient is alert and able to manage the mechanics of chewing and swallowing. Consultation with and input from speech-language pathologists can help clinicians identify the presence of dysphagia early in the transition process. Once a patient is cleared to safely consume a specific diet consistency (eg, blended foods), he or she should be encouraged to choose appropriate foods at meals and snacks. Enteral tube feedings can be held for approximately 1 hour before scheduled meals to stimulate appetite. Nocturnal infusion of tube feedings can also provide supplemental nutrition for patients who do not yet meet nutrition needs via oral intake during the day. When voluntary intake approaches 50% of nutrient requirements for more than 2 to 3 consecutive days, either the infusion rate of tube feedings can be slowed or the number of feedings each day can be progressively decreased.

Another method to help patients transition to oral intake is to use postmeal bolus feedings. To take advantage of the hunger drive, oral intake is optimal when the stomach is not full. Administering a feeding immediately after a meal therefore reduces the impact that EN has on the patient's appetite. The feedings can be varied according to the adequacy of each meal. For example, suppose a patient would need 480-mL boluses of enteral formula 3 times daily when consuming no food orally. If he or she does not eat a meal or eats very little, a 480-mL bolus feeding should be administered. If the patient eats about half of a "usual" meal (as based on the patient's or caregiver's opinion of what is normal for the patient), 240 mL of formula should be administered. The entire bolus feeding could be omitted if the patient eats all or most of a "usual" meal. Clinical trials are needed to confirm the efficacy of this type of schedule; however, anecdotal reports suggest that this system helps the patient who is transitioning back to oral intake by providing a way to promote adequate nutrition.[1]

Transitioning Hospitalized Patients to Other Settings

When a hospitalized patient is expected to need EN for a prolonged period, the nutrition support clinician may be in a position to oversee the patient's transition to receive EN at home or in a long-term care or rehabilitation setting. An important aspect of transition planning is to establish a feeding schedule that is safe and meets nutrition goals while being as convenient for the patient's lifestyle as possible. At this juncture, reimbursement issues may influence the choice of enteral formulation or the type of equipment available for use at home or in a long-term care/rehabilitation facility.

Communication with the home care provider or facility nursing staff regarding the patient's nutrition care plan is essential for success in achieving therapeutic goals. To promote a seamless transition to home, the clinician may also assist with supply acquisition and patient/family teaching in preparation for discharge. Smooth transition to home for pediatric patients with complex medical needs and enteral feeds requires contributions from a multidisciplinary team, including care coordinators, nurses, physicians, dietitians, and speech therapists.[46]

The EN regimen should be well tolerated before a patient is discharged from the hospital. The feeding schedule and method of feeding should be adjusted and simplified to accommodate individual and/or caregiver schedules. Gravity bag or syringe may be the preferred method to administer gastric feedings in the home setting.[33] If an EN feeding pump is needed to administer gastric feedings at home, insurance providers may require supportive documentation of the need.[33]

Patients receiving EN at home and their caregivers will need ongoing education on the feeding regimen and possible complications. Feeding tolerance and the adequacy of the nutrition goals should be routinely monitored by home care providers. See Chapter 11 for a detailed review of EN in the home setting.

Termination of Nutrition Support

The ASPEN standards of practice for hospitalized patients recommend that hospitals develop protocols to address the termination of nutrition support therapy.[32] These protocols should be designed to allow clinicians to use clinical judgment in accordance with accepted standards of medical ethics, institutional policies, and state and federal laws. Nutrition support may be modified or discontinued when there are disproportionate burdens on the patient or when feedings are no longer beneficial to the patient. Functionally competent patients of all ages, parents/guardians, and/or the legal surrogates of minor or incompetent patients should be involved in any decisions regarding the withholding or withdrawing of nutrition support. A patient's wishes for care should be considered in making decisions to withhold or withdraw EN. Refer to Chapter 2 for a more detailed discussion of this issue.

References

1. Boullata JI, Carrera AL, Harvey L, et al. ASPEN safe practices for enteral nutrition therapy. *JPEN J Parenter Enteral Nutr.* 2017;41(1):15–103. doi:10.1177/0148607116673053.

2. Lyman B, Williams M, Sollazzo J, et al. Enteral feeding set handling techniques: a comparison of bacterial growth, nursing time, labor and material costs. *Nutr Clin Pract.* 2017;32(2): 193–200.

3. Perry J, Stankorb SM, Salgueiro M. Microbial contamination of enteral feeding products in thermoneutral and hyperthermal ICU environments. *Nutr Clin Pract.* 2015;30(1):128–133.

4. Hsu TC, Chen NR, Sullivan MM, et al. Effect of high ambient temperature on contamination and physical stability of one-liter ready-to-hang enteral delivery systems. *Nutrition.* 2000;16:165–167.

5. Areval-Manso JJ, Martinez-Sanchez P, Juarez-Martin B, et al. Preventing diarrhoea in enteral nutrition; the impact of the delivery hang set hang time. *Int J Clin Pract.* 2015; 69(8): 900–908.

6. Neely AN, Mayes T, Gardner J, Kagan RJ, Gottschlich MM. A microbiologic study of enteral feeding hang time in a burn hospital: can feeding costs be reduced without compromising patient safety? *Nutr Clin Pract.* 2006;21:610–616.

7. Jalali M, Sabzghabaee AM, Badri SS, Soltani HA, Maracy MR. Bacterial contamination of hospital-prepared enteral tube feeding formulas in Isfahan, Iran. *J Res Med Sci.* 2009; 14(3):149–156.

8. Mathus-Vliegen EM, Bredium MWJ, Binnekade JM. Analysis of site of bacterial contamination in an enteral feeding system. *JPEN J Parenter Enteral Nutr.* 2006;30(6):519–525.

9. Bobo E. Reemergence of blenderized tube feedings: exploring the evidence. *Nutr Clin Pract.* 2016;31(6):730–735.

10. US Food and Drug Administration. Compliance program guidance manual: medical foods program—import and domestic. Chapter 21: food composition, standards, labeling and economics, program 7321.002. Implementation date: August 24, 2006, completion date: September 30, 2008. https://www.fda.gov/downloads/food/complianceenforcement/ucm073339.pdf. Accessed December 16, 2018.

11. Bankhead R, Boullata J, Brantley S, et al. Enteral nutrition practice recommendations. *JPEN J Parenter Enteral Nutr.* 2009;33(2):122–167.

12. Centers for Disease Control and Prevention. *Enterobacter sakazakii* infections associated with the use of infant formula—Tennessee 2001. *MMWR Morb Mortal Wkly Rep.* 2002; 51(14):298–300.

13. Centers for Disease Control and Prevention. *Cronobacter* species isolation in two infants—New Mexico, 2008. *MMWR Morb Mortal Wkly Rep.* 2009;58(42):1179–1183.

14. Payne-James JJ, Rana SK, Bray JM, McSwiggan DA, Silk D. Retrograde (ascending) bacterial contamination of enteral diet administration sets. *JPEN J Parenter Enteral Nutr.*1992;16(4):369–373.

15. Hurrell E, Kucerova E, Loughlin M, et al. Neonatal enteral feeding tubes as loci for colonisation by members of the *Enterobacteriaceae. BMC Infect Dis.* 2009;9:146.

16. Mehall J, Kite C, Gilliam C, Jackson R, Smith S. Enteral feeding tubes are a reservoir for nosocomial pathogens. *J Pediatr Surg.* 2002;37(7):1011–1012.

17. Juma N, Forsythe S. Microbial biofilm development on neonatal enteral feeding tubes. *Adv Exp Med Biol.* 2015;830: 113–121.

18. Vieira MMC, Santos VFN, Bottoni A, Morais TB. Nutritional and microbiological quality of commercial and home-made blenderized whole food enteral diets for home-based enteral nutritional therapy in adults. *Clin Nutr.* 2018;37(1): 177–181. doi:10.1016/j.clnu.2016.11.020.

19. Gallagher K, Flint A, Mouzaki M, et al. Blenderized enteral nutrition diet study: feasibility, clinical and microbiome outcomes of providing blenderized feeds through a gastric tube in a medically complex pediatric population. *JPEN J Parenter Enteral Nutr.* 2018;42(6):1046–1060.

20. Tutor S, Bennett K. Blenderized tube feeding. In: Steele C, Collins E, eds. *Infant and Pediatric Feedings: Guidelines for Preparation of Human Milk and Formula in Health Care Facilities.* 3rd ed. Chicago, IL: Academy of Nutrition and Dietetics; 2019: 173–183.

21. White H, King L. Enteral feeding pumps: efficacy, safety, and patient acceptability. *Med Devices.* 2014;7:291–298.

22. McClave SA, Taylor BE, Martindale RG, et al. Guidelines for the provision and assessment of nutrition support therapy in the adult critically ill patient: Society of Critical Care Medicine (SCCM) and American Society for Parenteral and Enteral Nutrition (ASPEN). *JPEN J Parenter and Enteral Nutr.* 2016;40(2):159–211.

23. Scott R, Bowling TE. Enteral tube feeding in adults. *J R Coll Physicians Edinb.* 2015;45:46–54.

24. Walker R, Probstfeld L, Tucker A. Hang height of enteral nutrition influences the delivery of enteral nutrition. *Nutr Clin Pract.* 2018;33(1):151–157. doi:10.1177/0884533617700132.

25. Hutsler D, Szekely L. Delivery and bedside management of feedings. In: Steele C, Collins E, eds. *Infant and Pediatric Feedings: Guidelines for Preparation of Human Milk and Formula in Health Care Facilities.* 3rd ed. Chicago, IL: Academy of Nutrition and Dietetics; 2019:201–215.

26. Hockenberry MJ, Wilson D, eds. *Wong's Nursing Care of Infants and Children.* 9th ed. St. Louis, MO: Elsevier; 2011.

27. Bowden VR, Greenberg CS. Feeding, enteral. In: Bowden VR, Greenberg CS, eds. *Pediatric Nursing Procedures.* 4th ed. Philadelphia, PA: Wolters Kluwer; 2016:301–309.

28. Lord LM. Restoring and maintaining patency of enteral feeding tubes. *Nutr Clin Pract.* 2003;18:422–426.

29. Lord LM. Enteral access devices: types, function, care, and challenges. *Nutr Clin Pract.* 2018;33(1):16–38.

30. Garrison CM. Enteral feeding tube clogging: what are the causes and what are the answers? A bench top analysis. *Nutr Clin Pract.* 2018;33(1):147–150.

31. Dandeles LM, Lodolce AE. Efficacy of agents to prevent and treat enteral feeding tube clogs. *Ann Pharmacother.* 2011; 45:676–80.

32. Ukleja A, Gilbert K, Mogensen K, et al. Standards for nutrition support: adult hospitalized patients. *Nutr Clin Pract.* 2018;33(6):906–920.

33. Kozeniecki M, Fritzshall R. Enteral nutrition for adults in the hospital setting. *Nutr Clin Pract.* 2015;30(5):634–651.

34. Doley J, Phillips W. Overview of enteral nutrition. In: Mueller CM, ed. *The ASPEN Adult Nutrition Support Core Curriculum.* 3rd ed. Silver Spring, MD: American Society for Parenteral and Enteral Nutrition; 2017:214–225.

35. Matarese L, Charney P. Capturing the elusive diagnosis of malnutrition. *Nutr Clin Pract.* 2017;32(1):11–14.

36. Weckwerth J. Monitoring enteral nutrition support tolerance in infants and children. *Nutr Clin Pract.* 2004;19(5):496–503.

37. Adam S, Batson S. A study of problems associated with the delivery of enteral feeding in critically ill patients in five ICUs in the UK. *Intensive Care Med.* 1997;23:261–266.

38. Rice TW, Swope T, Bozeman S, Wheeler AP. Variation in enteral nutrition delivery in mechanically ventilated patients. *Nutrition.* 2005;21:786–792.

39. Ibrahim EH, Mehringer L, Prentice D, et al. Early versus late enteral feeding of mechanically ventilated patients: results of a clinical trial. *JPEN J Parenter Enteral Nutr.* 2002;26:174–181.

40. Krishnan JA, Parce PB, Martinez A, et al. Caloric intake in medical ICU patients: consistency of care with guidelines and relationship to clinical outcomes. *Chest.* 2003;124:297–305.

41. Sudenis T, Hall K, Carlotto R. Enteral nutrition: what the dietitian prescribes is not what the burn patient gets! *J Burn Care Res.* 2015;36(2):297–305.

42. Taylor B, Brody R, Denmark R, Southard R, Byham-Gray L. Improving enteral delivery through the adoption of the "feed early enteral diet adequately for maximum effect (FEED ME)" protocol in a surgical trauma ICU: a quality improvement review. *Nutr Clin Pract.* 2014;29:639–648.

43. Kudsk KA, Minard G, Croce MA, et al. A randomized trial of isonitrogenous enteral diets after severe trauma: An immune-enhancing diet reduces septic complications. *Ann Surg.* 1996;224:531–543.

44. Taylor S, Fettes S, Jewkes C, et al. Prospective, randomized, controlled trial to determine the effect of early enhanced enteral nutrition on clinical outcome in mechanically ventilated patients suffering head injury. *Crit Care Med.* 1999;27:2525–2531.

45. Worthington P, Balint J, Bechtold M. When is parenteral nutrition appropriate? *JPEN J Parenter Enteral Nutr.* 2017; 41: 324–377.

46. Sevilla W, McElhanon B. Optimizing transition to home enteral nutrition for pediatric patients. *Nutr Clin Pract.* 2016; 31(6):762–768.

CHAPTER 9

Complications of Enteral Nutrition

Introduction

Enteral nutrition (EN) therapy is the preferred feeding modality when the gastrointestinal (GI) tract is functional but the patient is unable to orally consume adequate nutrients. The enteral route is promoted as an efficacious and cost-effective method of providing nutrients to patients, compared to the parenteral route. However, EN is not without its challenges and risks for serious complications. This chapter reviews selected GI and metabolic complications of EN that can contribute to a patient's morbidity and mortality (Table 9-1). Chapter 3 examines complications specific to feeding tubes, and formula-related issues (eg, microbial contamination) are addressed in Chapter 7. Most EN-related complications can be prevented with planning and bedside care using best-practice protocols. Ongoing

> **TABLE 9-1.** Selected Medical Complications Related to Enteral Nutrition[a]
>
> **Gastrointestinal-related complications**:
> - Nausea and vomiting
> - Abdominal distention
> - Maldigestion and malabsorption
> - Diarrhea
> - Constipation
> - Gastroesophageal reflux
> - Pulmonary aspiration
>
> **Metabolic alterations**:
> - Refeeding syndrome
> - Electrolyte and mineral imbalances
> - Vitamin deficiencies
> - Fluid imbalances
> - Hypercapnia
> - Glucose intolerance
> - Essential fatty acid deficiency

[a]Refer to Chapter 3 for information on complications related to enteral access devices, such as tube misplacement, occlusion, or migration; buried bumper syndrome; and site irritation/ulceration.

monitoring and reassessment should be a standard component of follow-up care (see Chapter 8).

Gastrointestinal-Related Complications

Nausea and Vomiting

Nausea and/or vomiting occur in approximately 12% to 26% of patients who receive EN,[1–3] and in up to 46% of critically ill patients.[4] Vomiting, especially in minimally responsive patients, may increase the risk of pulmonary aspiration, pneumonia, and sepsis, although evidence in support of this hypothesis is weak.

Multiple etiologies for nausea and vomiting are associated with EN. Delayed gastric emptying, or gastroparesis, is most often blamed.[5,6] Potential causes of and interventions for slowed emptying are listed in Table 9-2.[3–11]

Nausea and vomiting in critically ill patients may be caused by something other than delayed gastric emptying, such as adverse effects of medication, soy allergy, or lactose

---

TABLE 9–2. Possible Causes of and Interventions for Delayed Gastric Emptying

Causes:
- Hypotension
- Hypokalemia
- Sepsis
- Medications (eg, anesthesia, anticholinergics, opioids)
- Diabetes mellitus and other metabolic diseases (eg, hypothyroidism, electrolyte disorders, renal failure)
- Surgery (including vagotomy)
- Formula-related issues:
  - Excessively rapid infusion of formula
  - Use of cold formula
  - Use of formula with a high fat content

Interventions:
- Reducing or discontinuing opioid and anticholinergic medications and finding substitutes for other problematic medications when clinically appropriate
- Improving glucose control
- Positioning the feeding tube in a postpyloric location, although this may not resolve vomiting and may require concomitant gastric drainage
- Switching to a low-fat and/or isotonic formula (low fiber)
- Administering the feeding solution and all flushes at room temperature
- Reducing the rate of infusion
- Administering a prokinetic agent (eg, metoclopramide, erythromycin)

Source: Information is from references 3–11.

intolerance. (Note: Enteral formulas administered to critically ill patients are lactose free.) The etiology of nausea should be identified, if possible, instead of assuming that it is related to EN.

If nausea or vomiting occur as the rate of administration or bolus volume of the EN increases, one approach is to decrease the rate or volume to the last tolerated amount, with an attempt to increase the rate again after symptoms abate. Closed-system delivery methods and selection of a polymeric formula, rather than peptide-based or elemental formula, may reduce nausea associated with formula smell and appearance.[8,9] Evidence-based, nurse-driven protocols can standardize approaches to GI complications and may result in timely delivery of nutrition and achievement of feeding goals.[12,13]

The presence of abdominal distention in a patient with nausea indicates a need to perform more detailed abdominal assessments. Obstipation or fecal impaction may also lead to abdominal distention and nausea, particularly in the institutionalized or chronically critically ill patient. The development of abdominal distention during EN in conjunction with other symptoms, such as early satiety, vomiting, lack of flatus, and no bowel movements, may be suggestive of severe constipation or fecal impaction or the more serious postoperative ileus or paralytic ileus, which can lead to delays in feeding and extended hospital stay.[9,14,15]

One of the adverse consequences of ileus is intestinal dilatation and increased abdominal pressure, which in turn may increase gastric residual volume (GRV) and the risk for vomiting.[14] Postoperative ileus usually resolves without intervention within 24–72 hours of surgery, but it may last for days to weeks. It is important to rule out ileus or other type of GI pathology (eg, acute megacolon, acute colonic pseudo-obstruction) that could lead to enteric ischemia, intestinal perforation, and increased mortality.[14]

Current evidence-based guidelines suggest omitting use of routine GRV assessment because GRVs do not correlate with EN intolerance and do not decrease the incidence of ventilator-associated pneumonia.[8,16] If GRV is evaluated and measurements are low (<300–500 mL) and yet nausea persists, antiemetic medications may resolve the problem. While GRV is not useful in determining aspiration risk, this bedside assessment technique can be a valuable tool for detecting early signs of GI dysfunction and feeding intolerance, thus allowing for prompt intervention.[8]

Abdominal Distention

Abdominal distention is a common reason why EN is interrupted.[8] Distention (with or without elevated GRV) and its associated symptoms of bloating and cramping may be the result of ileus, obstruction, obstipation, ascites, lactose intolerance, or diarrheal illness.[14,15]

As previously mentioned, excessively rapid formula administration, infusion of cold formula, or initial use of a fiber-containing formula may occasionally contribute to abdominal distention.[8,17] Abdominal distention is diagnosed by visual inspection and palpation, as well as from patient report. Evidence is lacking regarding how to define a significant increase in abdominal girth. Therefore, careful clinical and radiological evaluation remain the most practical means of assessment.

Distention caused by ileus or mechanical bowel obstruction may be diagnosed from a flat and upright abdominal X-ray or abdominal computed tomography scan. Obtaining upper GI radiology with small bowel follow-through, along with observation of intestinal anatomy and motility, can provide additional insights into the clinical situation. If intestinal integrity and function are normal, EN may be continued so long as the patient is closely monitored.

Guidelines support enteral feeding through mild to moderate ileus.[16] However, the discontinuation of feedings may be necessary if motility is poor or if the bowel is markedly dilated. Parenteral nutrition (PN) may be considered if the GI tract will be inaccessible or the patient will be unable to tolerate EN while awaiting return of bowel function.[8]

Maldigestion and Malabsorption

Maldigestion refers to impaired breakdown of intact macronutrients (eg, lactose) into absorbable forms. *Malabsorption* is defective mucosal uptake and transport of nutrients (fat, carbohydrate, protein, vitamins, electrolytes, minerals) or water from the small intestine.

Disorders that lead to carbohydrate maldigestion and malabsorption are commonly divided into primary and secondary forms.[18] Primary forms include rare congenital defects in specific brush-border enzymes or transport mechanisms, and secondary are those that arise from any condition affecting structural integrity or function of the pancreas and small intestine.

It is extremely important to not confuse disaccharidase deficiency, malabsorption, and intolerance as these are distinctive conditions and are not treated in the same manner.[18] Similarly, carbohydrate intolerance, which is a common condition, must be differentiated from carbohydrate malabsorption, which involves deficiencies in various enzymes and transporters.[18]

Absorption depends on many factors, including gastric emptying, small intestinal motility and transit, presence of pancreatic enzymes, contact surface area, and depth of the diffusion barrier of the absorptive epithelium.[5] General clinical manifestations of malabsorption include abdominal pain, unexplained weight loss, flatulence, bloating, steatorrhea, and diarrhea.[18] Other documented problems associated with malabsorption are related to vitamin or mineral deficiencies; these conditions include anemia, tetany, bone pain and pathologic fractures, bleeding, dermatitis, neuropathy, glossitis, and edema.[19]

Screening and diagnosis of malabsorption may include the following:

- Gross and microscopic examination of the stool to determine fat and protein content of a random stool collection (in a qualitative study) and measure serum carotene concentration.
- Imaging studies of intestinal transit time and motility.
- Evaluation of intake-output balance: A quantitative fecal fat study is the most traditional test used in an inpatient or ambulatory setting to diagnose pancreatic exocrine insufficiency. For this test, the patient consumes a diet containing 100 g of fat and stool is collected for 72 hours. Modifications can be made to this procedure for patients unable to tolerate such a high fat content. In general, if more than 7% of the total amount of fat consumed is obtained from the stool collection, that indicates fat malabsorption. A result of 15 g/d or greater indicates severe steatorrhea.[20]
- Assessment of maldigestion/malabsorption of specific nutrients: Evaluation may include lactose tolerance tests, the Schilling test to screen for abnormal absorption of vitamin B_{12}, and various radioisotopic methodologies for identification of iron, calcium, various amino acids, folic acid, pyridoxine, and vitamin D malabsorption. Hydrogen and methane concentrations in breath samples can help diagnose lactose, fructose, sucrose, and sorbitol malabsorption.[18]

- Endoscopic small bowel biopsy: This test is helpful in diagnosing various mucosal disorders such as celiac disease, tropical sprue, inflammatory bowel disease, and Whipple's disease.

Causes of maldigestion/malabsorption include gluten-sensitive enteropathy, Crohn's disease, diverticular disease, radiation enteritis, enteric fistulas, HIV infection, pancreatic insufficiency, short bowel syndrome, and numerous other disorders. The rate and extent of glucose absorption are greatly reduced in the critically ill population.

Knowledge of the patient's medical history and selection of an appropriate enteral product should help minimize the likelihood of malabsorption and maldigestion during enteral feeding. The use of a semi-elemental or elemental formula with a greater percentage of medium-chain triglycerides or structured lipids may improve tolerance.[8] It is best practice in the intensive care unit (ICU) to initiate feedings early. Although early feeding has not been shown to affect subsequent gastric emptying or GI hormones, it may improve subsequent nutrient absorption.[21] PN may be necessary in patients who do not respond to efforts to improve GI tolerance of EN.

Diarrhea

Diarrhea is a commonly reported problem in patients receiving EN.[22] Estimates of its incidence in enterally fed patients range from 2% to 95%.[23,24] The variation in estimates is related to the lack of a common definition of diarrhea. It can be defined as stool weight of more than 200 g/d, but it is frequently defined clinically as 3 or more watery or loose stools in a 24-hour period.[15,25,26] Stool volume can be measured by placing a collection device in the toilet or by using a bedpan. In incontinent patients, volume can be estimated by measuring rectal tube or rectal pouch output or weighing the soiled pad beneath the patient after each stool (assuming 1 g = 1 mL of stool).

Diarrhea can be categorized as motility-related, malabsorptive, inflammatory/exudative, secretory, or osmotic. A systematic approach is required to identify the underlying cause and implement appropriate treatment strategies.[15,26] Clinicians should always thoroughly investigate the etiology of diarrhea while initiating appropriate medical and nutrition-related interventions to address the problem (see Table 9-3).[9,15,16,26] Diarrhea may be caused by intolerance of specific components in enteral formula (eg, lactose, sucrose, fructose, soy), or it may be related to the characteristics of the formula (eg, high osmolality, low fiber content, high amounts of fermentable oligosaccharides, disaccharides, monosaccharides, and polyols)[15,22,24] However, most standard 1 kcal/mL formulas are now lactose free and isotonic and contain only a moderate amount of fat. Consequently, formula intolerance is a less common cause of diarrhea than some might assume. More common causes include medications (eg, antibiotics, liquid medications in a sorbitol base, glucose-lowering agents, stool softeners, prokinetics, proton pump inhibitors) and infection (eg, *Clostridium difficile*). Other possible etiologies include steatorrhea, small intestine bacterial overgrowth (SIBO), and various GI diseases such as short bowel syndrome (SBS).

When diarrhea occurs, the patient's medication regimen should be among the first areas of investigation. Antibiotics can cause diarrhea without necessarily causing *Clostridium difficile* overgrowth. Any drug given via a jejunal feeding tube should be appropriately diluted with water to avoid a dumping-like syndrome associated with hyperosmolality.

TABLE 9-3. Selected Options for Addressing Clinically Significant Diarrhea in Patients Receiving Enteral Nutrition

Option	Comments
Medical assessment	Before assuming diarrhea is related to enteral nutrition, rule out infectious or inflammatory causes, fecal impaction, or known problematic medications.
Consider changes to the medication regimen if drugs are the suspected cause of diarrhea	Consultation with a pharmacist may help the clinician determine whether discontinuing, reducing, or reformulating medication is an option.
Administer an antidiarrheal agent (eg, loperamide, diphenoxylate) once an infectious etiology has been ruled out or is being treated	Carefully choose agents that are not hyperosmolar or in a sorbitol base; these may worsen diarrhea. Consult with a pharmacist regarding sorbitol content of liquid medications because the sweetener is not always listed as an ingredient.[9]
Use an enteral formula with a blend of soluble and insoluble fiber[15,26]	In the hemodynamically stable ICU patient specifically, the routine use of a soluble fiber additive should be considered as a prophylactic measure to help maintain commensal microbiota and promote bowel health. The recommended dose is 10–20 g given as a supplement in divided doses over 24 hours.[16]

(continued)

TABLE 9-3. *(Continued)*

Option	Comments
Switch the patient from a hyperosmolar enteral formula to a more isotonic formula	Consider a small-peptide formulation if the patient has persistent diarrhea or suspected malabsorption, or if he or she does not respond to fiber supplementation.[15,16,26]
Consider administering probiotics to patients with specific clinical conditions if randomized controlled trials have demonstrated both safety and outcome benefits[16]	For example, in trials, *Lactobacillus GG* has been associated with improved outcomes in patients with antibiotic-associated diarrhea.[16]

For example, some drugs, such as potassium chloride liquid, should be mixed with a minimum of 30 to 60 mL per 10 mEq dose to avoid direct irritation of the gut.[9] Refer to Chapter 10 for additional information on medication administration in patients receiving EN.

Microbial contamination of the enteral feeding solution can cause infectious diarrhea or other problems and is a particular risk for vulnerable hosts such as neonates, critically ill patients, and immune-suppressed patients. Additionally, proton pump inhibitors and histamine$_2$ receptor antagonists diminish the gastric acid microbial barrier; therefore, patients taking these drugs may be at increased risk of enteric infections, which may predispose them to greater risk of morbidity related to formula contamination.[27] The risk of EN contamination is less when closed enteral formula systems are used and greater when open systems are used.[8,28] Refer to Chapter 7 for additional information on closed vs open systems and the prevention of microbial contamination.

Patients receiving EN who have malabsorptive conditions (eg, SBS, pancreatic insufficiency) may experience steatorrhea (the malabsorption of fat), which is made clinically obvious by frothy, odoriferous stools. The condition is confirmed by a fecal fat analysis (quantitative or qualitative). A lower-fat enteral formula may reduce the symptoms of fat malabsorption. Enteral formulas with fat in the form of medium-chain triglycerides may provide an alternative source of energy in the presence of fat malabsorption. Inclusion of pancreatic enzymes in the patient's drug regimen may help if pancreatic dysfunction is present.[20]

Bacterial overgrowth in the GI tract can cause severe enteritis with marked diarrhea, fever, and even sepsis. Conditions that predispose patients to SIBO include intestinal stasis and low acid states due to gastric resection or possibly the use of proton pump inhibitors, which are common in GI surgical patients and those with chronic pancreatitis. Up to 40% of patients with pancreatic insufficiency will develop SIBO.[20] Symptomatic patients should receive oral antimicrobial therapy that targets both aerobic and anaerobic organisms, as well as interventions to decrease bacterial colonization.[20]

Many primary diseases of the intestine, including inflammatory bowel disease, SBS, gluten-sensitive enteropathy, and acquired immunodeficiency syndrome, may result in malabsorption or secretory diarrhea. Recognition and treatment of these diseases can minimize diarrhea. In some patients with GI disease, the use of elemental or semi-elemental products with a greater percentage of fat from medium-chain triglycerides may facilitate absorption.[16]

In patients with SBS, malabsorption can lead to severe diarrhea or significant ostomy losses. Whether the overall bowel functions as if it is shortened or it has actually been resected, patients may require relatively large doses of antimotility medications to control stool output. If all strategies to promote EN tolerance have been exhausted, patients with SBS may require PN to supplement enteral nutrient delivery.

Although lactase deficiency is common in illness, lactose intolerance is not a significant issue with EN therapy because, as previously noted, most formulas are lactose free. However, a patient may have diarrhea associated with lactose intolerance during the transition from EN to oral intake. It may be prudent to reduce or eliminate milk products from the diet, provide lactose-reduced dairy products or oral lactase, or advance to a low-lactose solid diet.

A potential consequence of diarrhea occurring with EN is incontinence-associated dermatitis, which can lead to excoriation and skin breakdown. In situations where stool may come into prolonged contact with the skin, measures should be taken to prevent skin breakdown. One option is the topical application of skin protectants such as a moisture barrier cream or liquid protectant film.[29] Another option is the application of a stool collection apparatus such as a rectal pouch. The perineal skin should be inspected frequently, treated with gentle cleaning, and kept as dry as possible.

Constipation

Defining constipation is difficult because normal defecation varies from person to person.[30] The best clinical definition of constipation is the accumulation of excess waste in the colon, often to the transverse colon or even the cecum, associated with infrequent and difficult defecation.[8]

Constipation is a common problem for enterally fed patients, particularly those who are elderly and/or bedridden.[8] Multiple observational studies in critically ill patients defined constipation as the inability to pass stool within 72 hours of admission; applying this definition, the incidence of constipation in the ICU is as high as 50%–83%. In the critically ill patient, constipation is associated with early satiety and feeding intolerance, and it may increase intra-abdominal pressure, making weaning from a ventilator more difficult; for these reasons, constipation can interfere with nutrition goals in critically ill patients.[31] Other symptoms associated with constipation include abdominal distention, bloating, and vomiting; consequences of severe constipation may include fecal impaction or bowel perforation requiring urgent nursing, medical, or pharmaceutical interventions.[8,32]

In patients receiving EN, the residue and extent of absorption of an EN product are factors to consider when investigating the occurrence of constipation. A predigested, low-residue product may be completely absorbed, resulting in a stool frequency of less than once a week. A plain abdominal X-ray may be ordered for diagnosis to clearly differentiate constipation from small bowel obstruction or ileus.

With uncomplicated constipation, there is rarely any small bowel dilatation. A variant of constipation is impaction of stool in the rectal vault. Impaction can be diagnosed and treated by rectal exam. Enemas, cathartics, and even endoscopy may be required to treat severe impaction. Impaction should also be considered in patients, particularly those who are elderly or bed-bound, when stool volumes have been small and then become liquid. Liquid stool will seep around an impaction (obstipation). In addition, impaction may be the cause of delirium and agitation in older adults.

Common causes of constipation in patients receiving EN include specific medications (eg, benzodiazepines and opioids), inadequate fluid intake or dehydration, inadequate fiber intake, and lack of physical activity.[8,33] To avoid dehydration, it is important to provide adequate fluid during EN. Hydration may be problematic when a concentrated formula is needed for fluid restriction. If usual hydration guidelines are contraindicated, consider a stool softener and/or a laxative or cleansing enema.[28,32,33]

Inadequate fiber intake results in infrequent bowel movements without significant buildup of waste in the colon. Fiber propels waste through the colon; use of a fiber-containing formula may be particularly important for the patient who requires long-term tube feeding.[8,30] If fiber is added to the enteral regimen, patients must receive a minimum of 1 mL of fluid per kcal to prevent solidification of waste in the colon and constipation. Given that isotonic EN formulas contain only 80%–85% of water by volume, additional fluid is often needed to facilitate regular stool output and minimize the chance of impaction.[8,28,30,32,33]

Inadequate physical activity contributes to constipation. Patients should be encouraged and/or assisted to ambulate whenever possible.

Of note, a systematic review and meta-analysis of the use of bowel protocols in ICU patients found a lack of significance for unit bowel protocols to reduce either the occurrence of constipation and feeding intolerance or days on mechanical ventilation.[30] Feeding protocols that provide evidence-based guidance for early identification of and intervention for constipation are recommended.[9,16,33]

Gastroesophageal Reflux

In healthy individuals, physiological reflux is cleared by a peristaltic wave, assisted by gravity in the erect person, and acid is neutralized by swallowed saliva, which is high in bicarbonate.[14] Delayed gastric emptying raises intragastric pressure and threatens the integrity of the gastroesophageal barrier. Medications commonly administered in the hospital and ICU settings (eg, opioids, nitrates, calcium channel blockers, theophylline, diazepam, and barbiturates) have the potential to relax the lower esophageal sphincter and contribute to reflux.[14]

Percutaneous endoscopic gastric tubes have been found to reduce, although not completely prevent, occurrence of reflux in both ventilated and nonventilated patients.[34] Postpyloric feeding reportedly minimizes microaspiration and pneumonia; however, duodenogastric reflux has been documented in patients fed in this manner.[14] A duodenal feeding tube may be inserted at the bedside using blind insertion techniques or newer electromagnetic placement devices, whereas jejunal tube placement is most reliably achieved with endoscopic or fluoroscopic techniques.[8,28] Distal jejunal placement beyond the ligament of Treitz is recommended for patients with gastric outlet obstruction, gastroparesis, gastric fistula, pancreatitis, and known reflux and aspiration of gastric contents.[8,28]

Controversy exists as to whether postpyloric feeding is associated with improved tolerance, fewer complications, or favorable patient outcomes. The most recent nutrition therapy guidelines published concluded that small bowel feeding may reduce regurgitation, aspiration, and pneumonia; however, no difference has been found between small bowel and gastric feedings in mortality, hospital or ICU length of stay, duration of mechanical ventilation, or time to achieve goal EN.[16] Best practices to minimize gastroesophageal reflux in patients receiving EN include elevating the head of the bed at least 30°, altering the EN delivery method from bolus or intermittent to continuous, using prokinetic agents as appropriate for gastric feeding, diverting the level of feeding to a postpyloric location, and transitioning to oral nutrition as quickly and safely as possible.[8,16]

Pulmonary Aspiration

Aspiration can be defined as the inhalation of material into the airway. This material may include nasal and oral pharyngeal secretions as well as reflux of liquids, food, and other gastric contents.[35] Symptoms associated with clinically significant aspiration include dyspnea, tachypnea, wheezing, frothy or purulent sputum, rhonchi and rales, tachycardia, fever, cyanosis, anxiety, and agitation. Pulmonary aspiration of tube feeding formula can also be asymptomatic (ie, silent aspiration). In fact, aspiration of saliva is a normal phenomenon during sleep. Pneumonia can result from pulmonary aspiration of tube feeding formula; however, aspiration of very small amounts of fluid alone is insufficient to cause pneumonia.[17]

Despite correlations between aspiration and tube feeding, causal relationships have not been established. The progression of pulmonary aspiration of feeding formula to aspiration pneumonia is hard to predict and may depend on the quantity and acidity of the formula in addition to the particulates and contaminants in the formula. Age, immune status, and comorbidities also influence the tendency toward aspiration pneumonia development. When the quantity and acidity of the formula overwhelm either the patient's natural defense mechanisms or the patient's altered pulmonary defense mechanisms, pneumonia is more likely to occur.

Aspiration pneumonia is estimated to account for 5%–15% of pneumonia in hospitalized patients.[36] However, unless a patient is discovered regurgitating and then develops a new pulmonary infiltrate on radiographic film, proving that aspiration was the cause of the pneumonia is difficult.[37,38] The incidence of pulmonary aspiration in tube-fed patients varies depending on the patient population studied and the technique used to identify aspiration. In the critically ill patient population, the risk for pulmonary aspiration is thought to be increased because patients are in a prolonged supine position and are likely to have endotracheal intubation, delayed gastric emptying, and a decreased level of consciousness. Risk factors for aspiration include sedation, the use of paralytic agents, supine patient positioning, gastric tube feedings, malpositioned feeding tubes, mechanical ventilation, vomiting, gastroesophageal reflux disease, transportation within the hospital, staffing level of nursing, and advanced patient age.[39,40]

Methods to Determine Aspiration Risk

Patients at risk for aspiration should be identified based on their diagnosis, clinical factors, and physical findings. Any clinical signs of sepsis, the level of sedation, and the influence of vasopressor agents should be closely monitored.[39] The patient should be assessed for level of consciousness, feelings of fullness, nausea, and abdominal distention, and vital signs should be routinely evaluated.

Historically, measurement of GRV has been used to monitor patients for the risk of aspiration. However, although much research has been conducted to define an acceptable range for GRVs, investigators have not been able to identify the precise level of GRV that places the patient at greatest risk for obvious GI intolerance. Therefore, it is unclear how GRV values might best be applied in decision-making about when to advance or discontinue feedings. In clinical guidelines on nutrition support for critically ill patients, the Society of Critical Care Medicine and American Society for Parenteral and Enteral Nutrition suggest that GRVs should not be used as part of routine care to monitor mechanically ventilated patients in the ICU receiving EN. The rationale for this recommendation is that the procedure may have adverse outcomes and GRVs do not correlate with incidence of pneumonia, regurgitation, or aspiration.[16] If ICUs do use GRVs to assess aspiration risk, the guidelines recommend that clinicians should not hold EN if a patient's GRV is less than 500 mL unless there are other signs of intolerance.[16] It is appropriate to abruptly cease enteral feeding upon overt regurgitation or aspiration.

If GRVs are assessed and a patient's GRVs are in the range of 250 to 500 mL, clinicians may want to consider a stepwise approach to assess the potential for GI intolerance. Elevated and increasing GRVs may be a symptom of another underlying problem manifesting itself as delayed gastric emptying. If serial measurements reveal a change in GRV, other potential causes of the change must be investigated.[41]

Even if the GRV is less than 250 mL, assessment of aspiration risk should continue.[42] Just as high GRVs should not automatically result in holding of enteral feedings, low GRVs should not result in decreased vigilance in the monitoring of signs and symptoms of GI intolerance.

When clinicians choose to assess GRVs, they must understand that procedures for measuring GRVs are poorly defined and not standardized. Unreliable methods are often used to detect aspiration. For example, using a syringe to withdraw gastric contents will not consistently result in aspiration of the total volume of fluid present in the stomach.[43]

Furthermore, many variables can affect the accuracy of bedside GRV measurements. These include the type of feeding tube used when performing the measurement, the position of the feeding tube ports in the GI tract, and the patient's position.

Large GRVs are detected more often when large-bore sump tubes are used for the measurement. Using small-bore tubes can underestimate the GRV. A study of 645 dual measurements made by using small-bore feeding tubes and large-bore sump tubes concurrently present in the stomach of 62 critically ill patients indicated that large GRVs were detected 2 to 3 times more often with large-bore sump tubes.[44] Regardless of the size of the feeding tube used, ports positioned at the gastroesophageal junction will result in a negligible GRV in most cases.[45]

Patient positioning may reasonably be assumed to affect the amount of GRV obtained; this factor may be of greater significance in infants than in adults.[45,46] In a study of 10 critically ill patients, McClave and associates found no difference in GRVs obtained when the patients were supine vs in a right lateral decubitus position;[45] similarly, van der Voort and Zandstra reported that GRVs were similar when 19 critically ill patients were prone as opposed to supine.[47] In contrast, Malhotra and coauthors reported significantly higher GRVs from 27 preterm babies when they were supine as opposed to prone.[48]

Finally, there is no established consensus about how frequently to monitor GRVs, if they are monitored. Numerous studies have documented evaluation of GRV from every 4 to every 12 hours, depending on when the feedings were initiated and the previous GRV obtained.[45]

Methods to Detect Aspiration

There is no validated method currently in clinical use to detect aspiration of tube feeding formula. In the past, blue food coloring was added to enteral formula to attempt to detect aspiration of gastric feedings. However, in 2003, the US Food and Drug Administration issued a public health advisory describing the association between FD&C Blue #1 dye and patient fatalities from hypotension and metabolic acidosis, as well as blue discoloration of the skin, organs, and body fluids.[49] Given these safety concerns, the blue dye method is no longer used. Notably, it was also shown to be ineffective in detecting aspiration.[50]

The use of glucose oxidase strips to test tracheal secretions for glucose from enteral formula is also problematic because investigators have found glucose in tracheal secretions of unfed patients.[43] Because there are no reliable methods to detect formula aspiration in tube-fed patients, clinicians should prioritize strategies to minimize risk factors for delayed gastric emptying, aspiration, and aspiration pneumonia.

Strategies to Prevent Aspiration

Because pulmonary aspiration can have life-threatening complications, prevention of aspiration and the identification of high-risk patients are crucial. During gastric feedings, it is extremely important to raise the head of the bed to 30°–45° or position the patient upright in a chair, if possible.[28] The patient should be monitored at least every 4 hours for proper positioning.[28] This simple measure has been associated with decreased esophageal and pharyngeal reflux of gastric contents and a decreased incidence of aspiration pneumonia.[51] If head-of-the-bed (HOB) elevation is contraindicated, the reverse Trendelenburg position should be considered for patients receiving gastric feeds.[28]

The National Pressure Ulcer Advisory Panel recommends limiting the HOB elevation to 30° for patients on bedrest, unless contraindicated, to reduce the risk for pressure ulcers, which are more likely to occur with higher HOB elevations.[52] Schallom and colleagues reviewed research aimed at lowering aspiration risk as well as that directed at preventing pressure ulcers and recommend that HOB elevation decisions should be made in the context of each patient's overall condition.[53] Critically ill patients who require mechanical ventilation and heavy sedation are at the highest risk for aspiration and may benefit more from the 45° HOB elevation with periodic lowering of the head of the bed to 30°. HOB elevation of 30° is recommended for critically ill patients at less risk for aspiration and patients who are not critically ill. Infants under 1 year of age should sleep on their back and not have the head of the bed elevated.[28] In all cases, pressure-relieving measures should be employed.

When tube-fed patients are unable to effectively clear their airway secretions, additional precautions must be taken. Sedative use should be minimized; feeding tube placement and GI intolerance should be assessed at 4-hour intervals; bolus feedings should be avoided; endotracheal cuff pressures should be maintained at appropriate levels; and secretions above cuff should be cleared before deflation.[54] Oral care at least twice daily helps decrease the bacterial load of the oral cavity.[55]

If patients experience feeding intolerance involving high GRVs or emesis, interventions to consider include a slower infusion rate, use of a prokinetic agent (metoclopramide or low-dose erythromycin), or switching to small bowel tube feedings. The possibility that the feeding tube is malpositioned should also be considered when nausea and emesis occur. In 1 investigation, 25 of 201 critically ill patients were found to have malpositioned feeding tubes that increased the risk for aspiration.[56] If the open ports within the tube tip lie in the esophagus, the risk of regurgitation and aspiration likely increases. After a feeding tube is placed in the antrum of the stomach or the small bowel, the feeding tube should be marked at the exit site or the tube length should be measured and documented so that placement can be checked every 4 hours or per the institution's protocol.[28] Obtaining a residual from a nasally or orally placed small bowel feeding tube or from the jejunal port of a transgastric jejunal feeding tube is a useful technique to detect inadvertent upward dislocation of the tip of the feeding tube into the stomach. Residual volumes from the small bowel are typically quite low (eg, <10 mL); a sudden sharp increase in residual volume (eg, ≥100 mL) is a good indication that the tube has migrated up into the stomach.[57]

The use of care protocols may minimize aspiration risk. Metheny and colleagues compared usual care of critically ill, tube-fed patients to care guided by an aspiration risk-reduction protocol (ARRP), which called for HOB elevation of at least 30° (unless contraindicated) and an algorithmic approach for elevated GRVs that directed small bowel feeding tube placement.[58] In the usual care group, 88% aspirated and 48% developed pneumonia. In the ARRP group, 39% aspirated and 19% developed pneumonia. The authors concluded that strict HOB elevation when appropriate and the use of an ARRP to manage elevated GRVs in critically ill, tube-fed patients can significantly lower the incidence of aspiration and aspiration-related pneumonia.

In a randomized, controlled, double-blind trial comparing the efficacy of combination therapy with erythromycin and metoclopramide to erythromycin alone, Nguyen and associates defined feeding intolerance as (a) 2 or more GRVs ≥250 mL within the first 24 hours, or (b) any 6-hour GRV ≥250 mL thereafter while receiving EN at a rate of ≥40 mL/h. They used the 250-mL threshold for the GRV as an indication for therapy, not for holding enteral feeds. They found that the combination therapy was more effective in improving the outcomes of enteral feedings in critically ill patients.[59]

Metabolic Alterations

With the exception of refeeding syndrome, EN by itself is unlikely to be the cause of significant metabolic derangements or specific nutrition deficiencies. However, many patients undergoing EN support have underlying conditions that predispose them to metabolic derangements.

Malnourished children are at increased risk for metabolic problems. All moderately to severely malnourished children should have serum potassium, phosphorus, magnesium, and glucose levels checked at least daily during the first week of initiation of nutrition support, as well as periodically during the gradual advancement of feedings.[60]

Refeeding Syndrome

Re-initiation of carbohydrate-containing feeding of severely malnourished patients may result in refeeding syndrome, in which there are acute intracellular shifts of electrolytes as cell anabolism is stimulated.[61–65] Refeeding syndrome can affect the cardiac, respiratory, hepatic, and neuromuscular systems, possibly leading to various clinical complications, including hematologic, neuromuscular, cardiac, and respiratory dysfunction and even death.

Refeeding syndrome can result in acute decreases in circulating levels of potassium, magnesium, and phosphorus. Serum levels should be monitored very closely, and deficiencies should be treated as needed to maintain normal circulating levels. Many patients with refeeding syndrome also require thiamin and folate supplementation.[63–66]

Patients at high risk for refeeding syndrome and other metabolic complications should be followed closely, and depleted levels of minerals and electrolytes should be corrected before feedings are initiated.[28] When monitoring metabolic parameters prior to the initiation of enteral feedings and periodically during EN therapy, clinicians should follow protocols and consider the patient's underlying disease state and length of therapy.

Prevention of refeeding syndrome is of utmost importance.[67] Stanga and colleagues highlighted 7 cases that exhibited 1 or more features of refeeding syndrome, including deficiencies and low plasma levels of potassium, phosphorous, magnesium, and thiamin. These metabolic issues were compounded further by salt and water retention.[68] The aforementioned hallmarks of refeeding syndrome responded to specific interventions. In most cases, these abnormalities could have been anticipated and prevented.[67,68]

For at-risk patients, nutrition support should be initiated at approximately 25% of the estimated energy goal and advanced over 3 to 5 days to the goal rate.[28] Serum electrolytes and vital signs should be monitored carefully after nutrition support is started.[28,66]

Electrolyte and Mineral Imbalances

Electrolytes are lost via stool, ostomies, fistulas, emesis, venting gastrostomy tubes, urine, and skin. Patients with excessive losses may need increased intake of various electrolytes. Potassium, magnesium, and phosphorus are required for optimal protein synthesis. The kidneys are primarily responsible for excretion of potassium, magnesium, and phosphorus; intake of these may need to be restricted in patients with renal insufficiency or failure. Serum concentrations should be monitored at intervals based on patient acuity, and electrolytes and minerals should be replaced as needed to keep serum levels within the normal range.[69]

Sodium

Sodium is the primary extracellular cation in the body and the major controller of osmolality. Clinical features of hyponatremia and hypernatremia relate to the nervous system and include the following: depressed mentation, confusion, irritability, obtundation, coma, seizures, nausea, vomiting, anorexia, and headache. Serum sodium represents a ratio of sodium to water.[69]

Abnormal circulating levels of sodium primarily reflect the status of body water. A relative excess of water compared with sodium results in hyponatremia, while a relative excess of sodium compared with water results in hypernatremia. A common cause of hyponatremia in hospitalized patients is the excessive effect of arginine vasopressin ("antidiuretic hormone") as with the syndrome of inappropriate antidiuretic hormone secretion (SIADH), which results in retention of water in excess of sodium. SIADH can result from a variety of causes, including intracranial hemorrhage, trauma, tumor, or encephalitis; carcinoma of the lung, duodenum, pancreas, thymus, or lymph nodes; pneumonia; tuberculosis; lung abscess; cystic fibrosis; or certain medications. The most common cause of hypernatremia in tube-fed patients is dehydration due to water losses in excess of sodium (eg, excess sweating, osmotic diuresis causing exorbitant urinary losses, limited water intake). Thus, hypernatremia is treated primarily by administration of fluid, and hyponatremia is treated by fluid restriction.[69]

Hypernatremia and hyponatremia also can be caused by high and low sodium intake, respectively, in relation to output. Most enteral formulas contain low amounts of sodium. Patients with increased sodium losses require sodium replacement. Sodium chloride may be judiciously included in the flush solution. The amount of salt used is based on the sodium deficit, the volume of fluid losses, and the organ from which the fluids originated. Conversely, the sodium content of intravenous (IV) fluids needs to be calculated when hypernatremia is evaluated. See Tables 9-4 and 9-5 for additional information on hypo- and hypernatremia.[17,69]

Potassium

Potassium is the primary intracellular cation in the body and the major determinant of electrical membrane potential. Decreased concentrations of potassium (ie, hypokalemia) result in cardiac arrhythmias, muscle weakness, impaired protein synthesis, and impaired insulin secretion. Potassium deficiency results from losses in the stool, GI secretions, and urine (especially with diuretics). Elevated serum potassium (hyperkalemia) is often caused by poor

TABLE 9-4. Hyponatremia

Possible EN-Associated Causes	Preventive or Therapeutic Measures
• SIADH causing water retention and dilution of sodium	• Restrict fluid.
• Hepatic, cardiac, or renal insufficiency	• Monitor sodium level daily. • Assess fluid status.
• Reduced sodium intake relative to output	• Provide diuretic therapy, if indicated. • Restrict fluid and/or sodium.
• High gastrointestinal output (vomiting, diarrhea)	• Provide sodium-containing replacement fluids to offset losses.

Abbreviations: EN, enteral nutrition; SIADH, syndrome of inappropriate antidiuretic hormone secretion.

Source: Information is from references 17 and 69.

TABLE 9-5. Hypernatremia

Possible EN-Associated Causes	Preventive or Therapeutic Measures
• Inadequate fluid intake with increased fluid loss (sweating, osmotic diuresis)	• Monitor daily fluid intake and outputs.
• Increased sodium intake (IV fluid)	• Monitor electrolytes, BUN, and Cr daily.
• Depletion of total body sodium, extracellular mass, extracellular fluid	• Monitor body weight daily; weight change >0.2 kg/d reflects change in ECF volume. • Estimate fluid loss. Mild loss is indicated by 3% decrease in body weight; moderate loss is indicated by a 6% decrease; and severe loss is a 10% decrease. • Replace fluid loss via enteral or parenteral route to replete ECF.

Abbreviations: BUN, blood urea nitrogen; Cr, creatinine; ECF, extracellular fluid; EN, enteral nutrition; IV, intravenous.

Source: Information is from references 17 and 69.

kidney function. Traumatic injuries that release potassium from injured cells can also cause hyperkalemia.[69] See Tables 9-6 and 9-7 for additional information on hypo- and hyperkalemia.[17,69]

Calcium

Calcium is the primary divalent cation of the extracellular fluid and is essential for regulating processes that require movement in the body (eg, excitation-contraction coupling

TABLE 9-6. Hypokalemia

Possible EN-Associated Causes	Preventive or Therapeutic Measures
• Effect of ADH and aldosterone • Diuretic therapy • Excessive losses (with diarrhea or via nasogastric tube) • Metabolic alkalosis • Insulin therapy • Dilution	• Supplement potassium to normal serum values before initiation of tube feeding. • Monitor serum potassium daily until levels are stable with patient at goal EN rate. • Supplement potassium and chloride. • Consider supplementation protocol.

Abbreviations: ADH, antidiuretic hormone; EN, enteral nutrition.

Source: Information is from references 17 and 69.

TABLE 9-7. Hyperkalemia

Possible EN-Associated Causes	Preventive or Therapeutic Measures
• Metabolic acidosis	• Correct acidosis, if possible; recheck serum potassium. • Correct serum potassium before initiation of EN, if possible. • Monitor serum potassium daily.
• Poor perfusion (eg, congestive heart failure)	• Treat cause of poor perfusion.
• Renal failure	• Administer potassium-binding resin, glucose, and/or insulin therapy.
• Excessive potassium intake from EN, IV fluid, oral diet	• Eliminate potassium from IV fluids; reduce potassium in EN and oral diet.

Abbreviations: EN, enteral nutrition; IV, intravenous.

Source: Information is from references 17 and 69.

in cardiac, smooth, and skeletal muscles; neurotransmission; hormonal secretion; ciliary motion; cell division).[70] Calcium circulates in the blood in 3 fractions: ionized, chelated, and protein bound. The ionized fraction is physiologically active and homeostatically regulated, and the best measure of circulating calcium status is the ionized calcium level. Total calcium levels, which are measured by most laboratories, do not accurately reflect ionized calcium status.[69]

Ionized calcium levels are usually obtained with a parathyroid hormone level when serum total calcium values are persistently low despite attempts to normalize them. In the absence of an ionized calcium measurement, clinicians often use the following equation to determine a corrected or adjusted value, although the reliability of this calculation has been questioned:

Adjusted Serum Calcium Value (mg/dL) = [Normal Serum Albumin (g/dL) − Observed Serum Albumin (g/dL) × 0.8] + Observed Serum Calcium (mg/dL)

If adequate dietary calcium is not received over the short term, it will be mobilized from bone and will not be immediately reflected in serum levels. Long-term depletion of calcium from bones may lead to osteopenia or osteoporosis. Conversely, excess calcium administration during ischemic and septic states can cause cellular injury.[69] Calcium should be administered to patients in the smallest amounts possible to maintain normal concentrations.

Phosphorus

Phosphorus is a source of cellular energy (eg, adenosine triphosphate, creatine phosphate), a component of cyclic adenosine monophosphate and cyclic guanosine monophosphate (important intracellular messengers), a component of 2,3-diphosphoglycerate (important for oxygen offloading from hemoglobin), and synthesis of nucleotides. Most circulating phosphorus is in the ionized form.[69,70]

Phosphorus depletion (hypophosphatemia) causes a sick-cell syndrome in which all cells of the body (eg, in the immune system, muscle, and liver) demonstrate diminished function. Respiratory arrest can occur with severe phosphorus depletion. Common causes of hypophosphatemia are administration of large amounts of carbohydrate (ie, phosphorus shifts intracellularly when glucose enters the cell), administration of drugs (eg, insulin, epinephrine, phosphate-binders, sucralfate), and phosphate losses from the GI tract and kidneys.[69]

Serum phosphorus concentrations should be monitored based on patient acuity and replacement provided as necessary. If levels are severely low, phosphorus should be administered intravenously. See Tables 9-8 and 9-9 for additional information on hypo- and hyperphosphatemia.[17,69]

TABLE 9-8. Hypophosphatemia	
Possible EN-Associated Causes	**Preventive or Therapeutic Measures**
• Refeeding syndrome • Excessive energy intake	• Supplement phosphorus to reach normal levels before initiation of tube feeding.
• Binding by sucralfate, antacids	• Monitor serum phosphorus daily and replete as necessary with changing clinical course.
• Insulin therapy	• Supplement phosphorus as sodium or potassium form, as clinically indicated, via enteral or parenteral route.

Abbreviation: EN, enteral nutrition.

Source: Information is from references 17 and 69.

TABLE 9-9. Hyperphosphatemia

Possible EN-Associated Cause	Preventive or Therapeutic Measures
• Renal insufficiency	• Administer phosphate-binder therapy. • Choose EN product with lower phosphorus content.

Abbreviation: EN, enteral nutrition.

Source: Information is from references 17 and 69.

Magnesium

Magnesium is an important cofactor for many essential enzymes. Magnesium depletion (hypomagnesemia) can result from urinary and GI losses or decreased dietary intake. Hypomagnesemia predisposes a patient to cardiac arrhythmias and cellular injury.[69] See Tables 9-10 and 9-11 for additional information on hypo- and hypermagnesemia.[17,69]

TABLE 9-10. Hypomagnesemia

Possible EN-Associated Causes	Preventive or Therapeutic Measures
• Excessive GI losses (diarrhea, high ostomy output) • Malabsorption	• Supplement magnesium to normal serum values before initiation of tube feeding. • Monitor serum magnesium daily until levels are stable with patient at goal EN rate. • Consider supplementation protocol.

Abbreviations: EN, enteral nutrition; GI, gastrointestinal.

Source: Information is from references 17 and 69.

TABLE 9-11. Hypermagnesemia

Possible EN-Associated Causes	Preventive or Therapeutic Measures
• Renal failure • Excessive magnesium intake from EN and/or oral diet	• Reduce magnesium in EN and oral diet.

Abbreviation: EN, enteral nutrition.

Source: Information is from references 17 and 69.

Zinc

Zinc plays important roles in immune function, wound healing, vitamin A metabolism, glucose control, cellular proliferation, and more. Table 9-12 reviews causes of and interventions for zinc deficiency (hypozincemia).[71]

Vitamin Deficiencies

Patients who receive nutrition support may develop vitamin deficiencies, which are often the result of inadequate

TABLE 9-12. Hypozincemia

Possible EN-Associated Cause	Preventive or Therapeutic Measures
• Excessive losses (via nasogastric tube, protein-losing enteropathy, ostomy, wound)	• Supplement zinc via enteral or parenteral route. • Monitor for signs and symptoms of zinc deficiency, such as hair loss.

Abbreviation: EN, enteral nutrition.

Source: Information is from reference 71.

vitamin intake (ie, intake that fails to match requirements or compensate for losses) or poor absorption. Malnourished patients are at increased risk of developing vitamin deficiencies while receiving EN therapy because of their depleted state when nutrition support is initiated.

Fat-soluble vitamins (vitamins A, D, E, and K) require pancreatic enzymes and bile for absorption. Concentrations of these vitamins may be low in patients with pancreatic insufficiency, cirrhosis, or malabsorption syndromes. Vitamin K is required for activation of coagulation proteins, and vitamin D is necessary for the maintenance of circulating calcium. Table 9-13 reviews causes and interventions for vitamin K deficiency.[71]

Common water-soluble vitamin deficiencies include folate, ascorbic acid, and thiamin. Humans are almost entirely dependent on dietary sources for these vitamins and require constant intake to maintain normal stores.[71] Thiamin is an essential vitamin for carbohydrate metabolism, including glucose. In the United States, chronic alcoholism, advanced age, long-term malnutrition, malabsorption syndromes, prolonged antacid therapy (thiamin is destroyed in

TABLE 9-13. Vitamin K Deficiency

Possible EN-Associated Causes	Preventive or Therapeutic Measures
• Inadequate vitamin K intake in diet • Prolonged use of low-fat or low–vitamin K formula • Cirrhosis, malabsorption, pancreatic insufficiency	• Supplement vitamin K. • Consider probiotic agents. • Measure prothrombin time and partial thromboplastin time or INR daily until stable.

Abbreviations: EN, enteral nutrition; INR, international normalized ratio.

Source: Information is from reference 71.

TABLE 9-14. Thiamin Deficiency

Possible EN-Associated Causes	Preventive or Therapeutic Measures
• Chronic alcoholism • Advanced age • Long-term malnutrition • Refeeding syndrome • Malabsorption • Antacid therapy • Dialysis, diuretic	• Thiamin supplementation for 3–7 days (IV for 3 days, *PO* for 7 days). • Consider addition of folate and multivitamin/mineral in cases of alcoholism, refeeding syndrome, malabsorption, or chronic disease.

Abbreviations: EN, enteral nutrition; IV, intravenous; *PO, per os* (by mouth).

Source: Information is from reference 71.

alkaline pH), and dialysis are common causes of thiamin deficiency. Thus, many of these patients are provided thiamin and folic acid upon hospital admission. See Table 9–14 for additional information on thiamin deficiency.[71]

Fluid Issues

Dehydration and overhydration are risks for patients receiving EN (see Tables 9-15 and 9-16).[17] All enteral prescriptions should include the patient's fluid requirements as calculated by a qualified clinician who has done a thorough review of the patient's current clinical status, including fluid losses that require replacement (see Chapter 1 for additional information on assessment). The risk for dehydration is higher in older adults because they have decreased lean body mass and therefore have diminished water reserves. Equations used to estimate fluid requirements should take into account the patient's weight, age, and clinical condition (see Chapter 6).[69]

TABLE 9-15. Dehydration	
Possible EN-Associated Causes	**Preventive or Therapeutic Measures**
• Excessive fluid loss (vomiting, diarrhea, gastric tube loss) • Inadequate fluid intake • Administration of formula concentrated in energy and protein to a patient who cannot express thirst	• Monitor daily fluid intake and output (urine, ostomy, fistula outputs). • Monitor body weight daily and assess for edema. Weight change >0.2 kg/d reflects a change in ECF volume. • Estimate fluid losses. Mild loss is indicated by 3% decrease in body weight; moderate loss is indicated by a 6% decrease; and severe loss is a 10% decrease. • Monitor serum electrolytes, urine-specific gravity, BUN, and Cr daily. BUN:Cr is usually 10:1 in state of normal hydration. • Provide enteral or IV fluid as indicated.

Abbreviations: BUN, blood urea nitrogen; Cr, creatinine; ECF, extracellular fluid; EN, enteral nutrition; IV, intravenous.

Source: Information is from reference 17.

Dehydration results when fluid needs are not being met. Treatment of dehydration is aimed at restoring intravascular volume.

Even though tube feeding formulas are liquid, they typically will not meet total fluid needs. Tube feeding formulas are approximately 67%–87% water. Most patients receiving EN will require the equivalent of about 15%–30% of

TABLE 9-16. Overhydration	
Possible EN-Associated Causes	**Preventive or Therapeutic Measures**
• Excessive fluid intake	• Monitor fluid intake and output daily. • Monitor edema.
• Rapid refeeding	• Assess fluid status daily.
• Catabolism of lean body mass with potassium loss	• Monitor body weight daily.
• Refeeding syndrome	• Monitor weight. Weight change >0.2 kg/d reflects a change in ECF volume. • Monitor aldosterone levels, which will be elevated with sodium retention. • Consider use of less-concentrated formula.
• Renal, hepatic, or cardiac insufficiency	• Provide diuretic therapy.

Abbreviations: ECF, extracellular fluid; EN, enteral nutrition.

Source: Information is from reference 17.

the formula volume in additional water to meet normal fluid requirements. Nutrition support clinicians must be mindful of other sources of fluids (IV fluids, oral intake, flushes after medication administration, etc) when managing EN regimens.

Dehydration also occurs when extra body fluid losses (eg, water loss from skin during fever, loose stools, emesis, large draining wounds, chronic drooling, drains, ostomy/fistula/ gastric outputs, paracentesis losses, losses through lactation and overuse of diuretics) are not met by fluid intake. The volume of these losses should be measured (if possible) or estimated and then repleted. Wound dressings could be weighed before and after placement to measure fluid loss from wounds. Excessive diaphoresis that soaks bed linens has been associated with the loss of 1 liter of fluid.[69,72]

The use of high-protein or concentrated formulas can increase dehydration risk. High-protein formulas may cause an osmotic diuresis due to the high renal solute load and loss of body water. Concentrated feeding formulas contain 67%–75% water and are used commonly for patients with advanced renal disease, those who are fluid overloaded, and those receiving intermittent feedings who are unable to handle a larger volume of feeding administered during a given time period. In the latter case, a lower volume of concentrated formula is given and the extra water needed is administered in between the feedings. See Chapter 4 for additional information on high-protein and concentrated formulas.

Early signs of dehydration include dry mouth and eyes, thirst, dark urine with a strong odor, lightheadedness upon standing, headache, fatigue, loss of appetite, flushed skin, and heat intolerance. Orthostatic hypotension (a drop in systolic blood pressure by ≥ 20 mmHg upon standing) is usually present in dehydrated patients. Dehydration can progress to include dysphagia, muscle cramps, painful urination, sunken eyes with dim vision, poor skin turgor (sternum: >2 seconds), clumsiness, and delirium.[69] An increasing serum sodium concentration, blood urea nitrogen (BUN) level, or BUN-creatinine ratio suggests dehydration. An elevated urine-specific gravity (>1.028) together with low urine output also points to dehydration.

Chronic overhydration may precipitate edema and congestive heart failure. Treatment is aimed at excess fluid removal through diuresis or dialysis.[69]

After the initial fluid prescription is documented, a patient's fluid status must be monitored closely and fluid intake adjusted based on intake and outputs, laboratory values, and clinical status. Patients and their caregivers should be educated on the signs and symptoms of dehydration and overhydration so that adjustments to the nutrition regimen can be made in a timely manner.

Hypercapnia and Acid-Base Disorders

Hypercapnia (elevated blood levels of carbon dioxide [CO_2]) with resultant respiratory acidosis is a theoretical nutrition concern in patients on ventilators or those retaining CO_2 (such as patients with markedly diminished pulmonary function). Because the metabolic by-products of carbohydrate metabolism are CO_2 and water, it was theorized that restricting dietary carbohydrate would decrease CO_2 production. However, this treatment approach has not resulted in a clinical benefit, and it is now recognized that CO_2 production is more affected by excess total energy. Perceived differences in CO_2 production between formulas with high vs lower fat content may be due to fat-induced slowing of gastric emptying.[73] See Table 9-17 for additional information on hypercapnia.[17]

Glucose Intolerance

Hyperglycemia is more common with PN than with EN. The enteral products developed to reduce hyperglycemia are higher in fat and contain fiber, both intended to slow gastric emptying. This may not be desirable in acutely ill patients in whom antropyloric dysfunction (poor gastric emptying, gastroparesis) commonly complicates gastric feeding. Slow advancement of the feeding formula and close collaboration with the medical team should

TABLE 9-17. Hypercapnia	
Possible EN-Associated Causes	**Preventive or Therapeutic Measures**
• Overfeeding of energy	• Use IC to measure energy requirement, if possible. • If IC is unavailable, provide only maintenance energy needs until hypercapnia resolves.
• Excessive carbohydrate provision in patient with respiratory dysfunction	• Provide appropriate balance of carbohydrate, protein, and fat. Consider providing fat to supply 30% of total energy.

Abbreviations: EN, enteral nutrition; IC, indirect calorimetry.

Source: Information is from reference 17.

allow adequate glucose control with standard feeding products.

Glycemic control should be considered a primarily medical issue in the acutely ill patient. Enteral products marketed for patients with diabetes may help improve the ease of glycemic control in chronic care, but they have not yet been proven effective in acutely ill patients.[74] See Tables 9-18 and 9-19 for further information on hyper- and hypoglycemia.[75] For further information on formulas marketed for glycemic control, refer to Chapter 4.

Essential Fatty Acid Deficiency

Patients receiving EN may be at risk for essential fatty acid deficiency. The EN prescription for the types and amount of lipids should be based on careful, individualized assessment. Essential fatty acid deficiency is further reviewed in Table 9-20.[76]

TABLE 9-18. Hyperglycemia

Possible EN-Associated Causes	Preventive or Therapeutic Measures
• Refeeding syndrome • Diabetes mellitus, sepsis, catabolism, trauma, or other disease states or conditions • Insulin resistance • Glucocorticoids • Excessive carbohydrate	• Correct serum glucose before initiation of EN, if possible. • Monitor serum glucose every 6 hours, or per protocol. • Treat underlying disease. • Maintain appropriate intervascular volume and hydration. • Provide appropriate pharmacological intervention. • Consider providing 30% of total energy as fat. • Consider use of an enteral product with fiber.

Abbreviation: EN, enteral nutrition.

Source: Information is from reference 75.

TABLE 9-19. Hypoglycemia

Possible EN-Associated Cause	Preventive or Therapeutic Measures
• Abrupt cessation of EN in a patient receiving insulin or other hypoglycemic drug	• Monitor serum glucose every 6 hours, or per protocol. • Treat with IV or enteral glucose to increase serum level to >100 mg/dL. • Taper EN gradually.

Abbreviations: EN, enteral nutrition; IV, intravenous.

Source: Information is from reference 75.

TABLE 9-20. Essential Fatty Acid Deficiency

Possible EN-Associated Causes	Preventive or Therapeutic Measures
• Inadequate linoleic acid intake • Poor absorption due to Crohn's disease, short bowel syndrome	• Provide at least 4% of energy needs as linoleic acid. • Add modular fat component to EN if needed. • Provide soybean oil via enteral route (1.1–1.6 g/d based on age, gender).

Abbreviation: EN, enteral nutrition.

Source: Information is from reference 76.

References

1. Montejo JC. Enteral nutrition-related gastrointestinal complications in critically ill patients: a multicenter study. The Nutritional and Metabolic Working Group of the Spanish Society of Intensive Care Medicine and Coronary Units. *Crit Care Med.* 1999;27:1447–1453.

2. Montejo JC, Grau T, Acosta J, et al. Multicenter, prospective, randomized, single-blind study comparing the efficacy and gastrointestinal complications of early jejunal feeding with early gastric feeding in critically ill patients. *Crit Care Med.* 2002;30:796–800.

3. Wasseem S, Moshiree B, Dragonov PV. Gastroparesis: current diagnostic challenges and management considerations. *World J Gastroenterol.* 2009;15(1):25–37.

4. Davies AR, Bellomo R. Establishment of enteral nutrition: prokinetic agents and small bowel feeding tubes. *Curr Opin Crit Care.* 2004;10:156–161.

5. Chapman MJ, Nguyen NQ, Deane AM. Gastrointestinal dysmotility: evidence and clinical management. *Curr Opin Clin Nutr Metab Care.* 2013;16(2):209–216.

6. Taylor SJ, Manara AR, Brown J. Treating delayed gastric emptying in critical illness: metoclopramide, erythromycin, and bedside (Cortrak) nasointestinal tube placement. *JPEN J Parenter Enteral Nutr.* 2010;34(3):289–294.

7. Sidery MB, Macdonald IA, Blackshaw PE. Superior mesenteric artery blood flow and gastric emptying in humans and the differential effects of high fat and high carbohydrate meals. *Gut.* 1994;35:186–190.

8. Kozeniecki M, Fritzshall R. Enteral nutrition for adults in the hospital setting. *Nutr Clin Pract.* 2015;30(5):634–651.

9. Btaiche IF, Chan L, Pleva M, Kraft MD. Critical illness, gastrointestinal complications, and medication therapy during enteral feeding in critically ill adult patients. *Nutr Clin Pract.* 2010;25(1):32–49.

10. Ali T, Hasan M, Hamadani M, Harty RF. Gastroparesis. *South Med J.* 2007;100(3):281–286.

11. Parkman HP, Hasler WL, Fisher RS, et al. American Gastroenterological Association technical review on the diagnosis and treatment of gastroparesis. *Gastroenterology.* 2004;127:1592–1622. doi:10.1053/j.gastro.2004.09.055.

12. Marshall AP, Cahill NE, Gramlich L, MacDonald G, Alberda C, Heyland DK. Optimizing nutrition in intensive care units: empowering critical care nurses to be effective agents of change. *Am J Crit Care.* 2012;21(3):186–194. doi:10.4037/ajcc2012697.

13. Williams TA, Leslie GD, Leen T, Mills L, Dobb GJ. Reducing interruptions to continuous enteral nutrition in the intensive care unit: a comparative study. *J Clin Nurs.* 2013; 22(19–20):2838–2848. doi:10.1111/jocn.12068.

14. Aderinto-Adike AO, Quigley EM. Gastrointestinal motility problems in critical care: a clinical perspective. *J Dig Dis.* 2014;15(7):335–344. doi:10.1111/1751-2980.12147.

15. Frazer C, Hussey L, Bemker M. Gastrointestinal motility problems in critically ill patients. *Crit Care Nurs Clin N Am.* 2018;30:109–121.

16. McClave SA, Taylor BE, Martindale RG, et al. Guidelines for the provision and assessment of nutrition support therapy in the adult critically ill patient: Society of Critical Care Medicine (SCCM) and American Society for Parenteral and Enteral Nutrition (A.S.P.E.N.). *JPEN J Parenter Enteral Nutr.* 2016;40(2):159–211. doi:10.1177/0148607115621863.

17. Malone AN, Seres DS, Lord L. Complications of enteral nutrition. In: Mueller CM, ed. *The ASPEN Adult Nutrition Support Core Curriculum.* 3rd ed. Silver Spring, MD: American Society for Parenteral and Enteral Nutrition; 2017:265–284.

18. Omer A, Quigley EMM. Carbohydrate maldigestion and malabsorption. *Clin Gastroenterol Hepatol.* 2018;16(8):1197–1199. doi:10.1016/j.cgh.2018.01.048.

19. Rezaie A, Buresi M, Lembo A, et al. Hydrogen and methane-based breath testing in gastrointestinal disorders: the North American consensus. *Am J Gastroenterol.* 2017;112:775–784.

20. Berry AJ. Pancreatic enzyme replacement therapy during pancreatic insufficiency. *Nutr Clin Pract.* 2014;29(3):312–321.

21. Nguyen NQ, Burgstad C, Bellon M, et al. Delayed enteral feeding impairs intestinal carbohydrate absorption in critically ill patients. *Crit Care Med.* 2012;40(1):50–54.

22. Chang S, Huang H. Diarrhea in enterally fed patients: blame the diet? *Curr Opin Clin Nutr Metab Care.* 2013;16:588–594.

23. Whelan K. Enteral tube feeding diarrhea: Manipulating the colonic microbiota with probiotics and prebiotics. *Proc Nutr Soc.* 2007;66:299–306.

24. Whelan K, Schneider SM. Mechanisms, prevention, and management of diarrhea in enteral nutrition. *Curr Opin Gastroenterol.* 2011;27:152–159.

25. Wierdsma NJ, Peters JH, Weijs PJ, et al. Malabsorption and nutritional balance in the ICU: fecal weight as a biomarker: a prospective observational pilot study. *Crit Care.* 2011; 15(6):R264.

26. de Brito-Ashurst I, Preiser JC. Diarrhea in critically ill patients: the role of enteral feeding. *JPEN J Parenter Enteral Nutr.* 2016;40(7):913–923.

27. Imhann F, Vich Vila A, Bonder MJ, et al. The influence of proton pump inhibitors and other commonly used medication on the gut microbiota. *Gut Microbes.* 2017;8:351–358.

28. Boullata JI, Carrera AL, Harvey L, et al. ASPEN safe practices for enteral nutrition therapy. *JPEN J Parenter Enteral Nutr.* 2017;41(1):15–103.

29. Brennan MR, Milne CT, Agrell-Kann M, Ekholm BP. Clinical evaluation of a skin protectant for the management of incontinence-associated dermatitis. *J Wound Ostomy Continence Nurs.* 2017;44(2):172–180.

30. Lord LM. Maintaining hydration and tube patency in enteral tube feedings. *Safe Pract Patient Care.* 2011;5(2):1–11.

31. Mostafa SM, Bhandari S, Ritchie G, Grotton N, Wenstone R. Constipation and its implications in the critically ill patient. *Br J Anaesth.* 2003;91(6):815–819.

32. Johanson JF. Review of the treatment options for chronic constipation. *Med Gen Med.* 2007;9(2):25–59.

33. Bittencourt AF, Martins JR, Logullo L, et al. Constipation is more frequent than diarrhea in patients fed exclusively by enteral nutrition: results of an observational study. *Nutr Clin Pract.* 2012;27(4):533–539.

34. Schallom M, Orr J, Metheny N, Pierce J. Gastroesophageal reflux in critically ill patients. *Dimens Crit Care Nurs.* 2013; 32:69–77.

35. Zaloga GP. Aspiration-related illnesses: definitions and diagnosis. *JPEN J Parenter Enteral Nutr.* 2002;26(6 Suppl):S2–S7.

36. Dibardino DM, Wunderink RG. Aspiration pneumonia: a review of modern trends. *J Crit Care.* 2015;30(1):40–48.

37. Hamaoui E. Gastroesophageal reflux during gastrostomy feeding. *JPEN J Parenter Enteral Nutr.* 1995;19:172–173.

38. Gustke RF, Varma RR, Soergel KH. Gastric reflux during perfusion of the proximal small bowel. *Gastroenterology.* 1970; 59:890–895.

39. Metheny N, Clouse RE, Chang YH, et al. Tracheobronchial aspiration of gastric contents in critically ill tube-fed patients: frequency, outcomes, and risk factors. *Crit Care Med.* 2006;34:1007–1015.

40. Kollef MH, von Harz B, Prentice D, et al. Patient transport from intensive care increases the risk of developing ventilator associated pneumonia. *Chest.* 1997;112:765–773.

41. McClave SA, Lukan JE, Stefater JA, et al. Poor validity of residual volume as a marker for risk of aspiration in critically ill patients. *Crit Care Med.* 2005;33:324–330.

42. McClave SA, Demeo MT, DeLegge MH, et al. North American Summit on Aspiration in the Critically Ill Patient: consensus statement. *JPEN J Parenter Enteral Nutr.* 2002;26 (6 Suppl):S80–S85.

43. Metheny NA, Dahms TE, Stewart BJ, Stone KS, Frank PA, Clouse RE. Verification of inefficacy of the glucose method in detecting aspiration associated with tube feedings. *Medsurg Nurs.* 2005;14:112–121.

44. Metheny NA, Stewart J, Nuetzel G, Oliver D, Clouse RE. Effect of feeding-tube properties on residual volume measurements in tube-fed patients. *JPEN J Parenter Enteral Nutr.* 2005;29:192–197.

45. McClave SA, Snider HL, Lowen CC, et al. Use of residual volume as a marker for enteral feeding intolerance: prospective blinded comparison with physical examination and radiographic findings. *JPEN J Parenter Enteral Nutr.* 1992;16: 99–105.

46. Metheny NA. Preventing respiratory complications of tube feedings: evidence-based practice. *Am J Crit Care.* 2006;15: 360–369.

47. van der Voort PH, Zandstra DF. Enteral feeding in the critically ill: comparison between the supine and prone positions: a prospective crossover study in mechanically ventilated patients. *Crit Care.* 2001;5:216–220.

48. Malhotra AK, Deorari AK, Paul VK, Bagga A, Singh M. Gastric residuals in preterm babies. *J Trop Pediatr.* 1992;38: 262–264.

49. US Food and Drug Administration. FDA Public Health Advisory: Reports of Blue Discoloration and Death in Patients Receiving Enteral Feedings Tinted With The Dye, FD&C Blue No. 1. https://www.fda.gov/forindustry/coloradditives/coloradditivesinspecificproducts/inmedicaldevices/ucm142395.htm. Published September 29, 2003. Accessed December 12, 2018.

50. Metheny NA, Dahms TE, Stewart BJ, et al. Efficacy of dye-stained enteral formula in detecting pulmonary aspiration. *Chest.* 2002;122:276–281.

51. Drakulovic MB, Torres A, Bauer TT, et al. Supine body position as a risk factor for nosocomial pneumonia in mechanically ventilated patients: a randomized trial. *Lancet.* 1999;354(9193):1851–1858.

52. National Pressure Ulcer Advisory Panel, European Pressure Ulcer Advisory Panel, Pan Pacific Pressure Ulcer Alliance. *Prevention and Treatment of Pressure Ulcers.* Perth, Australia: Cambridge Media; 2014.

53. Schallom M, Dykeman B, Metheny N, Kirby J, Pierce J. Head-of-bed elevation and early outcomes of gastric reflux, aspiration and pressure ulcers: a feasibility study. *Am J Crit Care.* 2015;24(1):57–66.

54. American Association of Critical-Care Nurses. AACN practice alert: prevention of aspiration in adults. https://www.aacn.org/clinical-resources/practice-alerts/prevention-of

-aspiration Published February 1, 2016. Accessed December 19, 2018.

55. American Association of Critical-Care Nurses. AACN practice alert: oral care for acutely and critically ill patients. https://www.aacn.org/clinical-resources/practice-alerts /oral-care-for-acutely-and-critically-ill-patients. Published June 2017. Accessed December 12, 2018.

56. Metheny NA. Preventing respiratory complications of tube feedings: evidence-based practice. *Am J Crit Care.* 2006;15(4): 360–369.

57. Braunschweig CL, Levy P, Sheean PM, Wang X. Enteral compared with parenteral nutrition: a meta-analysis. *Am J Clin Nutr.* 2001;74:534–542.

58. Metheny NA, Davis-Jackson J, Stewart BJ. Effectiveness of an aspiration risk-reduction protocol. *Nurs Res.* 2010;59(1): 18–25.

59. Nguyen NQ, Chapman M, Fraser RJ, Bryant LK, Burgstad C, Holloway RH. Prokinetic therapy for feed intolerance in critical illness: one drug or two? *Crit Care Med.* 2007; 35(11):2561–2567.

60. A.S.P.E.N. Board of Directors. Guidelines for the use of parenteral and enteral nutrition in adult and pediatric patients. *JPEN J Parenter Enteral Nutr.* 2002;26(1 Suppl):1SA–138SA.

61. Jolly AF, Blank R. Refeeding syndrome. In: Zaloga G, ed. *Nutrition in Critical Care.* St. Louis, MO: Mosby; 1994:765–782.

62. Bowling TE, Silk DB. Refeeding remembered. *Nutrition.* 1995;11:32–34.

63. Solomon SM, Kirby DF. The refeeding syndrome: a review. *JPEN J Parenter Enteral Nutr.* 1990;14:90–97.

64. Parli SE, Ruf KM, Magnuson B. Pathophysiology, treatment, and prevention of fluid and electrolyte abnormalities during refeeding syndrome. *J Infus Nurs.* 2014;37(3):197–202. doi:10.1097/NAN.0000000000000038.

65. Mehanna HM, Moledina J, Travis J. Refeeding syndrome: what it is, and how to prevent and treat it. *BMJ.* 2008; 336(7659):1495–1498. doi:10.1136/bmj.a301.

66. Kraft MD, Btaiche IF, Sacks GS. Review of the refeeding syndrome. *Nutr Clin Pract.* 2005;20:625–633.

67. Friedli N, Stanga Z, Sobotka L, et al. Revisiting the refeeding syndrome: results of a systematic review. *Nutrition.* 2017;35: 151–160. doi:10.1016/j.nut.2016.05.016.

68. Stanga Z, Brunner A, Leuenberger M, et al. Nutrition in clinical practice—the refeeding syndrome: illustrative cases and guidelines for prevention and treatment. *Eur J Clin Nutr.* 2008;62:687–694.

69. Canada TW, Lord LM. Fluids, electrolytes, and acid-base disorders. In: Mueller CM, ed. *The ASPEN Adult Nutrition Support Core Curriculum.* 3rd ed. Silver Spring, MD: American Society for Parenteral and Enteral Nutrition; 2017:113–138.

70. Zaloga GP, Chernow B. Divalent ions: calcium, magnesium, and phosphorus. In: Chernow B, ed. *The Pharmacologic Approach to the Critically Ill Patient.* 3rd ed. Baltimore, MD: Williams & Wilkins; 1994:777–804.

71. McKeever L. Vitamins and trace elements. In: Mueller CM, ed. *The ASPEN Adult Nutrition Support Core Curriculum.* 3rd ed. Silver Spring, MD: American Society for Parenteral and Enteral Nutrition; 2017:140–182.

72. Russell MK. Monitoring and complications. In: Charney P, Malone A, eds. *ADA Pocket Guide to Enteral Nutrition.* Chicago, IL: American Dietetic Association, 2005.

73. Akrabawi SS, Mobarhan S, Stoltz RR, Ferguson PW. Gastric emptying, pulmonary function, gas exchange, and respiratory quotient after feeding a moderate versus high fat enteral formula meal in chronic obstructive pulmonary disease patients. *Nutrition.* 1996;12:260–265.

74. Malone AM. Enteral formula selection: a review of selected product categories. *Pract Gastroenterol.* 2005;29:44–74. https://med.virginia.edu/ginutrition/wp-content/uploads/sites/199/2015/11/MaloneArticle-June-05.pdf. Accessed December 12, 2018.

75. Walker R, Tucker AM, Birtcher KK. Diabetes mellitus. In: Mueller CM, ed. *The ASPEN Adult Nutrition Support Core Curriculum.* 3rd ed. Silver Spring, MD: American Society for Parenteral and Enteral Nutrition; 2017:675–700.

76. Hise M, Brown JC. Lipids. In: Mueller CM, ed. *The ASPEN Adult Nutrition Support Core Curriculum.* 3rd ed. Silver Spring, MD: American Society for Parenteral and Enteral Nutrition; 2017:71–96.

CHAPTER 10

Medication Administration with Enteral Nutrition

Introduction

Patients receiving enteral nutrition (EN) often require administration of medications through that same enteral access device (EAD). By appreciating the complexity of drug administration through a feeding tube and using appropriate administration techniques, nutrition support clinicians can reduce the risk for obstructed tubes, reduced drug efficacy, and increased drug toxicity. To maximize the best use of medication in patients receiving EN, administration techniques should ensure bioavailability without further complicating the patient's overall care. See Table 10-1 for selected factors to review when considering administration of oral drug products through an enteral feeding tube.

Recommendations for administering medication via enteral feeding tubes are available.[1-9] However, since the 1980s, surveys of enteral drug administration practices

TABLE 10-1. Selected Factors to Review Before Administering Medications via an Enteral Feeding Tube

- Length of a patient's functional bowel beyond the tube's distal tip
- Internal diameter and length of the tube
- Composition of the tube
- Routine flushing regimen
- Location of the distal end of the feeding tube relative to the site of drug absorption
- Size of the opening(s) at the distal end of the feeding tube
- Need to keep a drug separate from a tube feeding formula
- Size of the enteral syringe [pressures]

and techniques have demonstrated a gap between best-practice recommendations and actual practice. These surveys suggest that only 5%–43% of practitioners flush tubes before or between the administration of medications, only 32%–51% administer drugs separately from one another, only 44%–64% dilute liquid medication, and 75%–85% avoid crushing modified-release dosage forms.[10–16] Some of these practices may contribute to measurable adverse outcomes—in particular, tube obstruction, reduced drug efficacy, and increased drug toxicity. Best-practice techniques for medication administration through a feeding tube are reviewed in this chapter.

Dissolution and Absorption of Drugs

Commercially available drugs that are intended for systemic effect after oral administration are designed with the physiology of the healthy, intact gastrointestinal (GI) tract in mind. Immediate-release dosage forms begin to disintegrate and dissolve in the stomach before entering the small bowel environment, where dissolution and absorption continue. Although some drug absorption may occur throughout the GI tract by mass effect, the sites of absorption for specific drugs are distinct and sometimes unknown.

Administration of a drug via an enteral feeding tube may bypass the required environment for optimal dissolution and absorption of the medication. For example, when administered as a medication, iron is predominantly absorbed in the duodenum following gastric dissolution. Thus, administration through a tube with the distal opening in the jejunum risks poor bioavailability of the iron.[9] Prior to administration of medication through a feeding tube, the location of the distal tube tip should be noted (see Chapter 3 for information on tube tip verification).

Enteral Access Devices and Medication Administration

For both accurate drug dosing and safe intraluminal pressures, only syringes manufactured and intended for enteral use should be used to measure and administer a medication through an enteral feeding tube. Only specially designed enteral syringes with ENFit® connectors will fit into ENFit enteral feeding devices, and those syringes should be used exclusively to deliver medications via a feeding tube. The Low-Dose Tip ENFit syringes have minimal dead space and have been shown to accurately deliver low-volume liquid medications.[17,18]

The ENFit connector is the new International Organization for Standardization (ISO) 80369-3 standard for enteral feeding device connectors. This connector is designed to prevent misconnection of enteral feeding lines to intravenous lines or other commonly encountered connectors not intended for enteral feeding delivery. Its unique design is only compatible with ENFit tubing, therefore promoting patient safety and reducing the risk for a severe or fatal administration error. For any EAD that does not yet have an ENFit connector, a temporary transition adapter is available to connect the traditional enteral port to the ENFit administration set until new ENFit tubing is available. Ultimately, all ENFit feeding tubes will use the ENFit connection. The ENFit syringe is available in 2 configurations—standard dose and low dose. ENFit-labeled enteral devices with medication or feeding ports are only compatible with ENFit medication syringes. ENFit syringes and connectors are available in a wide variety of sizes to allow for medication and formula delivery. Refer to Chapter 3 for illustrations of ENFit connectors.

Dosage Forms

Commercially available oral drug dosage forms are solids (eg, capsules, tablets) or liquids (eg, solutions, suspensions). Most tablets and capsules are immediate-release products (eg, compressed tablets, hard gelatin capsules), which contain the active drug molecule along with excipients (nontherapeutic ingredients required to formulate the product). These products are designed to allow the drug contents to be released within minutes of reaching the stomach following oral administration. Many drugs are also offered as modified-release products (eg, delayed- or extended-release), or as complex formulations.[19,20]

Solutions are homogeneous liquid mixtures in which the active medication is uniformly dissolved in the diluent. The diluent often contains water and a variety of other solvents (eg, ethanol); contents of the diluent are chosen based on the solubility of the active drug. The viscosity and osmolality of a solution vary with the drug and solvent. With regard to enteral administration, disadvantages of solutions include the increased potential for drug instability due to hydrolysis or oxidation.

Suspensions are heterogeneous liquids containing a poorly soluble active medication "floating" in a liquid medium that contains suspending or thickening agents. Disadvantages of suspensions for enteral administration include their viscosity and the potential that dispersed particles will settle, making it more difficult to deliver the medication to the site of drug absorption through an enteral feeding tube. Regardless of the container volume, suspensions should be shaken well immediately before the drug is administered via an EAD.

Crushing and Diluting Medications

Except for tablets that disperse easily when placed in an enteral syringe with water, contents of an appropriate tablet or capsule should be crushed to a fine powder before being dispersed, dissolved, or suspended in an appropriate volume of sterile water.[21] See Figure 10-1 for an example

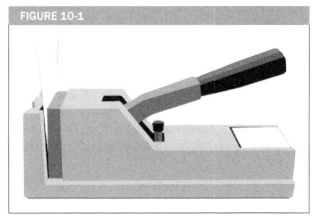

FIGURE 10-1

Example of a medication-crushing device. Illustration by Sarah Nishiura. Copyright © American Society for Parenteral and Enteral Nutrition.

of a medication-crushing device. Advantages of the smaller particle size are improved suspension and decreased likelihood that a tube or its distal exit site(s) will be obstructed. A disadvantage is increased risk of interaction with other medication particles found in the water if nonpurified water is used. Flushing the enteral feeding tube between medications decreases the incidence of enteral tube occlusions.[22]

Some tablets are very small, very hard, or film coated, making them difficult to crush. Enteric and film coatings do not crush well and tend to aggregate in clumps when diluted in water, thereby increasing the risk of clogging. Modified-release dosage forms should not be crushed for administration via feeding tubes because destroying the protective coating on a drug may make the medication much less effective or may result in an excessive—even fatal—dose of the drug being released at one time.[5,23] Instead, a more appropriate dosage form or therapeutic equivalent should be considered.

Interfering with the integrity of intact liquid-filled gel capsules poses another level of complexity as it is difficult to ensure accurate doses, so these forms of medication are also best avoided in enterally fed patients. Injectable dosage forms are generally not considered appropriate for administration through a feeding tube because they are designed for a physiological site with different characteristics.

Commercially available liquid formulations of a drug are not necessarily the best delivery option for a patient. The solvents, solubilizing agents, and excipients in such formulations may be factors that contraindicate enteral administration.[24] Also, in fluid-restricted patients, a balance between the patient's fluid requirements and the minimal volume required to dilute medications for enteral feeding tube administration must be realized.

Liquid dosage forms often must be further diluted with sterile water prior to administration through an enteral feeding tube. The viscosity and osmolality of the liquid dosage form, the internal diameter and length of the tube, and the location of the distal tip all must be considered when determining the final diluted volume of the liquid drug formulation. High-osmolality medicines may cause emesis and diarrhea; however, diluting medications to achieve a lower osmolality is not always possible.

Suspensions tend to have much higher viscosity than solutions. Some suspensions are granular and may contain modified-release particles. The resistance to flow through an enteral feeding tube can be reduced through dilution but still may not be adequate to overcome a narrow tube. Dilution of each liquid medication prior to administration is associated with improved delivery of the drug dose to the distal end of the tube.[25,26]

Liquid medication formulations may contain a number of excipients in addition to the drug and liquid. Several poorly absorbed sweeteners and stabilizers are used in liquid drug products; such additives invariably increase a product's osmolality and potential to cause diarrhea. Electrolyte-containing liquids also contribute to high osmolality.

Drug Interactions

Pharmacists and other clinicians do not routinely mix different medications in the same intravenous bag or syringe without first ensuring the stability and compatibility of the drugs. Similar precautions should be taken during preparation of medication for administration through enteral feeding tubes. Suboptimal drug administration has been identified as more common in patient care units that did not establish drug preparation and administration protocols.[27]

Interactions involving medication administered to patients receiving EN include those that pose a *compatibility* problem and those that influence the *stability* of the drug or nutrient. These interactions can result in feeding tube occlusion, altered drug or nutrient delivery and bioavailability, or altered GI tract function.

Occlusion of feeding tubes and altered clinical responses to drug therapy as a result of inappropriate enteral administration techniques are not routinely captured in medication error event rates. Regardless of etiology, obstruction ("clogging") of a feeding tube is both time- and resource-intensive to address; therefore, it is best to prevent clogs (see Chapter 3 for techniques to prevent feeding tube obstruction). Results of a national survey suggest that drug-related feeding tube obstruction exceeds 10% if modified-release dosage forms are routinely crushed.[15] Whenever a drug formulation is altered—whether by crushing, adding to fluid, or combining with other substances, drug stability may be compromised.

Drug Added to Enteral Nutrition

In patient care settings that do not use a closed EN feeding system, the opportunity to add medication to EN formulas may still exist. However, this practice is not recommended. There is a risk that the formula could be contaminated during the mixing process. Also, mixing medication with formula would require knowledge we generally do not have about the drug's compatibility with the formula, the stability of each component of the final mixture, and the therapeutic efficacy of the mixture.

Several older papers described the compatibility of a relatively small number of medications when admixed with a limited number of commercially available EN formulas.[28–33] This research shows that the type and concentration of protein, as well as the fiber and mineral content of the EN formula, are factors that influence compatibility, while drug product variables include pH, viscosity, osmolality, alcohol, and mineral content.[29,31] Few of these studies evaluated nutrient stability. Notably, 2 of the papers concluded that concentration of the medication may be significantly affected when mixed with formula,[30,32] and another reported that 95% of incompatible admixtures result in clogged feeding tubes, of which less than one-third could be resolved by flushing with water.[31]

The available data on compatibility and stability of formula-drug mixtures cannot be extrapolated to different forms of the same medication, different medications in the same drug class, or different enteral feeding formulas. For example, a liquid morphine product of lower concentration may result in phase separation and protein precipitation of an EN formula while a more concentrated version of the same drug may not.[28]

Drug Added to Drug

Combining drugs into one mixture for enteral administration is not recommended. The design of immediate-release oral products is based on the intended use through oral ingestion with 120–240 mL of water. Once in the gastric lumen, the water and endogenous secretions initiate the process of breaking down the tablet or capsule and dispersing the particles widely with continued dilution in the large volume of the stomach; subsequently, the broken-down and diluted drug empties into the duodenum and further disperses and dilutes in the large surface area of the small bowel. Combining 2 or more medications within the confined space of a mortar under a pestle or other tablet-crushing device may cause a chemical reaction much greater than the reaction that would occur when combining drugs orally. The applied force used in combining drugs before administration, and the resultant increase in particle surface area exposed, could accelerate changes in molecular structure and formation of complexes with subsequent changes in physical and chemical properties of each drug. When considering the various excipients also occupying that confined, nonphysiological space, the potential for chemical reactions increases even further. Any new dosage form created by crushing and mixing together 2 or more medications (and their excipients) must still be expected to release each drug in a known and consistent manner following administration.[21] This information is not available for most medications.

Combining liquid drug products requires knowledge of each solvent's physicochemical properties to minimize disruption of drug solubility and stability. Therefore, combining multiple liquid drug products can be quite complex, with the solubility of the products altered by each new additive in the mix. Again, the stability and compatibility of mixtures is impractical to predict.

Specific Drug-Nutrient Interactions

There are many potential drug-nutrient interactions involving EN therapy; however, a few drugs are particularly troublesome and generate more discussion than most. Four of these drugs are discussed here.

Phenytoin

Phenytoin is the most noteworthy drug for interaction with EN therapy. Many studies and case reports have been published, but findings from prospective, randomized controlled trials (RCTs) are limited. There are multiple theories regarding the interaction and many proposed solutions. Four RCTs of phenytoin and EN in healthy volunteers have been reviewed.[34,35] Only 1 RCT investigated whether EN formulation delivered through a feeding tube affects phenytoin; the others investigated the effect of oral EN on the drug. None of these RCTs documented an interaction between phenytoin and EN formulations. However, 25 reports and studies with less-rigorous designs (no randomization or placebo control) supported an interaction in patients.[34] Theories regarding the mechanism of interaction focus on issues related to pH and phenytoin binding, either to tubing or to an EN component.[36–40] Issues related to dosage form (eg, suspension, chewable tablets, capsule, parenteral solution), chemical form (eg, phenytoin acid vs phenytoin sodium), and solubility are encompassed in the discussion of pH.[36–38] Of the various methods proposed to manage the phenytoin-EN interaction, none are completely reliable, and monitoring of serum phenytoin concentrations and patient-specific pharmacokinetic parameters is highly recommended. Holding administration of the EN formulation for at least 1 hour, and possibly 2 hours, before and after phenytoin administration seems to produce the most consistent results.[41,42] However, some practitioners elect not to hold EN; they should monitor serum concentrations accordingly. Dilution of phenytoin suspension (1:1) is recommended when the suspension is administered through a feeding tube.[39] Regardless of the method used, consistency of administration is important to control 1 of the variables influencing the phenytoin concentration.

Carbamazepine

Carbamazepine is a relatively insoluble drug and is acid stable; thus, slow gastric emptying improves its bioavailability. Limited data suggest EN therapy reduces bioavailability, possibly by altering solubility. Relative bioavailability of 90% was reported in a randomized crossover study comparing administration of carbamazepine suspension via nasogastric tube with continuous EN and oral intake after an overnight fast in 7 healthy men.[43] Serum carbamazepine concentrations with tube feeding were significantly lower at 8 hours, and the lower maximum concentration approached statistical significance, although the small size of the study limited the ability of investigators to show significance. In an vitro study, recovery of carbamazepine was 58% when the drug was mixed with an intact protein enteral formulation, compared with 79% recovery after the drug was mixed with a simulated gastric juice.[44] Recovery when carbamazepine was mixed with the EN formulation and simulated intestinal juice was 59%. These findings suggest that postpyloric administration of carbamazepine may result in poor bioavailability. Binding of carbamazepine to a component of enteral formulations has not been demonstrated; thus, it is unclear if holding administration of the enteral formulation for 2 hours before and after the drug dose, as has been recommended, is the best method of mitigating this potential interaction.[45,46] Carbamazepine suspension should be diluted at least 1:1 with water if the medication is administered via a feeding tube because drug loss in the feeding tube seems to be reduced with dilution.[47]

Fluoroquinolones

Bioavailability of fluoroquinolone antibiotics seems to be reduced by enteral formulations. Studies in healthy volunteers reported a 25% to 28% decrease in ciprofloxacin bioavailability when the drug was administered with an enteral formulation, and decreases of 27% to 67% have been reported in hospitalized patients.[48–50] Reduced bioavailability has also been reported with repeated doses of ciprofloxacin via nasogastric tube in critically ill patients receiving continuous infusion of an enteral formulation.[51,52] Jejunal feeding has the greatest impact on reducing ciprofloxacin bioavailability and may increase the risk for treatment failure.[50,53] However, it is unclear whether reduced bioavailability with gastric feeding is clinically significant because serum drug concentrations above the minimum inhibitory concentration (MIC) for many pathogenic microorganisms have been reported.[54] This response will depend on the microorganism and its MIC given that the therapeutic effect of fluoroquinolones is driven by adequate peak-to-MIC or area under the drug-concentration curve (AUC)-to-MIC ratio.

Complexation of ciprofloxacin with divalent cations in the enteral formulation was initially thought to be responsible for reduced bioavailability. Fluoroquinolones are known to bind with divalent cations, and manufacturers of these medications advise separating drug administration from intake of foods, dietary supplements, or other drugs containing calcium, magnesium (eg, antacids), or iron. However, one in vitro study failed to find a correlation between cation content of the enteral formulation and the loss of different fluoroquinolones mixed into the formulation.[55] Ciprofloxacin loss was greatest (82.5%), followed by levofloxacin (61%) and ofloxacin (46%). The amount of loss seemed to increase with the degree of hydrophilicity of the individual drug. Better bioavailability of ofloxacin (90%) compared with ciprofloxacin (72%) has also been reported in healthy volunteers receiving the antibiotics with an enteral formulation.[48] The current recommendation is to hold administration of EN for at least 1 hour before a fluoroquinolone dose and 2 hours after the dose.[46] This approach seems to minimize effects of the interaction on ciprofloxacin and norfloxacin, and it is the safest approach for all fluoroquinolones unless drug-specific data clearly demonstrate an absence of a drug-nutrient interaction.

Warfarin

The interaction between warfarin and vitamin K in enteral formulations was a classic interaction of concern until the vitamin K content of most products was modified to ≤100 mcg/1000 kcal. Resistance to the anticoagulant effect of warfarin was still observed when the drug was coadministered with EN; the protein content of the formulation was suspected to be causative. However, warfarin resistance due to protein binding has not been adequately studied to confirm whether that is the mechanism of interaction.[56]

Clinicians may elect to manage the warfarin-EN interaction by separating the drug from the formula, increasing the warfarin dose, choosing an alternative anticoagulant therapy, or even using an elemental formula. (Note: Elemental formulas are costly and high in osmolality, and their use requires justification.) Holding administration of the EN formulation for at least 1 hour before and after the warfarin dose is expected to mitigate the interaction.[57] Nonetheless, response to warfarin therapy must be closely monitored when EN therapy is started, stopped, or altered. Interactions involving warfarin can be life threatening.

Planning the Patient's Medication Regimen

Each patient's medication regimen should be individualized. Pharmacists can provide necessary information on the physicochemical properties of a drug as well as interpretation of published stability and compatibility data. This guidance from the pharmacist can be applied to an individual patient's drug regimen and allow for more informed decision-making by the entire healthcare team.

A multidisciplinary intervention program involving guidelines, nurse education, and pharmacist recommendations has been shown to be effective in promoting the most appropriate drug administration practices and techniques, thereby reducing tube obstructions and drug errors.[27] Several strategies may help minimize the risk for adverse outcomes for patients receiving EN who are also being administered medications. For example, the entire medication regimen may be simplified, a medication that is not immediately needed may be temporarily discontinued, or dosing schedules may be altered to avoid administration of medications at the same time as enteral feedings.[5] Additionally, dosage forms or routes of administration may be altered, or the patient may be switched to a therapeutically similar drug product that is better suited for administration via the feeding tube.[5] The creation of extemporaneous medication formulas for individual patients may sometimes be the best option, particularly in pediatric practice settings.[58,59] Specific medication formulas may be found in the literature.[58–60] Aside from ensuring drug stability, the data should additionally reflect that the labeled drug dose can ultimately be delivered to the site at the distal end of the enteral feeding tube without significant loss.

Medication Administration Technique

To optimize therapeutic response of the medication and prevent complications such as tube occlusion, clinicians and caregivers should carefully follow documented procedures and guidelines for medication administration through an enteral feeding tube.[1] As discussed earlier, important concepts to consider include tube size and location of the tube tip. Administration of enteral formula is temporarily held while each medication is administered enterally. The period of time that the formula is held will depend on the interaction potential between the administered drug and the enteral formula. See Table 10-2 for practice recommendations and medication administration techniques.[1]

TABLE 10-2. Practice Recommendations and Procedures for Medication Administration Through an Enteral Access Device

1. Develop policies and procedures to ensure safe practices by staff across all departments involved with enteral medication preparation and administration.

2. Identify drug, dose, dosage form, route (ie, enteral), and access device (eg, nasoduodenal tube) in the prescriber's order.

3. Have a pharmacist review each medication order to determine whether the enterally administered medication will be safe, stable, and compatible as ordered.

4. Institute and follow nursing policies and procedures to prepare and administer each medication safely.

5. Provide nonsterile compounding pharmacy services to support medication preparation.

6. Use best practices as per USP <795> for any enteral drug preparations compounded in advance (ie, not for immediate use); these should include:
   a. Reference to published stability data clearly described with citations in the organization's master formulation records
   b. Documenting in a permanent compounding record
   c. Providing a beyond use date
   d. Storage in a container consistent with the stability/compatibility literature and USP <795>

7. Do not add medication directly to an enteral feeding formula.

8. Administer each medication separately through an appropriate access.

9. Avoid mixing together different medications intended for administration through the feeding tube, given the risks for physical and chemical incompatibilities, tube obstruction, and altered therapeutic drug responses.

(continued)

TABLE 10-2. *(Continued)*

10. Use available liquid dosage forms only if they are appropriate for enteral administration. If liquid dosage forms are inappropriate or unavailable, substitute only immediate-release solid dosage forms.

11. Prepare approved immediate-release solid dosage forms of medication for enteral administration according to pharmacist instructions. Techniques may include:
    a. Crush simple compressed tablets to a fine powder and mix with purified water.
    b. Open hard gelatin capsules and mix powder containing the immediate-release medication with purified water.

12. Use only appropriate instruments to measure and prepare enteral medication.

13. Use only clean enteral syringes ($\geq$20 mL with ENFit device) to administer medication through an EAD.

14. Provide appropriate tube irrigation around the timing of drug administration:
    a. Prior to administering medication, stop the feeding and flush the tube with at least 15 mL water.
    b. Administer the medication using a clean enteral syringe.
    c. Flush the tube again with at least 15 mL water, taking into account the patient's volume status.
    d. Repeat with the next medication.
    e. Flush the tube 1 final time with at least 15 mL water.

15. Restart the feeding in a timely manner to avoid compromising nutrition status. Hold the feeding by 30 minutes or more only if separation is indicated to avoid altered drug bioavailability.

16. Consult with an adult or pediatric pharmacist for patients who receive medications coadministered with EN.

Abbreviations: EAD, enteral access device; EN, enteral nutrition.

Source: Adapted with permission from reference 1: Boullata JI, Carrera AL, Harvey L, et al. ASPEN safe practices for enteral nutrition therapy. *JPEN J Parenter Enteral Nutr.* 2017;41:15–103.

Conclusion

Best practice in drug administration through enteral feeding tubes requires dedicated time and resources. Implementing standardized protocols for drug administration through an enteral feeding tube can reduce inconsistencies in practice that may otherwise interfere with appropriate medication delivery.[1,16,24] Such protocols, as well as clear communication among members of the interdisciplinary team and careful documentation of patient care (including medication and EN orders), are essential to the safe and effective delivery of drugs via EADs.

Practice Resources and Suggested Readings

Boullata JI. *Guidebook on Enteral Medication Administration.* Silver Spring, MD: American Society for Parenteral and Enteral Nutrition; 2018.

Boullata JI, Carrera AL, Harvey L, et al. ASPEN safe practices for enteral nutrition therapy. *JPEN J Parenter Enteral Nutr.* 2017;41:15–103.

Boullata JI. Drug administration through an enteral feeding tube. *Am J Nurs.* 2009;109(10):34–42.

Boullata JI, Armenti VT. *Handbook of Drug-Nutrient Interactions.* 2nd ed. New York, NY: Humana Press; 2010.

GEDSA. ENFit® medical guidelines: research and position statements. GEDSA website. http://stayconnected.org/enfit -medical-guidelines. Accessed October 22, 2018.

GEDSA. Procedure for inpatient settings: preparing and administering medications using ENFit®. GEDSA website. http://stayconnected.org/wp-content/uploads/2017/02 /medication-administration-poster.pdf. Accessed October 22, 2018.

Institute for Safe Medication Practices website. www.ismp.org. Accessed October 22, 2018.

McCabe BJ, Frankel EH, Wolfe JJ. *Handbook of Food-Drug Interactions.* Boca Raton, FL: CRC Press; 2003.

Mitchell J. Oral dosage forms that should not be crushed. Institute for Safe Medication Practices website. www.ismp.org/tools /donotcrush.pdf. Published November 20, 2016. Accessed October 22, 2018.

Williams NT. Medication administration through enteral feeding tubes. *Am J Health Syst Pharm.* 2008;65:2347–2357.

Wohlt PD, Zheng L, Gunderson S, Balzar SA, Johnson BD, Fish JT. Recommendations for the use of medications with continuous enteral nutrition. *Am J Health Syst Pharm.* 2009;66: 1458–1467.

References

1. Boullata JI, Carrera AL, Harvey L, et al. ASPEN safe practices for enteral nutrition therapy. *JPEN J Parenter Enteral Nutr.* 2017;41:15–103.

2. Lehmann S, Barber JR. Giving medications by feeding tube: how to avoid problems. *Nursing.* 1991;21(11):58–61.

3. McConnell EA. Giving medications through an enteral feeding tube. *Nursing.* 1998;28:66.

4. Gilbar PJ. A guide to enteral drug administration in palliative care. *J Pain Symptom Manage.* 1999;17:197–207.

5. Beckwith MC, Feddema SS, Barton RG, Graves C. A guide to drug therapy in patients with enteral feeding tubes: dosage form selection and administration methods. *Hosp Pharm.* 2004;39:225–237.

6. Dickerson RN. Medication administration considerations for patients receiving enteral tube feedings. *Hosp Pharm.* 2004;39:84–89,96.

7. Magnuson BL, Clifford TM, Hoskins LA, Bernard AC. Enteral nutrition and drug administration, interactions, and complications. *Nutr Clin Pract.* 2005;20:618–624.

8. Rollins C, Thomson C, Crane T. Pharmacotherapeutic issues. In: Rolandelli RH, Bankhead R, Boullata JI, Compher CW, eds. *Clinical Nutrition: Enteral and Tube Feeding.* 4th ed. Philadelphia, PA: Elsevier/Saunders; 2005:291–305.

9. White R, Bradnam V. *Handbook of Drug Administration via Enteral Feeding Tubes.* London, UK: Pharmaceutical Press; 2007.

10. Leff RD, Roberts RJ. Enteral drug administration practices: report of a preliminary survey. *Pediatrics.* 1988;81:549–551.

11. Mateo MA. Nursing management of enteral tube feedings. *Heart Lung.* 1996;25:318–323.

12. Belknap DC, Seifert CF, Peterman M. Administration of medications through enteral feeding catheters. *Am J Crit Care.* 1997;6:382–392.

13. Schmieding NJ, Waldman RC. Nasogastric tube feeding and medication administration: a survey of nursing practices. *Gastroenterol Nurs.* 1997;20:118–124.

14. Seifert CF, Johnston BA. Drug administration through enteral feeding catheters [letter]. *Am J Health-Syst Pharm.* 2002;59:378–379.

15. Seifert CF, Johnston BA. A nationwide survey of long-term care facilities to determine the characteristics of medication administration through enteral feeding catheters. *Nutr Clin Pract.* 2005;20:354–362.

16. Boullata JI, Hudson LM, Spencer CT, Preston AM, Oakes BA. Drug administration by feeding tube: results of a practice-based survey [abstract]. *Nutr Clin Pract.* 2007; 22:126.

17. Guenter P, Lyman B. ENFit enteral nutrition connectors. *Nutr Clin Pract.* 2016;31(6):769–772.

18. GEDSA. Reducing the risk of medical device tubing misconnections: ENFit® Low Dose Tip Syringe review. http://stayconnected.org/wp-content/uploads/2016/04/GEDSA-Low-Dose-Syringe-End-User-LDT-Preso-FINAL.pdf. Published 2016. Accessed October 22, 2018.

19. Franceschinis E, Voinovich D, Grassi M, et al. Self-emulsifying pellets prepared by wet granulation in high-shear mixer: influence of formulation variables and preliminary study on the in vitro absorption. *Int J Pharm.* 2005;291:87–97.

20. Matteucci ME, Brettmann BK, Rogers TL, Elder EJ, Williams RO, Johnston KP. Design of potent amorphous drug nanoparticles for rapid generation of highly supersaturated media. *Molec Pharm.* 2007;4:782–793.

21. USP. *USP-NF 41–NF 36.* Rockville, MD: United States Pharmacopeial Convention; 2018.

22. Scanlan M, Frisch S. Nasoduodenal feeding tubes: prevention of occlusion. *J Neurosci Nurs.* 1992;24:256–259.

23. Schier JG, Howland MA, Hoffman RS, Nelson LS. Fatality from administration of labetalol and crushed extended-release nifedipine. *Ann Pharmacother.* 2003;37:1420–1423.

24. Madigan SM, Courtney DE, Macauley D. The solution was the problem. *Clin Nutr.* 2002;21:531–532.

25. Clark-Schmidt AL, Garnett WR, Lowe DR, Karnes HT. Loss of carbamazepine suspension through nasogastric feeding tubes. *Am J Hosp Pharm.* 1990;47:2034–2037.

26. Seifert CF, McGoodwin PL, Allen LV. Phenytoin recovery from percutaneous endoscopic gastrostomy Pezzer catheters after long-term in vitro administration. *JPEN J Parenter Enteral Nutr.* 1993;17: 370–374.

27. van den Bemt PM, Cusell MB, Overbeeke PW, et al. Quality improvement of oral medication administration in patients with enteral feeding tubes. *Qual Saf Health Care.* 2006;15: 44–47.

28. Udeani GO, Bass J, Johnston TP. Compatibility of oral morphine sulfate solution with enteral feeding products. *Ann Pharmacother.* 1994;28:451–455.

29. Altman E, Cutie AJ. Compatibility of enteral products with commonly employed drug additives. *Nutr Support Serv.* 1984; 4(12):8,10,11,14.

30. Holtz L, Milton J, Sturek JK. Compatibility of medications with enteral feedings. *JPEN J Parenter Enteral Nutr.* 1987;11: 183–186.

31. Burns PE, McCall L, Worsching R. Physical compatibility of enteral formulas with various common medications. *J Am Diet Assoc.* 1988;88:1094–1096.

32. Strom JG, Miller SW. Stability of drugs with enteral nutrient formulas. *Ann Pharmacother.* 1990;24:130–134.

33. Crowther RS, Bellanger R, Szauter KE. In vitro stability of ranitidine hydrochloride in enteral nutrient formulas. *Ann Pharmacother.* 1995;29:859–862.

34. Au Yeung SC, Ensom MH. Phenytoin and enteral feedings: does evidence support an interaction? *Ann Pharmacother.* 2000;34:896–905.

35. Doak KK, Curtis EH, Dunnigan KJ, et al. Bioavailability of phenytoin acid and phenytoin sodium with enteral feedings. *Pharmacotherapy.* 1998;18:637–645.

36. Splinter MY, Seifert CF, Bradberry JC, et al. Recovery of phenytoin suspension after in vitro administration through percutaneous endoscopic gastrostomy Pezzer catheters. *Am J Hosp Pharm.* 1990;47:373–377.

37. Fleisher D, Sheth N, Kou JH. Phenytoin interaction with enteral feedings administered through nasogastric tubes. *JPEN J Parenter Enteral Nutr.* 1990;14:513–516.

38. Hooks MA, Longe RL, Taylor AT, Francisco GE. Recovery of phenytoin from an enteral nutrient formula. *Am J Hosp Pharm.* 1986;43:685–688.

39. Cacek AT, DeVito JM, Koonce JR. In vitro evaluation of nasogastric administration methods for phenytoin. *Am J Hosp Pharm.* 1986;43:689–692.

40. Guidry JR, Eastwood TF, Curry SC. Phenytoin absorption on volunteers receiving selected enteral feedings. *West J Med.* 1989;150:659–661.

41. Gilbert S, Hatton J, Magnuson B. How to minimize interaction between phenytoin and enteral feedings: two approaches—therapeutic options. *Nutr Clin Pract.* 1996;11:28–31.

42. Bauer LA. Interference of oral phenytoin absorption by continuous nasogastric feedings. *Neurology.* 1982;32:570–572.

43. Bass J, Miles MV, Tennison MB, et al. Effects of enteral tube feeding on the absorption and pharmacokinetic profile of carbamazepine. *Epilepsia.* 1989;30:364–369.

44. Kassam RM, Friesen E, Locock RA. In vitro recovery of carbamazepine from Ensure. *JPEN J Parenter Enteral Nutr.* 1989;13: 272–276.

45. Estoup M. Approaches and limitations of medication delivery in patients with enteral feeding tubes. *Crit Care Nurs.* 1994;14:68–79.

46. Engle KK, Hannawa TE. Techniques for administering oral medications to critical care patients receiving continuous enteral nutrition. *Am J Health Syst Pharm.* 1999;56: 1441–1444.

47. Clark-Schmidt AL, Garnett WR, Lowe DR, Karnes HT. Loss of carbamazepine suspension through nasogastric feeding tubes. *Am J Hosp Pharm.* 1990;47:2034–2037.

48. Mueller BA, Brierton DG, Abel SR, Bowman L. Effect of enteral feeding with Ensure on oral bioavailabilities of ofloxacin and ciprofloxacin. *Antimicrob Agents Chemother.* 1994;38: 2101–2105.

49. Piccolo ML, Toossi Z, Goldman M. Effect of coadministration of a nutritional supplement on ciprofloxacin absorption. *Am J Hosp Pharm.* 1994;51:2697–2699.

50. Healy DP, Brodbeck MC, Clendening CE. Ciprofloxacin absorption is impaired in patients given enteral feedings orally and via gastrostomy and jejunostomy tubes. *Antimicrob Agents Chemother.* 1996;40:6–10.

51. Mimoz O, Binter V, Jacolot A, et al. Pharmacokinetics and absolute bioavailability of ciprofloxacin administered through a nasogastric tube with continuous enteral feeding to critically ill patients. *Intensive Care Med.* 1998;24:1047–1051.

52. de Marie S, VandenBergh MFQ, Buijk SL, et al. Bioavailability of ciprofloxacin after multiple enteral and intravenous doses in ICU patients with severe gram-negative intraabdominal infections. *Intensive Care Med.* 1998;24:343–346.

53. Sahai J, Memish Z, Conway B. Ciprofloxacin pharmacokinetics after administration via a jejunostomy tube. *J Antimicrob Chemother.* 1991;28:936–937.

54. Cohn SM, Sawyer MD, Burns GA, et al. Enteric absorption of ciprofloxacin during tube feeding in the critically ill. *J Antimicrob Chemother.* 1996;38:871–876.

55. Wright DH, Pietz SL, Konstantinides FN, Rotschafer JC. Decreased in vitro fluoroquinolone concentrations after admixture with an enteral feeding formulation. *JPEN J Parenter Enteral Nutr.* 2000;24:42–48.

56. Penrod LE, Allen JB, Cabacungan LR. Warfarin resistance and enteral feedings: 2 case reports and a supporting in vitro study. *Arch Phys Med Rehabil.* 2001;82:1270–1271.

57. Dickerson RN, Garmon WM, Kuhl DA, Minard G, Brown RO. Vitamin K-dependent warfarin resistance after concurrent administration of warfarin and continuous enteral nutrition. *Pharmacotherapy.* 2008;28:308–313.

58. Trissel LA. *Trissel's Stability of Compounded Formulations.* 6th ed. Washington, DC: APhA Publications; 2018.

59. Jew RK, Soo-Hoo W, Erush SC, Amiri E. *Extemporaneous Formulations for Pediatric, Geriatric and Special Needs Patients.* 3rd ed. Bethesda, MD: American Society of Health-System Pharmacists; 2016.

60. Dansereau RJ, Crail DJ. Extemporaneous procedures for dissolving risendronate tablets for oral administration and for feeding tubes. *Ann Pharmacother.* 2005;39:63–67.

CHAPTER 11

Home Enteral Nutrition

Introduction

Home enteral nutrition (HEN) therapy delivers nutrients via a tube into the gastrointestinal (GI) tract to patients who are medically stable, living in the community, and unable to meet their nutrition needs orally. HEN may be appropriate for patients with neurological or neuromuscular dysfunction, head and neck or upper GI cancers, malabsorptive conditions, anorexia, failure to thrive, or other conditions.[1]

This chapter focuses on special issues associated with HEN. Enteral nutrition (EN) providers can play an important role in facilitating the transition from hospital to home by clarifying EN orders, educating patients and their caregivers, and arranging for timely delivery of supplies. Some home infusion and durable medical equipment (DME) companies have nutrition support clinicians who provide nutrition assessments and monitor patient progress. However, many patients are discharged home without such support.

Enteral access devices, EN formulas, administration schedules, and the frequency and intensity of laboratory and clinical monitoring can differ substantially from hospital to home. In the hospital, trained clinicians administer EN. In contrast, HEN is administered by the patient, family member, or other caregiver. The goal of care at the time of discharge and beyond is to provide appropriate, individualized, compassionate, cost-effective, and safe HEN support.

Benefits and Goals of Home Enteral Nutrition

Discharging a patient home on EN may have many advantages over prolonged hospitalization. Benefits include greater participation in activities of daily living, decreased cost of care, and reduced potential for hospital-acquired infection. Given current incentives to discharge patients from acute care settings as well as the aging of the US population, patients receiving EN are likely to have multiple chronic medical comorbidities that require home health care.[2,3] When indicated, HEN provides the most physiological mode of nutrient delivery for medically complex patients in the least restrictive environment.

Patient and home assessment, as well as proper management and monitoring, are essential to the safe and cost-effective delivery of HEN. Collaborative planning during the discharge process for a patient going home on EN should include attention to the HEN prescription, consideration of the patient's financial resources, the plan for follow-up, and education of the patient and/or caregiver.

Statistics on Enteral Nutrition in the Home Setting

Capturing demographic data on patients receiving HEN is difficult for a variety of reasons. There is no formal registry for patients receiving HEN; therefore, estimates regarding this population have largely been compiled based on data analysis of HEN studies.[4] In addition, patients receiving HEN may bypass traditional providers and obtain EN supplies and formula on their own.

In 2017, the American Society for Parenteral and Enteral Nutrition (ASPEN) published a comprehensive data analysis report regarding patients receiving EN.[4] This report focused on the use of EN across the care spectrum, including in the home setting, and it analyzed the number of patients receiving HEN, the types of formulas delivered, the types of feeding tubes placed, and routes of EN administration. As part of that EN market report, ASPEN conducted a survey of its members on a variety of EN practices and found that 44 of 492 survey respondents (8.9%) cared for patients receiving HEN. Survey respondents reported that their agency was caring for between 1 and 764 EN patients (average: 467 EN patients per agency). Of these patients, 75% were adults, 22% were pediatric patients, and 3% were infants or neonates.[4] In addition, about 23% of hospitalized EN patients were reportedly discharged home while receiving EN. Extrapolating from this information, it is estimated that approximately 50,000 US patients go home on EN per year.[4]

Regarding types of formulas used for HEN patients, the ASPEN survey found that most patients (59%) received standard intact nutrient formulas. The remaining patients received hydrolyzed protein/amino acid formulas (23%), disease-specific formulas (12%), formulas intended for patients with inherited diseases of metabolism (3%), and blenderized tube feedings (BTFs) (2%).[4] BTFs are discussed in greater detail later in this chapter. See Chapters 4 and 5 for additional information on types of formula.

ASPEN also collected survey data on the types of feeding tubes used. Respondents reported that most patients receiving HEN (75.4%) had gastrostomy tubes, 8.6% had gastrojejunostomy tubes, 8.1% had jejunostomy tubes, and 7.9% had short-term nasogastric or nasoenteric tubes. The ASPEN survey also found that 23% of patients in the home setting received continuous feedings via pump, 17% received intermittent feedings via pump, and 60% received bolus or intermittent feedings via gravity or syringe.[4]

Transition to Home

Patient Evaluation

Careful consideration must be taken when evaluating a patient for HEN. To successfully transition a patient to HEN, several criteria should be met. At the very minimum, the patient should be willing to enterally feed at home; the patient or a caregiver should be capable of administering EN; and the patient's tolerance to the prescribed enteral regimen should be evident. Table 11-1 provides a checklist of criteria that optimize a successful transition to home.[5] It is important to note that not all criteria may be met in every case.[5]

Selection of Providers of Supplies and Services

Providers of HEN supplies and services include DME companies, home infusion companies, and home health agencies. A DME company typically provides formula

TABLE 11-1. Discharge Preparation Checklist for Patients to Receive Home Enteral Nutrition

Category	Responsible Professionals
Patient assessment	
• Patient is deemed medically stable for discharge	• Primary medical team
• Patient exhibits tolerance of current feeding regimen	• Registered dietitian
	• Bedside nursing staff
• Patient is deemed able to tolerate planned home progression of feedings	• Case manager
	• Social worker
• Patient or caregiver exhibits willingness to continue administering enteral nutrition at home	• Home care company representative
Home environment	
• Adequate structure	• Case manager
• Electrical access	• Social worker
• Adequate physical access (bathroom/ramp)	• Home care company representative
• Heat and air conditioning	
• Clean water supply	
• Clean area for formula preparation	
• Road accessibility	
• Communication access: telephone or cell phone	
Caregiver education	
• Identification of caregivers	• Primary medical team
• Development of training schedule with identified caregivers	• Bedside nursing staff
	• Registered dietitian
• Education on feeding tube care and troubleshooting	• Home care company representative
	• Pharmacist
• Education on assessment of feeding tolerance	

(continued)

TABLE 11-1. *(Continued)*	
Category	**Responsible Professionals**
Caregiver education (continued)	
• Education on formula preparation and feeding schedule	
• Education on route of administration (bolus, gravity, pump)	
• Education on enteral medication administration	
Discharge planning	
• Identification of primary physician to manage enteral feedings	• Primary medical team
• Communication with primary physician about clinical status	• Inpatient care management team or professional who can coordinate insurance coverage and contact home care companies
• Initial postdischarge appointment set	
• Appointments for other subspecialty clinics as needed	• Case manager or care coordinator
• Coordination with home care company for feeding tube supply and formula	• Social worker
• Coordination with home nursing	

Source: Adapted with permission from reference 5: Sevilla WM, McElhanon B. Optimizing transition to home enteral nutrition for pediatric patients. *Nutr Clin Pract.* 2016; 31(6):762–768. doi:10.1177/0884533616673348.

and supplies, as well as medical equipment such as beds, walkers, wheelchairs, and respiratory equipment. Home infusion companies may provide not only formula and supplies but also medications administered intravenously and pharmacy and nursing services. Home health agencies may provide nursing services for education, training, and clinical monitoring.

The case manager, care coordinator, or social worker who is assisting in the transition to home is responsible for educating the patient regarding options for HEN providers. When selecting a provider, the following should be considered: the patient's insurance coverage, the availability of a registered dietitian and/or nutrition support team, the provider's hours of operation, its compliance with HEN standards of care, and whether it is accredited by an organization such as the Joint Commission, Accreditation Commission for Health Care, or Community Health Accreditation Program.[6,7]

Discharge Plan

The discharge process should begin as soon as the healthcare team determines that a patient may need HEN. The patient or caregiver is expected to become proficient in administering the formula, checking enteral access placement if needed, and maintaining skin integrity at the access site.[8] A collaborative approach from the multidisciplinary team and home care supplier is key to a safe and smooth transition. Table 11-2 lists ways that the multidisciplinary team can help facilitate the discharge process.[7]

In addition to the multidisciplinary team, the home care supplier plays an integral role in the discharge process. For example, the home care supplier may have a clinical representative meet with the patient prior to discharge to assist in evaluating the patient and educating the patient and family on how to use the feeding pump. The enteral supplier should also review the discharge order to verify that all equipment and supplies necessary to safely administer the feeding are on the prescription.

TABLE 11-2. Tips to Facilitate Discharge of Patients Who Will Receive Home Enteral Nutrition

- Obtain required diagnostic tests and procedures to demonstrate medical necessity and verify insurance coverage.
- Document the diagnosis requiring enteral nutrition for treatment.
- Establish feeding access.
- Determine the patient's tolerance to the enteral formulation.
- Explain to the patient and caregiver the risks and benefits of home nutrition support.
- Assess the patient's or caregiver's ability to perform activities of daily living and enteral nutrition–related tasks.
- Assess the learning needs of the patient and caregivers and provide appropriate patient education. If necessary, develop patient-specific learning materials to address literacy or language barriers.
- Engage the patient and family in a discussion about their expectations of involvement in daily care; include social workers or interpreters as needed in this discussion.
- Conduct psychosocial assessment of the patient.
- Identify caregiver(s).
- Determine the home care provider(s).
- Identify all necessary home infusion therapies and the follow-up communication required by each provider (blood samples for laboratory tests, wound care, etc).
- Identify who will prescribe the home enteral nutrition orders after discharge.
- Establish the type and amount of communication desired by the physician and nutrition support team after discharge.
- Educate the patient and family on how to contact the nutrition support team and reasons for urgent after-hours contact.

Source: Adapted with permission from reference 7: Konrad D, Mitchell R, Hendrickson E. Home nutrition support. In: Mueller CM, ed. *The ASPEN Adult Nutrition Support Core Curriculum.* 3rd ed. Silver Spring, MD: American Society for Parenteral and Enteral Nutrition; 2017:765–784.

Plans for the discharge home of pediatric patients receiving EN can vary significantly from plans used for the adult population. The coordination involved with discharging a medically complex child home can be especially challenging, and the risk for EN-related complications is considerable. Enteral devices used for children may vary from those of adults. For example, low-profile feeding devices (which require extension sets to feed) are commonly used. The pediatric patient may need to have their stomach vented or have gastric contents intermittently or continuously drained. Selection of an enteral provider with expertise in pediatric EN is imperative when dealing with this population.

Whether the patient is a child or an adult, patient and caregiver education is an important component of the transition to home. Education should begin as early as possible and include written and verbal forms of communication.[8] See the Patient Education section of this chapter for further discussion of this topic.

Insurance Coverage

HEN may be covered by Medicare, Medicaid/Medicaid managed care, private insurance plans, and other entities. Medicare covers HEN under Part B, the DME benefit. Patients who qualify for Medicare must meet specific criteria for HEN, as outlined here:[9]

- There is evidence of dysphagia.
- An emptying study for dysmotility and malabsorption is documented.
- Duration of EN is expected to last >90 days (continued need must be documented annually).
- EN is required to provide sufficient nutrients to maintain the patient's weight and strength commensurate with his or her overall health status.

- If oral intake continues, EN must constitute most of the patient's nutrition intake.
- Additional documentation is needed if the patient's EN requirement is <750 or >2000 kcal/d.

State Medicaid programs cover medical assistance for certain individuals and families with low incomes and limited resources. The rules for Medicaid reimbursement eligibility, payment rates, and types of reimbursement vary by state. The requirements should be reviewed on a case-by-case basis for each individual and state.

Some payers may require prior authorization for coverage of enteral formula and/or supplies—and coverage varies widely. Prior to discharge, it should be determined if formula and supplies are covered by the patient's individual health plan, and if medical justification or prior authorization is required. Ideally, HEN coverage should be evaluated before the enteral access device is placed. Insufficient insurance coverage for HEN may put undue financial burden on the patient or caregiver.

Patient Education

Clinicians involved in care of the patient receiving EN should contribute to the development and provision of a standardized patient nutrition education program (see Table 11-3).[8] Adequate education increases knowledge and may reduce therapy-related complications, improve clinical outcomes, bolster caregiver knowledge and confidence, and increase compliance with the treatment regimen.[10,11] It is beneficial to assess the patient's or caregiver's learning style and provide education in the most appropriate format for the individual learner (eg, use print material, audio recordings, videos, and/or teaching kits).[5] Printed material should be developed at a reading

TABLE 11-3. Practice Recommendations for Patient/ Caregiver Education About Home Enteral Nutrition

1. Begin the referral process once the decision for EN therapy is made.
2. Begin education for the patient receiving EN at home prior to placement of the EAD.
3. Provide patient and caregiver education that is comprehensive, includes education materials related to EN therapy, and uses a standard checklist.
4. Provide the patient and caregiver with verbal and written education that covers the following topics:
   ◦ Reason for EN and short-term and long-term nutrition goals (eg, weight goal)
   ◦ Feeding device, route, and method; formula; and feeding regimen
   ◦ Supplies needed to administer enteral tube feedings at home
   ◦ Use and cleaning of equipment, including administration/feeding set, infusion pump, and syringe
   ◦ Care of the feeding tube and access site, such as securing, flushing, and unclogging the tube and stoma care
   ◦ Nutrition and hydration guidelines: feeding plan/ regimen, water flushes, hydration monitoring
   ◦ Weight schedule, laboratory test recommendations
   ◦ Safe preparation and administration of formula
   ◦ Safe preparation and administration of medications
   ◦ Proper position during and after feedings
   ◦ Recognition and management of complications (mechanical, gastrointestinal, and metabolic)
   ◦ Available resources, emergency care plan, and healthcare contacts
5. Use demonstration and teach-back method of patient education to assess comprehension.
   ◦ Use various methods of education to take into account various learning styles.
   ◦ Implement an EN education checklist to assist with the discharge coordination process.

Abbreviations: EAD, enteral access device; EN, enteral nutrition.

Source: Adapted with permission from reference 8: Boullata JI, Carrera AL, Harvey L, et al. ASPEN safe practices for enteral nutrition therapy. *JPEN J Parenter Enteral Nutr.* 2017;41(1):15–103. doi:10.1177/0148607116673053.

level of fifth to sixth grade and avoid unnecessary use of medical and technical terms.[7]

Patient and caregiver instruction on the enteral access device is an important element of HEN education.[5] When discharged to home, some patients may require a combination of feeding methods, such as bolus feedings with a syringe during the day and continuous pump feeds at night. Specific print material regarding all the different routes of administration used (eg, bolus feeding, gravity feeding, or pump feeding) should be included in patient education. Education materials should detail the route of administration and the care and handling of the formula and the enteral access device (see Table 11-4).[5,7] Safety issues should

---

TABLE 11-4. Components of Patient Education about Using an Enteral Access Device

- Name and composition of enteral formula
- Methods for formula inspection, storage, preparation, and administration
- Formula hang time limits
- Infusion method (bolus, gravity, pump) and schedule
- Instructions for water flushes
- Instructions for administering medications via the feeding tube (if applicable)
- Identification of the type of tube, tube size (French), and date of placement
- Manufacturer's name and how to access manufacturer's information
- Enteral access device care
- Instructions for tube reinsertion (nasal) or instructions for securing the tube
- Signs and symptoms of complications
- Information for reordering supplies (company name and phone number)
- Contact name and phone number of the physician who ordered enteral nutrition

Source: Information is from references 5 and 7.

be reviewed repeatedly with patients and caregivers. After discharge to the home, ongoing education on safe handling techniques and the importance of a controlled, clean environment for HEN administration is imperative to avoid infectious complications.

Patient education materials should also include information regarding the patient's or caregiver's expectations and potential complications of HEN, with emphasis on problems that may require emergency interventions or rehospitalization. Tables 11-5 through 11-13 list selected

---

TABLE 11-5. Key Points for Patient Education on Nausea and Vomiting

Signs and symptoms:
- Abdominal distress, distention, feeling bloated
- Cramping
- Vomiting/dry heaves/retching
- Cold sweat

Possible causes:
- Feeding too quickly
- Formula is too concentrated
- Intolerance to formula ingredients
- Incorrect positioning of patient during feeds
- Contaminated formula
- Formula is too cold
- Constipation

Action steps:
- To lessen risk of nausea and vomiting, patient should sit up at $\geq 30°$ angle during feed and remain upright for 30 minutes after feeding.
- Discuss medication use with healthcare provider.
- Discuss formula and infusion rate with healthcare provider.
- Allow formula to reach room temperature prior to use.
- Verify proper storage and preparation of formula.
- If vomiting continues, stop feeding and call doctor.

Source: Information is from references 12 and 13.

TABLE 11-6. Key Points for Patient Education on Dehydration

Signs and symptoms:
- Excessive thirst
- Dry mouth, cracked lips
- Weight loss
- Fever
- Decreased urine output

Possible causes:
- Persistent diarrhea and/or vomiting
- Prolonged fever
- Insufficient fluid intake

Action steps:
- Administer fluids via tube.
- Call healthcare provider.

Source: Information is from references 12 and 13.

TABLE 11-7. Key Points for Patient Education on Constipation

Signs and symptoms:
- Infrequent and/or hard stool
- Bloating, gas
- Cramping or other pain

Possible causes:
- Inadequate fluid intake
- Medication side effect
- Inadequate fiber intake
- Decreased physical activity
- Dysmotility

Action steps:
- Ensure prescribed volume of formula and fluid is given.
- Discuss formula and medication use with healthcare provider.
- Increase physical activity if safe to do so.

Source: Information is from references 12 and 13.

TABLE 11-8. Key Points for Patient Education on Diarrhea

Signs and symptoms:
- Abdominal pain or cramping
- Frequent, loose, and/or watery stool

Possible causes:
- Side effect of medication
- Intolerance to formula
- Bowel disorder
- Infection

Action steps:
- Check with prescriber or pharmacist to evaluate whether medication is cause of diarrhea.
- Discuss formula and infusion rate with healthcare provider.
- Allow formula to reach room temperature prior to use.
- Follow recommendations for proper storage and preparation of formula.

Source: Information is from references 12 and 13.

complications that should be covered in patient/caregiver education for patients receiving long-term HEN.[12,13] The HEN provider as well as the home health nurse should instruct patients regarding these complications at the start of care and continually throughout the duration of therapy. Refer to Chapters 3 and 9 for additional information on EN complications.

Education may also include lists of resources and support organizations dedicated to tube feeding. Two of the largest patient support organizations are the Oley Foundation (www.oley.org) and Feeding Tube Awareness Foundation (www.feedingtubeawareness.org). Such organizations may provide education, consumer events, online communities, equipment/supply exchange programs, and a sense that others are undergoing the same issues related to HEN.

TABLE 11-9. Key Points for Patient Education on Aspiration

Signs and symptoms:
- Vomiting
- Heartburn
- Coughing or choking with difficulty breathing
- Chest pain
- Fever
- Shortness of breath
- Pneumonia

Possible causes:
- Diminished gag reflex
- Gastroesophageal reflux
- Swallowing disorder
- Silent aspiration
- Esophageal narrowing
- Decreased motility of esophagus and/or stomach
- Incorrect positioning of patient during feeds
- Tube migrated out of place

Action steps:
- Stop feeding, and open clamp to drain stomach contents if possible.
- Contact doctor.
- Patient should sit up ≥30° during feed and remain in an upright position for at least 30 minutes after feed.

Source: Information is from references 12 and 13.

Patient Monitoring

A major goal of monitoring patients who receive HEN is to prevent hospital readmission related to the enteral feeding. The appropriate type and amount of monitoring can vary widely and will depend on many factors, including the patient's age, medical condition, and insurance coverage. Pediatric patients may be regularly monitored by healthcare providers in an outpatient setting, such as a specialty

TABLE 11-10. Key Points for Patient Education on Site Irritation and/or Tube Leaking

Signs and symptoms:
- Irritated skin or rash around tube
- Burning pain
- Foul odor or local infection
- Sinus or ear infection (in patients using nasogastric or nasojejunal tubes)
- Granulation, or extra tissue built up around the insertion site
- Visible leakage from tube or around tube
- Multiple soaked dressings that require changing more than twice per day

Possible causes:
- Poorly fitting tube
- Tube tugging at exit site
- Improper skin care
- Broken tubing, cap, or antireflux valve
- Repeat clamping at same site
- Accidental cutting of the tube

Action steps:
- Stop feeding.
- If possible, clamp the tube between the patient's body and the problem area.
- Wash skin with warm water and mild soap, and pat dry. Apply a dry dressing as needed.
- Call doctor or home care nurse.
- Apply barrier cream to protect skin as needed.

Source: Information is from references 12 and 13.

clinic. This type of monitoring may be less common in the adult population.

The medical supply provider may also offer a degree of monitoring. This entity may have communication with the patient at least monthly for reorder of supplies. Some companies employ registered dietitians to assist in

TABLE 11-11. Key Points for Patient Education on Tube Displacement

Signs and symptoms:
- Tube has come out of body or has moved out of place
- Choking
- Difficulty breathing
- Nausea/vomiting
- Abdominal pain
- Diarrhea

Possible causes:
- Tube inadequately secured
- Accidental or excessive pulling of the tube
- Frequent vomiting
- Deflated balloon (if applicable)

Action step: Discontinue feeding and contact healthcare provider.

Source: Information is from references 12 and 13.

troubleshooting EN-related issues. Ultimately, however, patients/caregivers should refer to their healthcare providers for medical issues.

Patient Outcomes

The reporting and evaluation of outcomes is an important aspect of home care to promote continued quality improvement of HEN. ASPEN has established nutrition support standards for HEN that can be used as a guide for tracking patient outcomes.[6] If possible and practical, clinicians should utilize these standards as well as their organization's policies and procedures when developing tools to track outcomes. Ideally, data should be collected on mortality, hospital readmissions, complications, customer satisfaction, and problem reporting and resolution.[6]

TABLE 11-12. Key Points for Patient Education on Tube Obstruction/Blockage

Signs and symptoms:
- Inability to flush tube with water, infuse tube feeding, or administer medication via tube
- Bulging of tube when feeding or flushing

Possible causes:
- Medicine administered improperly
- Tube not flushed properly
- Putting soda through the tube
- Administering feedings or other substances that are too thick, sticky, or large to pass through tube
- Tube clamp is closed
- Infusion rate is too slow

Action steps:
- Make sure the tube clamp is open.
- Do not force formula or medication into a clogged tube.
- Try to flush the tube with a syringe filled with warm water. Pull the plunger back on syringe. Try flushing again with warm water.
- If flushing does not work, contact healthcare provider.

Source: Information is from references 12 and 13.

Blenderized Tube Feedings

An increasing number of families are preparing home-made BTFs or at least discussing them with their nutrition support clinicians. There has also been a sharp increase in the number of commercially available whole food–based formulas entering the market. These trends may reflect the desire of patients to reduce their intake of processed enteral formulas and consume more formulas prepared from whole foods, which patients may perceive to have emotional and nutritional benefits. Increased interest in BTFs may also stem from financial and nutrition-related

TABLE 11-13. Key Points for Patient Education on Pump or Power Failure

Signs:
- Unable to start pump
- Repeated alarms without obvious cause
- Excess formula left in the bag after recommended feeding time is complete

Possible causes:
- Power failure/low battery
- Pump charger parts are not properly connected
- Pump is unplugged
- Pump malfunction

Action steps:
- Check whether pump is plugged in.
- Check that the wall socket is functioning.
- Check that battery is charged.
- Stop pump, and check user's manual for instructions.
- If pump will not work, contact home care provider.

Source: Information is from references 12 and 13.

challenges associated with obtaining and using commercial formulas (eg, insurance limitations, gastrointestinal symptoms, intolerance of commercially prepared enteral formulas, or food allergies/intolerances).

Clinicians should therefore be prepared to educate patients and caregivers about the following aspects of using BTFs:[14,15]

- Safe food practices for preparation and storage of homemade BTFs
- The time and effort required by families to make and use BTFs

- Cost considerations (insurance companies do not usually cover the cost of food used in homemade BTFs)
- Methods to evaluate the nutrient content of BTFs
- How to choose homemade BTF recipes and plan for nutritionally complete feedings
- Whether BTFs can be administered via the patient's enteral access device:
  - Feeding tubes less than 10 Fr may be too small for blenderized formulas.
  - Diluting formulas to pass through tubes may diminish the amount of nutrients delivered.
  - Patients with a jejunostomy may not tolerate BTFs because the tubes are small in diameter and feedings are delivered into the small intestine; these patients should only use BTFs under medical supervision.
  - Homemade BTFs should not be kept at room temperature for more than 2 hours (unlike commercially prepared liquid formulas, homemade formula is not sterile); therefore, BTFs may not be safe for continuous feedings.
  - BTF infusion through an enteral feeding pump could block the pump's air sensors, which might allow air to enter the stomach.

Use of BTF does not have to be an all-or-none proposition, and combinations of commercial standard enteral formulas, commercial BTFs, and homemade BTFs may be used to meet all nutrition needs or to complement an existing feeding regimen. Several of the numerous resources on homemade blenderized diets to assist patients/caregivers and clinicians in meeting the nutrition needs of those who want to pursue this method are listed in the next section under Patient Education and Support.

Practice Resources

Professional Resources

- Agency for Clinical Innovation and the Gastroenterological Nurses College of Australia. *A Clinician's Guide: Caring for People With Gastrostomy Tubes and Devices.* Chatswood, Australia: Agency for Clinical Innovation; 2014.
- Boullata JI, Carrera AL, Harvey L, et al. ASPEN safe practices for enteral nutrition therapy. *JPEN J Parenter Enteral Nutr.* 2017;41(1):15–103. doi:10.1177/0148607116673053.
- Durfee SM, Adams SC, Arthur E, et al. A.S.P.E.N. standards for nutrition support: home and alternate site care. *Nutr Clin Pract.* 2014;29(4):542–555.
- Lyman B, Rempel G, Windsor K, Guenter P. Use of nasogastric feeding tubes for children at home: a template for caregiver education. *Nutr Clin Pract.* 2017;32(6):831–833.
- University of Virginia School of Medicine. GI Nutrition Support Team website. www.ginutrition.virginia.edu. Accessed November 15, 2018. (Go to Clinician Resources tab for blenderized recipes.)

Patient Education and Support

- Blenderized tube feeding (handout for parents). Seattle Children's website. www.seattlechildrens.org/globalassets/documents/for-patients-and-families/pfe/pe442.pdf. Accessed November 15, 2018.
- Complex Child website. GI section. www.complexchild.com/gi.html. Accessed November 15, 2018.
- Feeding Tube Awareness Foundation. www.feedingtubeawareness.org. Accessed November 15, 2018.

- Food for Tubies website. www.foodfortubies.org. Accessed November 15, 2018.
- Klein MD, Morris SE. *Homemade Blended Formula Handbook*. Tucson, AZ: Mealtime Notions; 2007. Available for purchase at www.mealtimenotions.com.
- Oley Foundation. www.oley.org. Accessed November 15, 2018.
- US Department of Agriculture. Choose My Plate website. www.choosemyplate.gov. Accessed November 15, 2018.

References

1. Delegge MH. Home enteral nutrition. *JPEN J Parenter Enteral Nutr*. 2002;26(5 Suppl):S4–S7.
2. McCall N, Petersons A, Moore S, Korb J. Utilization of home health services before and after the balanced budget act of 1997: what were the initial effects? *Health Serv Res*. 2003;38(1):85–106.
3. Castellanos VH, Silver HJ, Gallagher-Allred C, Smith TR. Nutrition issues in the home, community, and long-term care setting. *Nutr Clin Pract*. 2003;18(1):21–36.
4. Read J, Guenter P. *ASPEN Enteral Nutrition by the Numbers: EN Data Across the Healthcare Continuum*. Silver Spring, MD: American Society for Parenteral and Enteral Nutrition; 2017.
5. Sevilla WM, McElhanon B. Optimizing transition to home enteral nutrition for pediatric patients. *Nutr Clin Pract*. 2016; 31(6):762–768. doi:10.1177/0884533616673348.
6. Durfee SM, Adams SC, Arthur E, et al. A.S.P.E.N. standards for nutrition support: home and alternate site care. *Nutr Clin Pract*. 2014;29(4):542–555.
7. Konrad D, Mitchell R, Hendrickson E. Home nutrition support. In: Mueller CM, ed. *The ASPEN Adult Nutrition Support Core Curriculum*. 3rd ed. Silver Spring, MD: American Society for Parenteral and Enteral Nutrition; 2017:765–784.
8. Boullata JI, Carrera AL, Harvey L, et al. ASPEN safe practices for enteral nutrition therapy. *JPEN J Parenter Enteral Nutr*. 2017;41(1):15–103. doi:10.1177/0148607116673053.

9. Centers for Medicare & Medicaid Services. National coverage determination (NCD) for enteral and parenteral nutritional therapy (NCD 180.2). Medicare Coverage Database website. https://www.cms.gov/medicare-coverage-database/overview-and-quick-search.aspx. Published 1984. Accessed November 16, 2018.

10. Weston-Eborn R, Sitzman K. Selecting effective instructional resources. *Home Healthc Nurse*. 2005;23:402–403.

11. Schweitzer M, Aucoin J, Docherty SL, Rice HE, Thompson J, Sullivan DT. Evaluation of a discharge education protocol for pediatric patients with gastrostomy tubes. *J Pediatr Health Care*. 2014;28:420–428. doi:10.1016/j.pedhc.2014.01.002.

12. Agre P, Brown P, Stone K. Tube feeding troubleshooting guide. The Oley Foundation. https://cdn.ymaws.com/oley.org/resource/resmgr/Docs/TF_Troubleshooting_Guide_201.pdf. Updated May 2018. Accessed November 16, 2018.

13. Agency for Clinical Innovation. Feeding tubes—troubleshooting. https://www.aci.health.nsw.gov.au/__data/assets/pdf_file/0019/154801/feed_tube_troubleshooting.pdf. Updated August 2007. Accessed November 16, 2018.

14. Martin K, Gardner G. Home enteral nutrition: updates, trends, and challenges. *Nutr Clin Pract*. 2017;32(6):712–721. doi:10.1177/0884533617701401.

15. Escuro A. Blenderized tube feeding: suggested guidelines to clinicians. *Pract Gastroenterol*. 2014;38(12):58–64. https://www.practicalgastro.com/pdf/December14/Blenderized-Tube-Feeding-Suggested-Guidelines.pdf. Accessed November 16, 2018.

Index

Page numbers followed by *f* indicate figures, those followed by *t* indicate tables.